Ahmed Naji Al-Jamal

Medical Optical

AF773103

Ahmed Naji Al-Jamal

Medical Optical

Noor Publishing

Cover image: www.ingimage.com

Publisher:
Noor Publishing
is a trademark of
Dodo Books Indian Ocean Ltd. and OmniScriptum S.R.L publishing group

120 High Road, East Finchley, London, N2 9ED, United Kingdom
Str. Armeneasca 28/1, office 1, Chisinau MD-2012, Republic of Moldova, Europe
Managing Directors: Ieva Konstantinova, Victoria Ursu
info@omniscriptum.com

Printed at: see last page
ISBN: 978-620-9-23807-9

Medical Optics

Dr. Ahmed Naji Al-Jamal

University of Babylon-College of Engineering
Department of Biomedical Engineering

بسم الله الرحمن الرحيم

- فَافْتَحْ بَيْنِي وَبَيْنَهُمْ فَتْحًا وَنَجِّنِي وَمَنْ مَعِيَ مِنَ الْمُؤْمِنِينَ ﴿118﴾
- فَأَنْجَيْنَاهُ وَمَنْ مَعَهُ فِي الْفُلْكِ الْمَشْحُونِ ﴿119﴾

صدق الله العظيم

سورة الشعراء

Dedication

To the professors, whose passion for discovery illuminates the intricate machinery of life, and who tirelessly build bridges of understanding for the next generation.

And to the students, the future pioneers of science and medicine, whose curiosity will drive the next great revolutions in biology. May this book serve as a guide to the unseen world that awaits your exploration.

Author

ABSTRACT

Optics has, since ancient times, being used as aid for the examination of human patients and in some therapeutic treatments. Many of the optic medical instruments in use today were developed in the nineteenth century and, with the advent of optical fibers and laser light sources in the mid twentieth century, a new generation of medical devices, instruments, and techniques have been developed that have helped modernize medicine and perform task unimaginable only a few decades ago. This book illustrates—through several optical instrument and application examples—the uses, benefits, and future prospects that optics brings as an enabling technology to the medicine and the overall healthcare industry.

The book consists of twelve chapters: Chapter One: Terminology, Modeling, and Measurement , Chapter Two: Light in Medicine, Chapter Three: Optics in Medicine, Chapter Four: Endoscopy Device, Chapter Five: Optics and Human Vision, Chapter Six: Optical Properties of Tissues, Chapter Seven: Instrumentation in Photonics, Chapter Eight: Application of Radiation In Medicine, Chapter Nine: Laser in Medicine, Chapter Ten: Lasers with Biological Tissues, Chapter Eleven: Surgical Applications of Lasers, Chapter Twelve: Laser Application in Oral Surgery, Chapter Thirteen: Laser Applications in Otolaryngology, Chapter Fourteen: Non Thermal Diagnostic Applications, Chapter Fifteen: Therapeutic Applications.

My hope is that students and professors of the subspecialty of medical optics will benefit fully from this book.

Author

CONTUSES

CHAPTER 1
TERMINOLOGY, MODELING, AND MEASUREMENT

CHAPTER 2
LIGHT IN MEDICINE

CHAPTER 3
OPTICS IN MEDICINE

CHAPTER 7

INSTRUMENTATION IN PHOTONICS

CHAPTER 8

APPLICATION OF RADIATION IN MEDICINE

CHAPTER 9

LASER IN MEDICINE

CHAPTER 10

LASERS WITH BIOLOGICAL TISSUES

CHAPTER 11

SURGICAL APPLICATIONS OF LASERS

CHAPTER 12

LASER APPLICATION IN ORAL SURGERY

CHAPTER 13

LASER APPLICATIONS IN OTOLARYNGOLOGY

CHAPTER 14
NON THERMAL DIAGNOSTIC APPLICATIONS

CHAPTER 15
THERAPEUTIC APPLICATIONS

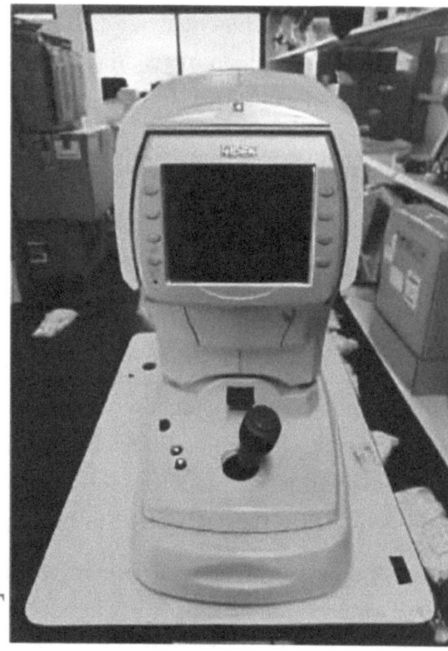

1

CHAPTER

TERMINOLOGY, MODELING, AND MEASUREMENT

1.1 TERMINOLOGY

Medical physics is the term of a science that overlaps with the two fields of medicine and physics, and it refers to the applications of physics to the function of the human body in health and disease.

i.e. physics of the body and the application of physics in the practice of medicine e.g.: laser in medicine, ultrasound in medicine, X-rays, sound, Computed Tomography (CT Scanner), Magnetic Resonance Imaging (MRI), sphygmomanometer Blood Pressure, Electrocardiography (ECG), Electromyography (EMG), Electroencephalogram (EEG), … etc.

In medicine the quantities are measured in nonstandard units e.g. pressure in mmHg or cmH_2O instead of N/m^2 or $dyne/cm^2$.

There are two groups of physics measurements in the body which are repetitive and non-repetitive functions.

The repetitive functions are the number of repetition per second, minute … e.g.: pulse rate (70/minute) breathing rate (16/min for men and 20/min for women), frequencies in the electrical signals from the brain, and food grind by stomach.

The non-repetitive functions mean that some movements in the body which are not repetitive uniformly, such as the time of the function of the kidney to remove the waste from the blood, food digestion in the body, time intervals of nerve signals, and eye movement.

The measurement in medicine should be very accurate, and the percentage of error should be as low as possible.

Diagnostic errors are not a result of measuring instruments only, because the error can be caused by a psychological reason, e.g. tabloidesque and pulse rate can be affected during the measurement by several reasons. The diagnostic errors can lead to wrong directions which are of two types:

i. A false negative error occurs when a patient is diagnosed to be free of disease when he/she does have it.

ii. A false positive error occurs when patient is diagnosed with a particular disease when he/she does not have it.

Examples:

- In Physiology: where law of physics can be applied to the function of the human body in health and disease.

- In Practice of medicine: the application of the physics of stethoscope, percussion and the application of sphygmomanometer, pacemaker, defibrillators and so forth.

- Biophysics: is the study of biological process using the theories and tools of physics.

- Biomedical engineering: they develop mechanical and electrical solutions to medical problems, such as developing diagnostic and imaging equipment and designing artificial organs.

- Health physics (Radiation protection): is the application of scientific principles to the protection of workers and public from the hazards of radiation.

Diagnostic positive and negative errors can be reduced by:

1- Research on the causes of misleading laboratory test values.

2- Development of new clinical tests.

3- Better instrumentation.

Most of the measurements are uncertain and inaccurate.

The uncertainties can be reduced by using:

1- Care in taking the measurement.

2- Repeating measurement.

3- Using reliable instruments.

4- Calibration of the instruments.

1.2 MODELING AND ANALOGY

1.2.1 Modeling

In general, it's the process of representing phenomenon as set of mathematical equations, to study the effect of changes on it.

Modeling often resorts to different ways to understand the phenomena, for example:

- To understand physical phenomena, use.
  - Simplification by selection of main features
  - Analysis
  - Qualitative or quantitative expression and verification

Analogies is used to understand the physical aspects of the body. (Not perfect), such as the eye analogous to camera.

MEDICAL OPTICS

To describe and explain phenomena that can't be experienced directly physicists employ models, using different types for different aims.

Example:

• Mechanical models are common in scientific activities, such as Quantum mechanical models and Bohr's atomic models.

• Electrical circuit model, which analogous the blood flow by the flow of electricity in wire.

• Mathematical model: consist of Equation and Function Equation such as Newton second law {F = **ma**}

Where: F: is the force, **m**: is the mass**, a**: is acceleration.

• Function models such as {R = f (p)} to indicate the heart rate R is the function of the power produced by the body.

• Feedback control (homeostasis): it is a control mechanism that uses information from measurement to manipulate a variable to achieve the desired result.

There are two types of feedback control

- Negative feedback
- Positive feedback

• Negative feedback helps the system toward equilibrium state.

Example:

- Home thermostat that maintains specified temperature, by increasing or decreasing the temperature to reach the setting temperature.
- Regulation of blood sugar level, by insulin secretion into the blood, when blood sugar levels reach homeostasis, the pancreas stops releasing insulin.

• Positive feedback is mechanisms that enhances the original stimulus,

Example:

Blood clotting, once the vessel is damaging the platelets start cling to the injured site and release chemicals that attract more platelets, the platelets continue to pile up until the clot is formed.

For Example: If you tore a small corner off this page and let it fall to the floor, it would go through various gyrations. Its path would be determined by the laws of physics, but it would be almost impossible to write the equation describing this path. Physicists would agree that the force of gravity would cause it to go in the general direction of the floor if some other force did not interfere. Air currents and static electricity would affect its path.

In trying to understand the physical aspects of the body, we often resort to analogies; physicists often teach and think by analogy. Keep in mind that analogies are never perfect.

For Example: In many ways the eye is analogous to a camera; however, the analogy is poor when the film, which must be developed and replaced, is compared to the retina, the light detector of the eye.

Some models involve physical phenomena that appear to be completely unrelated to the subject being studied.

For Example: A model in which the flow of blood is represented by the flow of electricity is often used in the study of the body's circulatory system. This electrical model can simulate very well many phenomena of the cardiovascular system. Of course, if you do not understand electrical phenomena the model does not help much. Also, as mentioned before, all analogies have their limitations.

Blood is made up of red blood cells and plasma, and the percentage of the blood occupied by the red blood cells (**the hematocrit**) changes as the blood flows toward the extremities. This phenomenon is difficult to simulate with the electrical model.

1.2.2 Analogy

It is how to express body organs or system functions:

a. Mechanical model: For hearing sound by the Ear.

b. Electrical circuit model: For blood flow circulation.

c. Optical model: For eye vision function.

1.2.3 Mathematics

a. Equation: For instance, the relation between heat, work and energy.

b. Function: for instance, on how blood pressure varies as a function of height.

1.2.4 Feedback control

a. Negative feedback: How to manipulate with negative results.

b. Positive feedback: How to manipulate with positive results.

1.3 MEASUREMENT

Are values which are made meaningful into specific units, its act as labels which make those value more useful in term of details, for example instead of saying that someone tall, we can say that the individual length is (6 feet).

Practice medical measurements can be divided into quantitative and qualitative measurements.

For Example: -Even though body temperature and pulse rate could be measured during the seventeenth century, these measurements were not routinely made until the nineteenth century. In this century there has been a steady growth of science in medicine as the number and accuracy of quantitative measurements used in clinical practice has increased.

The following figure 1.1 illustrates a few of the common measurements used in the practice of medicine. Some of these measurements are more reproducible than others.

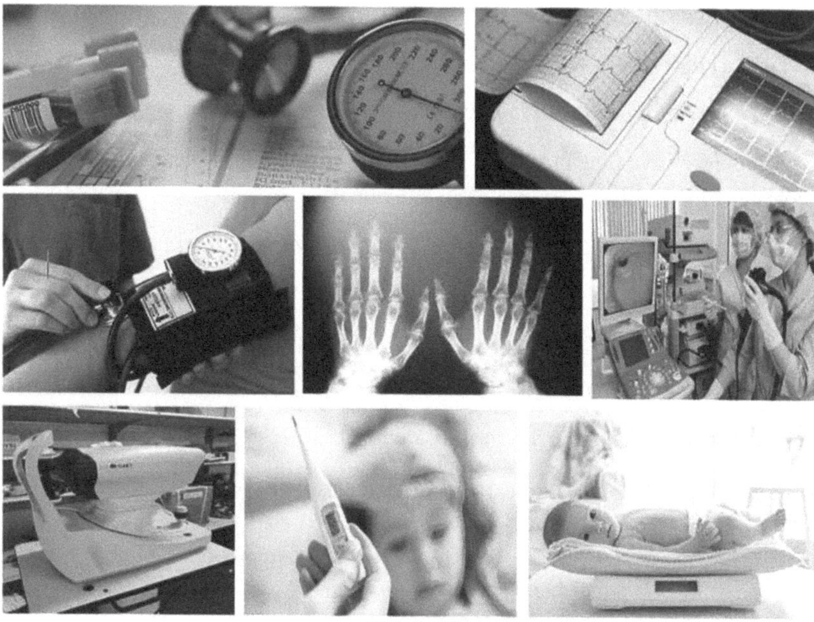

Figure1.1: illustrates a few of the common measurements used in the practice of medicine.

For Example: -An X-ray gives only qualitative information about the inside of the body; a repeat X-ray taken with a different machine may look quite different to the ordinary observer.

There are many other physical measurements involving the body and time. We can divide **them into two groups: -**

1. Measurements of repetitive processes, such as pulse.

2. Measurements of nonrepetitive processes, such as how long it takes the kidneys to remove a foreign substance from the blood.

Measurements of the repetitive processes usually involve the number of repetitions per second, minute, hour, and so forth.

For Example:

The pulse rate is about 70/min.

The breathing rate is about 15/min.

Nonrepetitive time processes in the body range from the action potential of a nerve cell (1msec) to the lifespan of an individual.

When must a physician decide if the patient is ill or not, and what the illness is?

After a physician has reviewed a patient's: -

1. Medical history.
2. The findings of the physical examination.
3. The results of the clinical laboratory measurements.

The decisions are two types:

1. Right decisions.
2. Wrong decisions.

It is not surprising that sometimes wrong decisions are made. These wrong decisions are of **two types:**

1. False Positives.
2. False Negatives.

*A **false positive*** error occurs when a patient is diagnosed with a particular disease when he or she does not have it.

*A **false negative*** error occurs when a patient is diagnosed to be free of a particular disease when he or she does have it.

Note: In some situations, a diagnostic error can have a great impact on a patient's life.

For Example:

A young woman was thought to have a rheumatic heart condition and spent several years in complete bed rest before it was discovered that a ***false positive diagnosis*** had been made-she really had arthritis, a disease in which activity should be maintained to avoid joint stiffening.

In the early stages of many types of cancer it is easy to make a false negative diagnostic error because the tumor is small. Since the probability of cure depends on early detection of the cancer, a ***false negative diagnosis*** can greatly reduce the patient's chance of survival.

Diagnostic errors (false positives and false negatives) can be reduced by:

1. Research into the causes of misleading laboratory test values.

2. Development of new clinical tests and better instrumentation.

Errors or uncertainties from measurements can be reduced by:

1. Using care in taking measurements.

2. Repeating measurements.

3. Using reliable instruments.

4. Properly calibrating the instruments.

Quantitative measurement includes:

1. Thermometer: which measures the temperature.
2. A weighing machine to measure the weight.
3. Sphygmomanometer measure blood pressure.
4. Syringes of different sizes for injection and aspiration of blood and fluid from the body.

Qualitative measurement gives information about the inside of the body, such as x- ray image, computed tomography (CT scan), ultrasound (US) image, magnetic resonance image (MRI) …

1.3.1 General structure:

a- Type of measurement.

b- Sensor or transducer: Use for detection.

c- Signal processing: Produced by the machine.

d- Output display: For diagnosis.

1.3.2 Units

There are several systems of units

- International system SI unit: it measures quantity such as length (meter) Mass (kilogram), time (second), current (ampere).
- Nonstandard unit: which is used in medicine such as blood pressure which is measured in millimeters of mercury (mmHg).
- Static characteristics that include accuracy and precision it is used in science and have different meanings.
- Accuracy: refers to the degree of correctness of measurement when compared to true or absolute value.
- Precision: refers to the degree of refinement of measurement.

After taking a lot of measurements, you notice that they are all close to each other this is precision, if they are degree with the true value this is accuracy.

a- Standard international units (SI).

b- Nonstandard units: As mentioned in sec. 1.

c- English units: Feet, pound, mile,etc.

1.3.3 static characteristics:

Using biostatistics to verify:

a- Accuracy of result.

b- Precision from standard.

c- Resolution among results.

d- Reproducibility of results.

1.3.4 Sources of error:

Defeats in one or more of the following:

a- Inherent variability of a poison.

b- Sensor or transducer fault.

c- Signal processing inaccuracy.

d- Output display inaccuracy.

e- Interconnection and feedback control: known or unknown.

f- Psychological effects.

g- Physical environment

h- Human factors: sensation, interpretation, mistakes, etc

Sources of error in medical measurements

1. Psychological effects

2. Human factors such as environmental and individual characteristics influence behavior.

3. Laboratory misleading test values, these errors can be reduced by Development of new clinical tests and better instrumentation.

Errors or uncertainties from measurements can be reduced by: -

1. Being Careful in taking the measurement.

2. Repeating measurements.

3. Using reliable instruments.

4. Properly calibrating the instruments.

The physician can decide if the patient is ill or not

After he or she has reviewed the patient's following information: -

1. Medical history.

2. The findings of the physical examination.

3. The results of clinical laboratory measurements

In summary

1. All measurements are uncertain and inaccurate.

2. With special effort we can reduce the error and the uncertainty.

3. In many cases there is no need to improve the measurement because the quantity being measured is variable.

2

CHAPTER

LIGHT IN MEDICINE

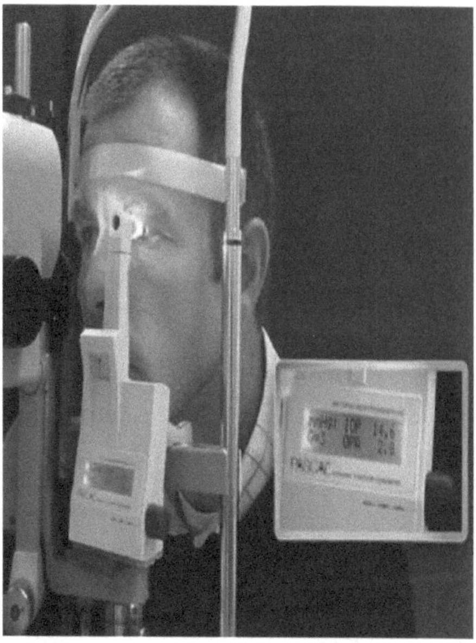

2.1 INTRODUCTION

Even though man is now very efficient at making artificial light, the sun is still the major source of light in the world. The sun is both beneficial and hazardous to our health.

Light has some interesting properties, many of which are used in medicine:

1.The speed of light changes when it goes from material into another. The ratio of the speed of light in a vacuum to its speed in each material is called the index of refraction. If a light beam meets a new material at an angle other than perpendicular, it bends or is refracted. This property permits light to be focused and is the reason we can read and see objects clearly.

2.Light behaves both as a wave and as a particle. As a wave it produces interference and diffraction, which are of minor importance in medicine. As a particle it can be absorbed by a single molecule. When a light photon is absorbed, its energy is used in various ways. It can cause a chemical change in the molecule that in turn can cause an electrical change. This is basically what happens when a light photon is absorbed in one of the sensitive cells of the retina (the light-sensitive part of the eye). The chemical change in a particular point of the retina triggers an electrical signal to the brain to inform it that a light photon has been absorbed at that point.

3.When light is absorbed, its energy generally appears as heat. This property is the basic for the use in medicine of IR light to heat tissues. Also, the heat produced by laser beams is used to "weld" a detached retina to the back of the eyeball and to coagulate small blood vessels in the retina.

4.Sometimes when photon is absorbed, a lower energy light photon is emitted. This property is known as fluorescence, it is the basis of the fluorescent light bulb. Certain materials fluoresce in the presence of UV light, sometimes called "black light", and give off visible light. The amount of fluorescence and the color of the emitted light depend on the wavelength of the UV light and on the chemical composition of the material that is fluorescing. One way fluorescence is used in medicine is in the detection of porphyria, a condition in which the teeth fluoresce red when irradiated with UV light. Another important application is in fluorescent microscopes.

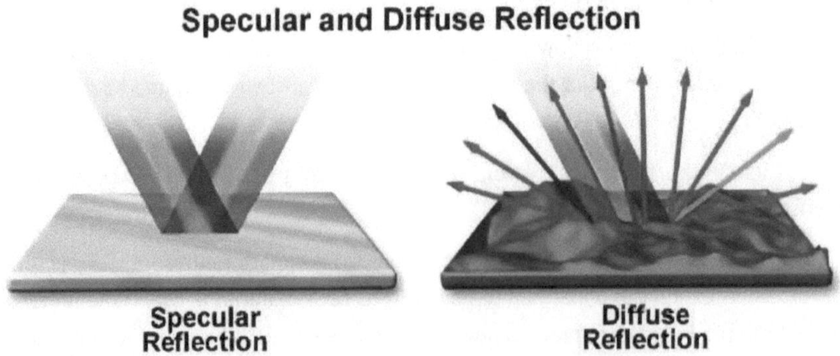

Figure 2.1: There are two types of reflection. Diffuse reflection and Specular reflection.

5.Light is reflected to some extent from all surfaces. There are two types of reflection. **Diffuse reflection** occurs when rough surfaces scatter the light in many directions. **Specular reflection** is more useful type of reflection; it is obtained from very smooth shiny surfaces such as mirrors where the light is reflected at an angle that is equal to the angle at which it strikes the surface. Mirrors are used in many medical instruments.

2.2 MEASUREMENT OF LIGHT AND ITS UNITS

The three general categories of light UV, visible, and IR are defined in terms of their wavelengths. Wavelengths of light used to be measured in microns ($1\mu=10^{-6}m$) or in angstroms ($1Å=10^{-10}m$), but at present the recommended unit is the nanometer ($1nm=10^{-9}m$). Ultraviolet light has wavelengths from about 100 to 400 nm; visible light extends from about 400 to 700 nm; and IR light extents from about 700 to over 10^4nm.

Visible light is measured in photometric units that relate to how light is seen by the average human eye. In photometry the quantity of light striking a surface is called illuminance and the intensity of a light source is called its luminance. All light radiation, including UV and IR radiation, can be measured in radiometric units. In radiometry the quantity of light striking a surface is called irradiance and the intensity of a light source is its radiance.

The wavelengths of light fit into the whole spectrum of electromagnetic radiation. Note that light has wavelengths much shorter than TV and radio waves but much longer than X-rays and gamma rays.

- Ultraviolet light has wavelengths from 100 to 400nm

- Visible light has wavelengths 400 to 700nm

- IR light has wavelengths from 700 to 104nm.

Each of these categories are subdivided according to wavelength. Ultraviolet

UV-A has wave lengths from 320 – 400nm

UV-B has wavelengths from 290 -320nm

UV-C has wavelengths from 100 – 290nm Visible light is measured in photometric units

Medical Optics

Illuminance the quantity of light striking a surface

Luminesce the intensity of a light source.

UV and IR radiation can be measured in radiometric units

Irradiance the quantity of light striking the surface.

Radiance the intensity of a light source

2.3 APPLICATIONS OF VISIBLE LIGHT IN MEDICINE

An obvious use of visible light in medicine is to permit the physician to obtain visual information about the patient regarding, ***for example***, the color of his skin and the presence of abnormal structures in or on his body. It is quite easy for a physician to examine the skin under normal lighting conditions, but when he wishes to look into a body opening, he is faced with the practical problem of getting light into the opening without obstructing the view. Like a lot of tricks, this one is done with mirrors.

The curved surface focuses the light at the region of interest. More sophisticated instruments, such as the **ophthalmoscope** for looking into the eyes and the **otoscope** for looking into the ears, use basically the same principle.

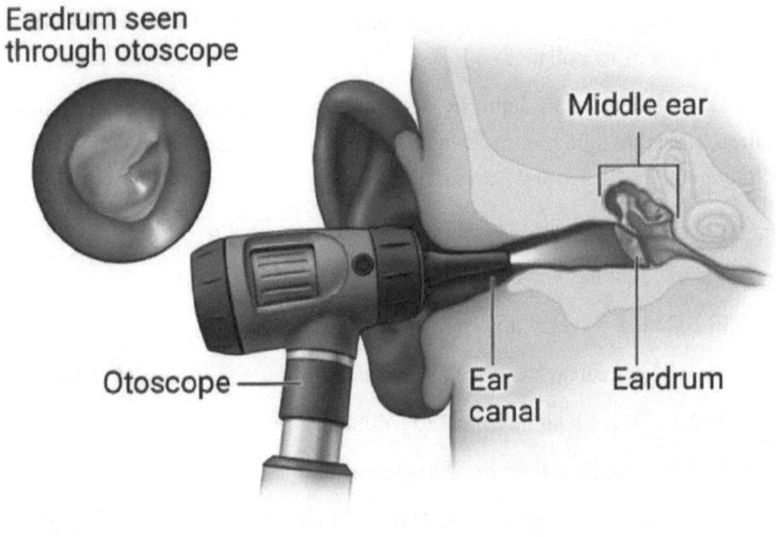

Figure 2.2: Illustrator the otoscope for looking into the ears.

A few instruments, called **endoscopes**, are used for viewing internal body cavities. Special purpose **endoscopes** are often given names indicating their purpose. *For example*, **cystoscopes** are used to examine the bladder, **proctoscopes** are used for examining the rectum, **enteroscopy** are used to examine small intestine, **colonoscopy** used to examine large intestine/colon, **hysteroscopy** used to examine the uterus and **bronchoscopes** are used for examining the air passages into the lungs. Some **endoscopes** are rigid tubes with a light source to illuminate the area of interest. Many of them are equipped with optical attachments to magnify the tissues being studied.

The development of fiber optic techniques permitted the construction of flexible endoscopes. Flexible endoscopes can be used to obtain information from regions of the body that cannot be examined with rigid endoscopes, such as the small intestine and much of the large intestine. Some flexible endoscopes are over a meter in length. The image obtained with a flexible endoscope is not as good as that obtained with a rigid endoscope, but often the only alternative to a flexible endoscopic examination is exploratory surgery.

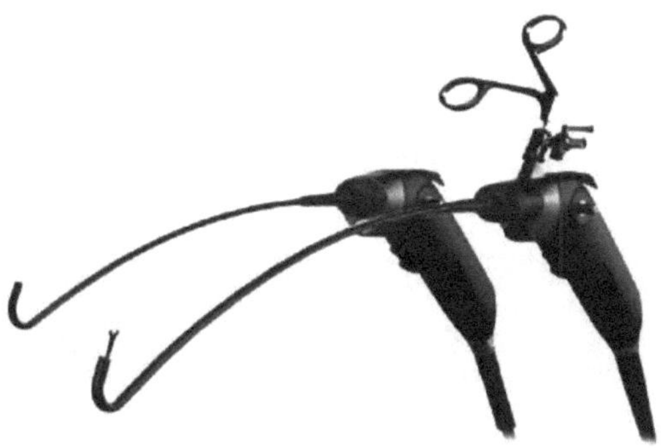

Figure 2.3: Flexible endoscopes usually have an opening or channel that permits the physician to take samples of the tissues (biopsies) for later microscopic examination.

Since light contains energy that largely appears as heat when it is absorbed, there is a limit on the amount of light that can be used in endoscopy. For endoscopy, the heating can be reduced by reducing the IR light from the source with special IR absorbing glass filters. In this cold-light endoscopy the light source contains very little IR radiation, and the heating of tissues is minimized.

Medical Optics

Transillumination is the transmission of light through the tissues of the body. Most of us have at one time or another shone a flashlight through our fingers to see the red glow that is produced. The glow is primarily red because most of the other colors in the beam are absorbed by the red blood cells; the red light is the only important component that is transmitted.

Transillumination is used clinically in the detection of hydrocephalus (water-head) in infants. Since the skull of young infants is not fully calcified, light is able to penetrate to the inside of the skull; if there is an excess of relatively clear cerebrospinal fluid (CSF) in the skull, light is scattered to different parts of the skull producing patterns characteristic of hydrocephalus. The special transilluminating device uses a 150W projection bulb as the light source.

The device has a two-position trigger switch. The infant is taken into a dark room for the study; after a few minutes of dark adaptation the physician pulls the trigger to its first position, which turns on a red light that permits him to find the patient. The physician then points the barrel at the part of the head to be studied and pulls the trigger to the second position, which turns off the red light and turns on the intense white light used for the study. Infrared absorbing glass in the beam removes almost all the IR radiation so that the light striking the infant is primarily visible light.

Transillumination is also used to detect pneumothorax (collapsed lungs) in infants. The bright light penetrates the thin front chest wall and reflects off the back chest wall to indicate the degree of pneumothorax.

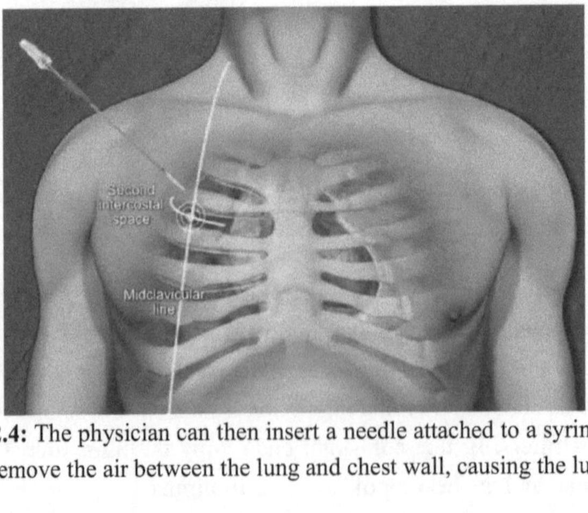

Figure 2.4: The physician can then insert a needle attached to a syringe into the area of collapse to remove the air between the lung and chest wall, causing the lung to reinflate.

The sinuses, the gums, the breasts, and the testes have also been studied with transillumination.

Visible light has an important therapeutic use. Since light is a form of energy and is selectively absorbed in certain molecules, it should not be surprising that it can cause important physiological effects. Many premature infants have jaundice, a condition in which an excess of bilirubin is excreted by the liver into the blood. Relatively recently (1958) it was discovered that most premature infants recover from jaundice if their bodies are exposed to visible light (phototherapy).

2.4 APPLICATIONS OF ULTRAVIOLET AND INFRARED LIGHT IN MEDICINE

The wavelengths adjacent to the visible spectrum also have important uses in medicine. Ultraviolet photons have greater energies than visible photons, while IR photons have lower energies. Because of their higher energies, UV photons are more useful than IR photons.

Ultraviolet light with wavelengths below about 290nm is germicidal-that is, it can kill germs-and it is sometimes used to sterilize medical instruments. Ultraviolet light also produces more reactions in the skin than visible light. Some of these reactions are beneficial, and some are harmful. One of the major beneficial effects of UV light from the sun is the conversion of molecular products in the skin into vitamin D. Dermatologists have also found that UV light improves certain skin conditions.

Ultraviolet light from the sun affects the melanin in the skin to cause tanning. However, UV light can produce sunburn as well as tan the skin. The wavelengths that produce sunburn are around 300nm, just at the edge of the solar spectrum. The amount of 300nm light in the sun's spectrum depends on the amount of atmosphere that the sunlight must pass through. Ordinary window glass permits some near UV to be transmitted but absorbs the sunburn component.

Solar UV light is also the major cause of skin cancer in humans. The high incidence of skin cancer among people who have been exposed to the sun a great deal, such as fishermen and agricultural workers, may be related to the fact that the UV wavelengths that produce sunburn are also very well absorbed by the DNA in the cells. Skin cancer usually appears on those portions of the body that have received the most sunlight, such as the tip of the nose, the tops of the ears, and the back of the neck.

You probably know that the sky is blue because light of short (blue) wavelengths is scattered more easily than light of long wavelengths. Ultraviolet light has even shorter wavelengths than blue light and is scattered even more easily. About half of the UV light hitting the skin on a summer day comes directly from the sun and the other half is scattered from the air in other parts of the sky. Thus you can get sunburned even when you are sitting in the shade under a small tree. Even when the sky is completely covered with clouds about one half of the UV light gets through.

Ultraviolet light cannot be seen by the eye because it is absorbed before it reaches the retina. The large percentage of near-UV light absorbed by the lens may be the cause of some cataracts (opacities of the lens).

About half of the energy from the sun is in the IR region. The warmth we feel from the sun is mainly due to the IR component. The IR rays are not usually hazardous even though they are focused by the cornea and lens of the eye onto the retina. However, looking at the sun through a filter (e.g., plastic sunglasses) that removes most of the visible light and allows most of the IR wavelengths through can cause a burn on the retina. Some people have damaged their eyes in this way by looking at the sun during a solar eclipse. Dark glasses absorb varying amounts of the IR and UV rays from the sun.

Heat lamps that produce a large percentage of IR light with wavelengths of 1000 to 2000 nm are often used for physical therapy purposes. Infrared light penetrates further into the tissues than visible light and thus is better able to heat deep tissues.

Two types of IR photography are used in medicine: reflective IR photography and emissive IR photography. The latter, which uses the long IR heat waves emitted by the body that give an indication of the body temperature, is usually called thermography. Reflective IR photography, which uses wavelengths of 700 to 900 nm to show the patterns of veins just below the skin. Some of these veins are visible, but many more can be seen on a near-IR photograph of the skin. Since the temperature on the skin depends on the local blood flow, a thermogram with good resolution shows the venous pattern much like a near-IR photograph.

There is considerable variation in the venous patterns of normal individuals.

Even in the same individual the venous patterns in the two breasts may be quite different. Cancer and other diseases can cause changes in the venous pattern, but these changes can be masked by the normal variations. Also, a layer of fat beneath the skin can reduce the appearance of the venous pattern.

Infrared can also be used to photograph the pupil of the eye without stimulating the reflex that changes its size.

2.5 LASERS IN MEDICINE

A laser is a unique light source that emits a narrow beam of light of a single wavelength (monochromatic light) in which each wave is in phase with the others near it (coherent light). Laser is an acronym for Light Amplification by Stimulated Emission of Radiation. While the basic theory for lasers was proposed by Albert Einstein in 1917, the first successful laser was not made until 1960, when T. H. Maiman produced a laser beam from a ruby crystal. Since 1960 scientists have made many types of lasers using gases and liquids as well as solids as laser materials.

In a laser, energy that has been stored in the laser material (e.g., ruby) is released as a narrow beam of light-either as a steady beam continuous wave (CW) or as an intense pulse. The beam remains narrow over long distances and can be thought of as an ideal "spot" light. A laser beam can be focused to a spot only a few microns in diameter. When all the energy of the laser is concentrated in such a small area, the power density (power per unit area) becomes very large. The total energy of a typical laser pulse used in medicine, which is measured in millijoules (mJ), can be delivered in less than a microsecond, and the resultant instantaneous power may be in megawatts. The output of a pulsed laser is usually measured by the heat produced in the detector (calorimetric method). The output of a low-power CW laser is often measured with a photodetector such as a silicon photocell (often called a solar cell).

Since in medicine lasers are used primarily to deliver energy to tissue, the laser wavelength used should be strongly absorbed by tissue. The short wavelengths (400 to 600 nm) are always absorbed better than the long wavelengths (~700nm).

Laser energy directed at human tissue causes a rapid rise in temperature and can destroy the tissue. The amount of damage to living tissue depends on how long the tissue is at the increased temperature. *For example*, tissue can withstand 70°C for

1sec. However, not all laser damage is due to heat. It also produces noticeable damage due to photochemical effects.

The laser is routinely used in clinical medicine only in ophthalmology. Its effectiveness in treating certain types of cancer and its usefulness as a "bloodless knife" for surgery are under active investigation. Lasers are also being used in medical research for special three-dimensional imaging called holography.

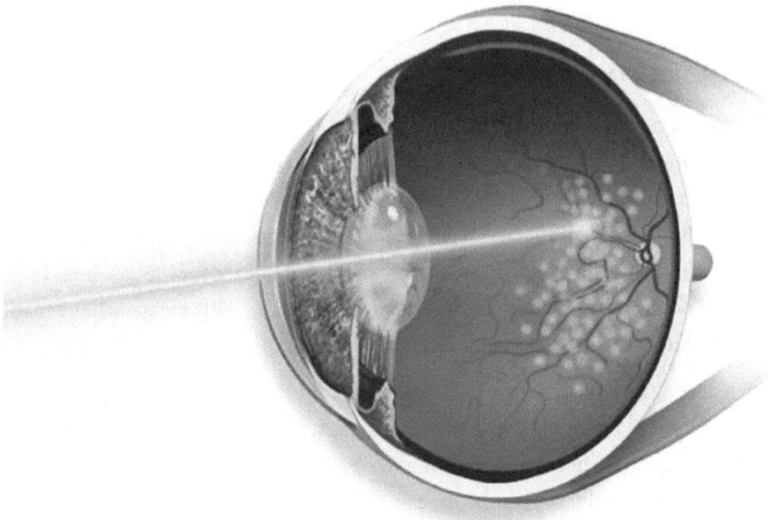

Figure 2.5: In ophthalmology lasers are primarily used for photocoagulation of the retina, that is, heating a blood vessel to the point where the blood coagulates and blocks the vessel.

The amount of laser energy needed for photocoagulation depends on the spot size used. In general, the proper dose is determined visually by the ophthalmologist at the time of the treatment. The minimum amount of laser energy that will do observable damage to the retina is called the Minimal Reactive Dose (MRD). *For example*, the MRD for 50μm spot in the eye is about 2.4mJ delivered in 0.25sec.

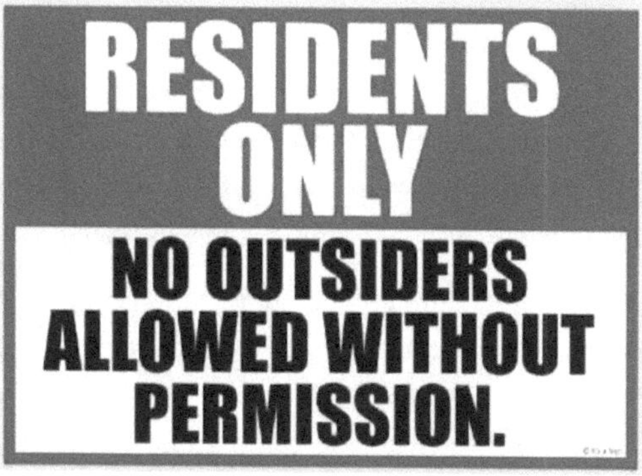

Figure 2.6: The area should have adequate warning signs and a system that prevents outsiders from entering while lasers are in use.

Photocoagulation is useful for repairing retinal tears or holes that develop prior to retinal detachment. When the retina is completely detached, the laser is of no help. A complication of diabetes that affects the retina, called diabetic retinopathy, can also be treated with photocoagulation.

Protective glasses must be worn in medical laser areas to protect the eyes of the patient and the workers. Since laser energy is concentrated in a narrow beam for long distances, even a reflected beam can be a hazard; thus, the walls and other surfaces in a laser installation should have low reflectivity (e.g., flat black paint).

2.6 APPLICATIONS OF MICROSCOPES IN MEDICINE

There have been few breakthroughs in science that have had as great an impact as the invention of the microscope by Leeuwenhoek (~1670). The use of the microscope in the pathology laboratory is as common as the use of the thermometer in the clinic.

The standard light microscope usually can be set at any of several magnifications by changing the power of the eyepiece or of the objective lens. The highest magnification that can be obtained is limited by the wavelength of visible light. Since the wavelengths of visible light range from 400 to 700 nm (0.4 to 0.7 μm), the smallest object that can be resolved is about 1μm in diameter. Since most cells are 5 to 50 μm in diameter, this type of microscope is adequate for resolving all but subcellular objects.

If you put a thin slice of tissue under a microscope you will not see much because most cells are transparent to all wavelengths of visible light-red blood cells are an exception. To distinguish different cells, it is usually necessary to stain them with a chemical that strongly absorbs certain visible wavelengths.

Other techniques in addition to staining are useful in microscopy. One technique takes advantage of the different indexes of refraction of different cell parts. Since light travels at different speeds in the various parts of a cell, the phase relationships of the light waves change in passing through a specimen. The phase-contrast microscope takes advantage of this phenomenon to allow cell structures to be seen without the use of stain. In this type of microscope, a light beam that passes through the tissue is combined with a reference beam directed through an optically uniform zone. The combined beams interfere, producing dark areas where there is destructive interference and light areas where there is constructive interference. The darkness depends on the degree of interference.

2.7 LIGHT-ACTIVATED THERAPIES

Light-activated therapeutic applications harness the versatility of light in manipulating photoactive molecules, proteins and cells. Phototherapies, which require only an appropriately selected light source, are commonplace in the clinic and are first-line treatments for some conditions.

For instance, since the 1960s, blue-light photo- therapy has been used to treat severe hyperbilirubinemia in millions of infants. More broadly, the use of exogenous photosensitizers offers capabilities beyond intrinsic light-induced signaling, such as oxidative killing of unwanted cells in photodynamic therapy (PDT). Today, PDT is an established modality used in oncology, dermato- ogy, ophthalmology, dentistry, cosmetics and other fields. The com- binned global markets for drugs and devices used in phototherapy and PDT were estimated to be US$630 million in 2014 (Fig. 2.7 b).

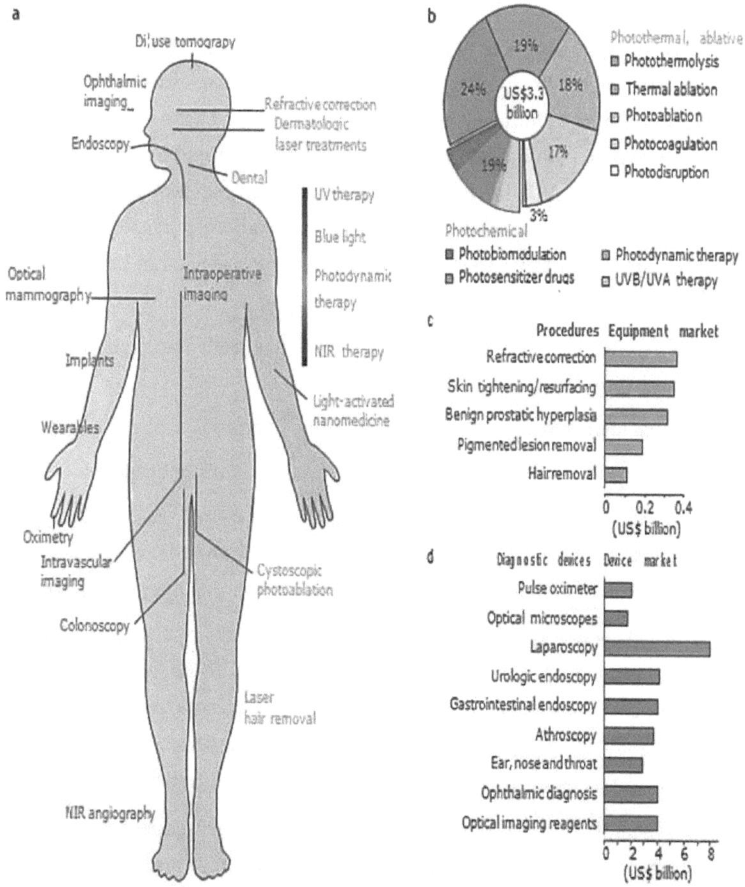

Figure 2.7: Medical application areas of light.

Ultraviolet light (100–400 nm). Exposure to the Sun's UV radiation, consisting of 95% UVA (320–400 nm) and 5% UVB (290–320 nm), is a major environmental risk factor for skin cancer, which afflicts more than 2 million people worldwide every year. UVB radiation can directly damage DNA and thus is particularly carcinogenic. UVA can also cause cancer via the generation of DNA-damaging free radi- calls. Despite the harmful effects, UV-light exposure may have poteen- tail beneficial effects through the modulation of immune responses. Indeed, UVB radiation can activate innate immune responses via release of antimicrobial peptides and vitamin D production, which may play a role in Finsen's phototherapy for lupus vulgaris. UVB light also suppresses the adaptive immune system by activation of regulatory T cells, B cells and mast cells. UVA light can also be immunosuppressive through the upregulation of the alternative complement pathway. These mechanistic findings have suggested a physiological role for low, non-carcinogenic doses of UV light: induce- Tion of innate immunity to protect against microbial attacks, and suppression of adaptive immunity to inhibit autoimmune or allergic responses. The latter mechanism forms the basis of UV phototherapy, which is used to treat a wide range of dermatomes in the clinic.

a, Representative applications of light in the human body for diagnosis and imaging (green), surgery (pink) and therapy (blue).

b, Global market in 2014 for medical lasers by therapeutic application.

c, Equipment spending in 2013 for leading laser-treatment procedures.

d, Global market in 2013–2014 for several major diagnostic devices. Data from BCC Research reports HLC093C, HLC072C and HLC172A (with permission of BCC Research).

Narrow-band UVB therapy. For over 90 years, UVB radiation has been used to treat psoriasis, a chronic, immune-mediated inflammatory disorder affecting tens of millions of people worldwide. It is also used to treat vitiligo, atopic dermatitis and other inflammatory dermatoses. With emission at 311 ± 2 nm, narrow- band UVB is preferable to standard broadband UVB (290–320 nm) because of improved efficacy and the reduced risk of erythema (superficial reddening of the skin).

Psoralen and UVA therapy (PUVA). This is another frequent treatment for psoriasis and vitiligo. It requires oral or topical administration of psoralen, exposure to UVA light, and is commonly used to treat patients for whom narrow-band UVB is unsuccessful. The therapy also works through immunosuppressive and antiproliferative effects.

Other effects. Several epidemiology studies have noted that increased sun exposure is associated with decreased risk of multiple sclerosis. A study in mice substantiated these findings, showing that UVB radiation suppresses the progression of experimental autoimmune encephalomyelitis. Another mouse study suggested that UVB radiation may suppress the development of obesity and metabolic syndrome independent of vitamin D supplementation.

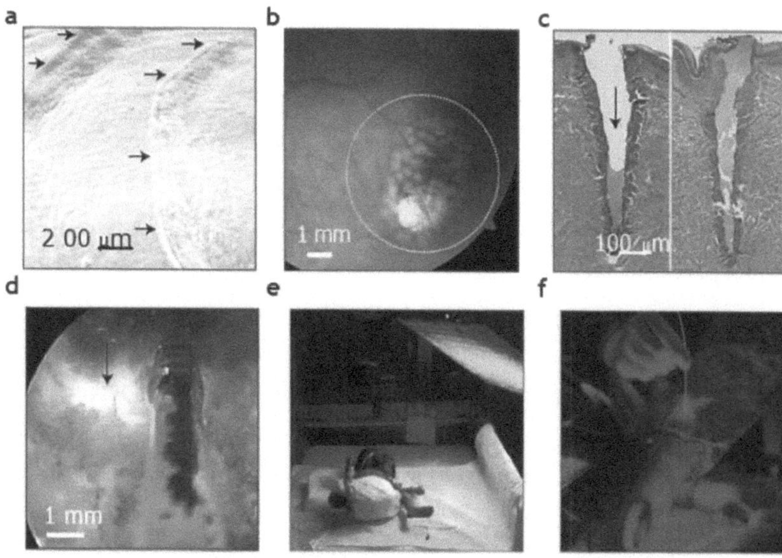

Figure 2.8: Surgical and therapeutic applications of light.

Visible light (400–700 nm). *Phototherapy for neonatal jaundice.* Jaundiced infants are commonly treated with phototherapy at 460–490 nm, preventing serious sequelae of hyperbilirubinemia, such as permanent neurological damage (Fig. 2.8e). Blue light isomerizes bilirubin to facilitate its excretion. In the United States, 0.5–4% of term and late-preterm infants receive phototherapy before discharge from the nursery. In low-resource settings, filtered sunlight using canopies is a promising and affordable option for treating neonatal jaundice.

Bright light therapy for mood disorders. Seasonal affective disorder is a common form of depression that coincides with shorter days during the winter months and has a prevalence of 0.4–9.9% in the Northern Hemisphere. This disorder and other conditions involving irregular light exposure, such as jet lag, have been linked to mood and cognitive alterations either by modulation of sleep and circadian rhythms, or by direct activation of neural pathways. These mechanisms are Medi- acted by intrinsically photosensitive retinal ganglion cells that express the photopigment melanopsin. Bright-light therapy has proven to be as effective as most antidepressant drugs for treating seasonal affective disorder. In fact, activation of the ganglion cells by bright blue light (480 nm) conveys signals to the brain that suppress melatonin secretion and reset circadian rhythms. Bright-light therapy has also shown promise for the treatment of non-seasonal major depressive disorder, but the mechanism of action is still unclear.

a, Photoablation. The scanning electron micrograph shows stepwise ablated patterns (arrows) in an experimental cornea by excimer laser irradiation.

b, Photocoagulation. Laser-induced damage spots around a retinal tear region7 (dashed circle).

c, Photothermal ablation. Histology of porcine skin tissues harvested 0 min (left) and 60 min (right) after fractional, pulsed CO2 laser exposure in vivo16. The arrow indicates the laser channel, which is filled with a fibrin plug within minutes.

d, Photothermal ablation (vaporization). A fiber-optic catheter delivers high-power continuous- wave laser light (arrow) to remove excess prostate tissue in a patient with benign prostate hyperplasia (www.youtube.com/watch?v=jAbSwtSN9xE).

e, Blue-light therapy for the treatment of neonatal jaundice.

f, Photodynamic therapy. Close-up image of a surgeon's hands in an operating room. Figure reproduced with permission from: a, ref. 4, Elsevier; b, ref. 7, Digital Journal of Ophthalmology; c, ref. 16, Wiley; d, Creative Commons license CC BY 3.0; e, VT Bijoy, Creative Commons license CC BY-SA 3.0; f, John Crawford, National Cancer Institute.

Antimicrobial treatment. Antibiotic resistance increasingly threatens the ability to effectively treat bacterial infections. Blue light at 405–470 nm has been effective in treating a broad range of bacterial infections, including Propionibacterium acnes-associated acne vulgaris and Helicobacter pylori gastritis in humans, as well as wound infections with methicillin-resistant Staphylococcus aureus (MRSA) and Pseudomonas aeruginosa in mouse models. The antimicrobial effect of blue light is thought to arise from the excitation of endogenous porphyrins within the bacterial cells. Before it is accepted for mainstream clinical practice, however, the possible development of microbial resistance to phototherapy needs to be evaluated.

Other effects. Insufficient outdoor exposure to sunlight has been implicated with the growing prevalence of myopia58 (an estimated 2.5 billion people worldwide will be affected by the condition by 2020). Supporting this observation, high ambient lighting was found to prevent the development of myopia in macaque models. Another potential application is the use of non-ablative lasers to adjuvant vaccines. Pre-treatment of the site of vaccine administration with visible or NIR light significantly enhanced vaccine efficiency and augmented immune responses in mouse models.

Near-infrared light (700–1,800 nm). *Photobiomodulation.* Also known as low-level laser-light therapy (LLLT), photobiomodulation uses red and NIR light at 600–1,000 nm, at fluences of 1–10 J cm^{-2} with intensity of 3–90 mW cm^{-2}. Clinical studies have suggested that light can stimulate epidermal stem cells in the hair follicle bulge to promote hair growth. Photobiomodulation for wound healing, tissue repair and anti-inflammatory therapy has been shown to be efficacious in animal models. Results from clinical trials have been mixed yet have shown therapeutic potential for neck pain and chronic traumatic brain injury. Because its underlying mechanisms are not well understood, adoption of photobiomodulation has been controversial, and its use largely empirical. The mechanisms are largely attributed to the absorption of NIR light by cytochrome C oxidase in mitochondria. This triggers the dissociation of inhibitory nitric oxide from the protein complex, thus increasing adenosine triphosphate synthesis, which can have direct beneficial effects on compromised and hypoxic cells. Therapeutic effects of photobiomodulation may also be mediated by the generation of reactive oxygen species (ROS) and the induction of gene transcription. In fact, photobiomodulation on tooth pulps in rats with 810 nm continuous-wave light at a total dose of 3 J cm^{-2} was shown to form tertiary dentin via direct dental stem cell differentiation through light-induced generation of ROS.

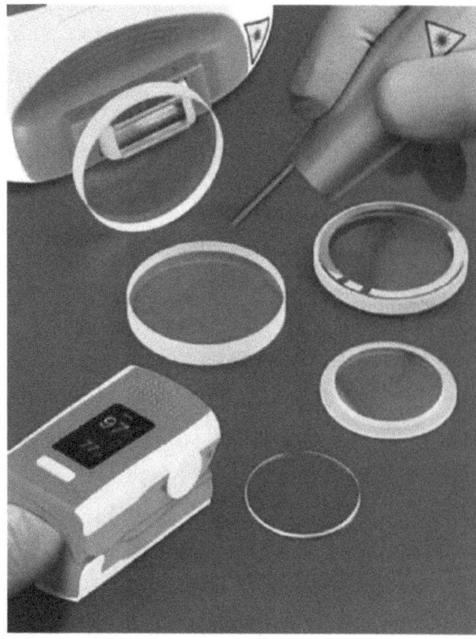

3 CHAPTER

OPTICS IN MEDICINE

3 INTRODUCTIONS

3.1 WHY OPTICS IN MEDICINE?

Unlike the present time, medical practitioners of the ancient world did not have the benefit of sophisticated instrumentation and diagnostic systems, such as X-rays, ultrasound machines, or CT scanners. Visual and manual auscultations were the tools of the day. Hence, since the early days of medicine, optics has been a useful and powerful technology to assist doctors, and all forms of healthcare practitioners carry out examination and diagnosis of their patients. This is so because one of the fundamental aspects of medicine is observation and physical examination of patience's general appearance. Hence, anything that can help "see" better the condition of a patient will be of aid. As such, optics, as the science that studies the behavior and manipulation of light and images, is an ideal tool to assist doctors gain better visual examination capabilities by providing improved illumination, magnification, access to small or internal body cavities, among others. But it is light and its interaction with living tissues is at the center of what makes optics in medicine possible. Light possesses energy and can interact with biological cells, tissues, and organs. Such interaction can be used to probe the state of such living matter for diagnostics and analytical purposes or, it could be used to induce changes on the same living systems and be exploited for therapeutic purposes. The science of light generation, manipulation, transmission, and measurement is known as *photonics*. The application of photonics technologies and principles to medicine and life sciences is known as *biophotonics*.

Nowadays, it is not only optics but also photonics that are used extensively in a myriad of medical applications, from diagnostics, to therapeutics, to surgical procedures. Hence, when we use the term medical optics, we are referring to biomedical optics and biophotonics as well. The interrelation between optics and light in medicine is ever present and it could be said that more significant advances in biophotonics are now due to the availability of more powerful, concentrated, and multi-spectral light sources which have been available only in the last 50 years. Historically, ambient light was the illumination source, which precluded performing exams late in the day or during certain hours in the wintertime. Oil candles in the ancient world gave way to wax ones and alcohol burning lamps in the fifteenth through the nineteenth centuries until the development of electricity and the introduction of the electric lamp by Edison. Then, in the 1960s, with the development of semiconductor lasers, light emitting diodes (LEDs) and lasers, modern medical optics began to take shape and coupled with the availability of optical fibers, a new generation of medical instruments and techniques began to be developed.

Fiber optics have been used in the medical industry even before their adoption and subsequent explosion as the technology of choice for long haul data communications. The advantages of optical fibers have been recognized by the medical community long ago. Optical fibers are thin, flexible, dielectric (non-conductive), immune to electromagnetic interference, chemically inert, non-toxic, and of course, small. They can also be sterilized using standard medical sterilization techniques. Their major advantage lies in the fact that they are thin and flexible so they can be introduced into the body for both remote sense, image and treat. Their initial and still most successful biological/biomedical application has been in the field of endoscopic imaging. Prior to the development of such devices, the only method of inspecting the interior of the body was through invasive surgery. Many patients owe their lives today to the existence of fiberoptic endoscopes. Optical fibers are not only useful for endoscopes but can also be used to transmit light to tissue regions of interest either to illuminate the tissue so that it can be inspected, or if much higher power laser light is used, to directly cut or ablate it. Hence, they are used extensively as laser-delivery probes, as well as imaging conduits in optical coherence tomography (OCT).

Optical fibers have revolutionized medicine in many ways and continue to do so thanks to the advent of new surgical trends, as summarized in Table 3.1. One such trend is the advent of minimally invasive surgery (MIS) where the trend now is to avoid cutting open patients and instead, perform small cuts and incisions through which a variety of different surgical instruments, such as catheters and probes, are inserted through these small openings, thus minimizing the postoperative pain and discomfort. Furthermore, there is today growing use of surgical robots where a surgeon operates them remotely using control arms to do a surgical procedure from the comfort of his office while the patient is at a remote hospital location.

Table 3.1: Medical industry trends that promote the use of optical fibers.

- Drives towards minimally invasive surgery (MIS) ! Need for disposable probes and catheters
- Miniaturization, Automation and Robotics ! Need for instrumented catheters

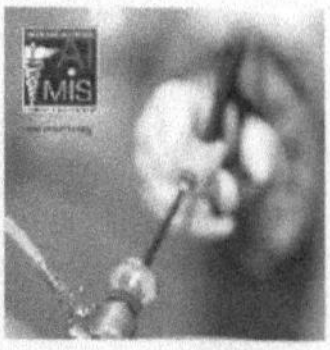

- Sensors compatible with MRI, CT, PET equipment as well as thermal ablative treatments involving RF or microwave radiation ! Need for fiber sensors

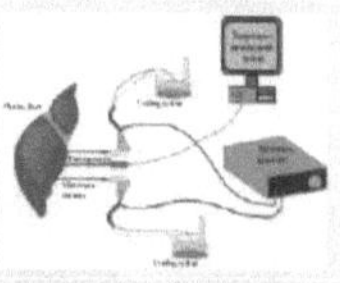

- Increased user of lasers ! Need for fiber delivery devices
- Increased use of optical imaging and scanning techniques ! Need for fiber OCT probes

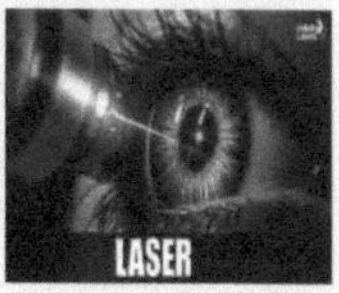

MEDICAL OPTICS

However, one of the issues with these types of systems is the fact that the surgeon loses the actual manual feedback and does not have sensitivity of the force needed to apply to a scalpel or other surgical tools. This is called *haptic* feedback. These "robotic surgeons" operate using very small tools and catheters, and in order to make sensing elements compatible with such slender instruments, fiber optics represent an ideal solution to provide shape, position, as well as force-sensing information to the remote surgeon's controls.

Fiber optic and photonic devices are also being exploited as sensing devices for patient monitoring during medical imaging and treatment using radiation devices such as MRI, CT, and PET type scan systems that involve the use of high-intensity electromagnetic fields, radiofrequencies, or microwave signals. Because the patient's risk of an electric shock conventional electronic monitoring devices and instrumentation cannot be used in these applications. Instead, patient monitoring is performed using optical fiber sensors.

Table 3.2: Typical applications of optics in medicine.

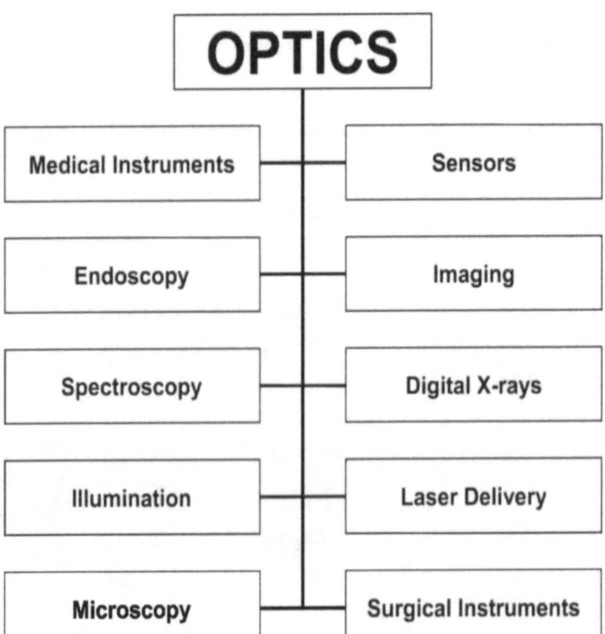

Based on the above arguments, the need for and benefits of optics (and photonics) in medicine becomes evident. Table 3.2 summarizes the key general applications for optics in medicine. In general, it could be said that optics has been and will continue to be an enabling technology to further the development and advancement of medicine and the healthcare industry.

3.2 GLOBAL HEALTHCARE NEEDS AND DRIVERS

We all need medical care from the day we are born, until the day we die. However, this need for medical care has now been affected and accentuated by a convergence of social, demographic, economic, environmental, and political global trends that have been developing over the last few decades. It is a world full of challenges that impact how to effectively deliver healthcare in an effective, affordable, and sustainable fashion. On one hand, average lifestyles have changed drastically in the past century resulting in a more sedentary lifestyle with lack of exercise, poor diet, smoking, and excessive alcohol consumption that have resulted in a growing number of chronic diseases such as obesity, arteriosclerosis, diabetes, and cancer that have become leading causes of death and disability. On the other hand, the entire global population keeps growing.

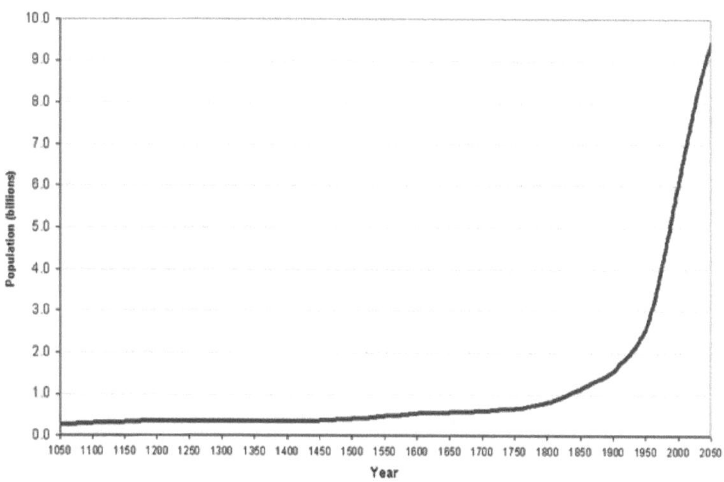

Figure 3.1: Historical global population growth.

MEDICAL OPTICS

According to a recent United Nations Department of Economic and Social Affairs (DESA) report the world's population is estimated to be more than 7.3 billion and growing at ~1.1 % annual rate, and expected to reach 8.5 billion by 2030, 9.7 billion in 2050, and 11.2 billion in 2100. As illustrated in Fig. 3.1, the world population has experienced continuous growth since the end of the Great Famine and the Black Death back in 1350, when the total population stood at merely 370 million. Nowadays, total annual births are approximately 135 million/year, while deaths are around 56 million/year, but are expected to increase to 80 million/year by 2040.

Add to this the fact that in certain parts of the world the population is aging, including the USA, Japan, and parts of Europe. Globally, the number of persons aged 65 or older is expected to reach nearly 1.5 billion by 2050. An aging population puts additional demands on healthcare since older people are more vulnerable to illness and chronic diseases. Furthermore, life expectancy at birth has increased significantly. The UN DESA estimates a 6-year average gain in life expectancy among the poorest countries, from 56 years in 2000–2005 to 62 years in 2010–2015, which is roughly double the increase recorded for the rest of the world. Another key trend and global challenge are the expected shortage of medical doctors and physicians available to meet the healthcare needs of a growing world population.

A large global population requires more doctors, medical devices, medical supplies, clinics, hospitals, and overall healthcare infrastructure to address the needs of people needing immunization or getting sick or injured. Hence, there is and will continue to be an overall growth and expansion of the health care industry on a global basis, that continuously demanding more medical instruments and technical innovations that can facilitate and expedite medical examinations, while reducing costs. Historically, optics has been an enabling technology for the design and development of such medical devices and instruments.

Another relevant and converging present trend is how biomedical devices and instruments are so extremely pervasive across the healthcare industry today. We may not realize it, but whenever we get our blood pressure tested, monitor our blood sugar, or when a expectant mother is being monitored by her doctor, an instrument or sensing device is needed which, often, is based on the use of an optical technique or based on the use of optical components. Couple this with the fact that in many parts of the underdeveloped world there is not enough doctors, hospitals, clinics, and instrumentation available to support local populations. Hence, it becomes critically important to develop simple, practical, effective, and inexpensive medical devices that can be used in rural and remote areas by non-professionals to examine and treat patients.

3.3 HISTORICAL USES OF OPTICS IN MEDICINE

Mankind has always been fascinated with light and the miracle of vision, dating back to the first century when the Romans were investigating the use of glass and how viewing objects through it, made the objects appear larger. However, most of the significant developments of optics for medical diagnosis and therapy started occurring in the nineteenth century. Before that, most of the known published works on optics and medicine dealt mostly with the anatomy and physiology of the human eye. For instance, the Greek anatomist, Claudius Galen (130–201) provided early anatomical descriptions of the structure of the human eye, describing the retina, iris, cornea, tear ducts, and other structures as well as defining for the first time the two eye fluids: the vitreous and aqueous humors. Subsequently, Arab scholars Yaqub ibn Ishaq al-Kindi (801–873) and Abu Zayd Hunayn ibn Ishaq alIbadi (808–873) provided a more comprehensive study of the eye in the ninth century in their *Ten Treatises on the Eye and the Book of the Questions of the Eye*. In the eleventh century Abu Ali al-Hasan ibn al-Haytham (965–1040)—known as Alhazen—also provided descriptions of the eye's anatomy in his Book of Optics (Kitab al-Manazir).

It is around this time that the so-called reading stones are being used as magnifying lenses to help read manuscripts. The English philosopher Robert Bacon (1214–1294) described in 1268 in his *Opus Majus* the mechanics of a glass instrument placed in front of his eyes. Then, in the thirteenth century, Salvino D'Armate from Italy made the first eye glass, providing the wearer with an element of magnification to one eye.

With the advent of the optical telescope optics took a significant step forward towards the development of one of the first early medical instruments, the microscope. The compound microscope was developed around the late 1590s by Hans and Zacharias Janssen, a father and son team of Dutch spectacle makers, who experimented with lenses by placing them in series inside a tube and discovered that the object near the end of the tube appeared greatly enlarged see Fig. 3.2.

Figure3.2: Photograph of the Jansen compound microscope (c. 1595).

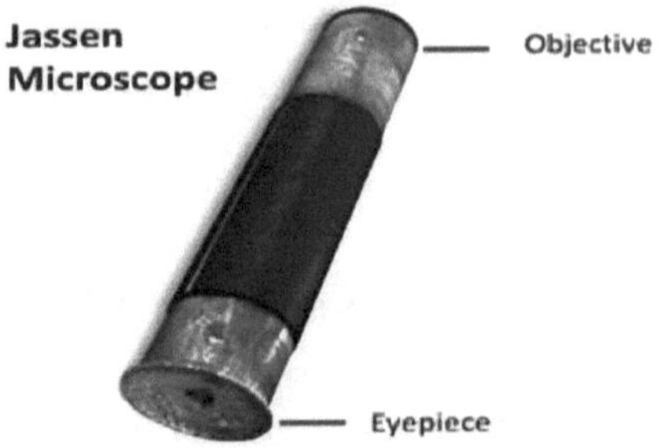

A seminal optical medical instrument development came in 1804 when the German born physician Philipp Bozzini (1773–1809) developed and first publicized his so-called light conductor (*Lichtleiter*), which enabled the direct view into the living body. The *lichtleiter* was an early form of endoscope which consisted of an open tube with a 45° mirror mounted at the proximal end with a hole in it. Illumination was provided by a burning alcohol and turpentine lamp was shone to a speculum mounted on the distal end and made to fit to the specific anatomy of the desired body opening to be inspected see Fig. 3.3. In December 1806 Bozzini's light conductor was presented to the professors of the Josephinum, the "Medical-Surgical Joseph's Academy" in Vienna.

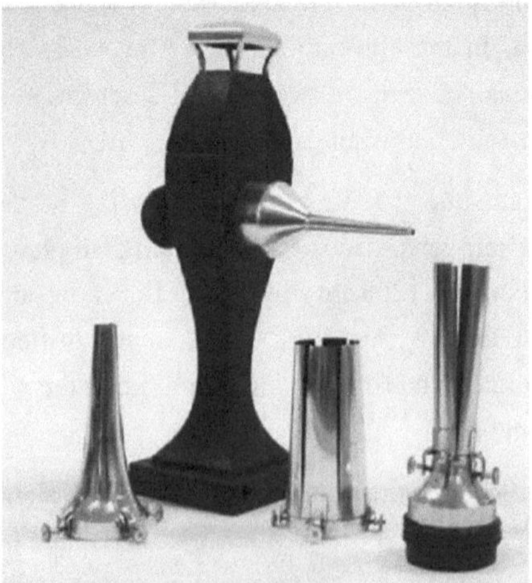

Figure 3.3: Bozzini's original light conductor with specula (c. 1806).

A period of significant activity and innovation in medical optics occurred from the mid-1800s through the early 1900s, when a variety of early medical instruments such as otoscopes, ophthalmoscopes, retinoscopes, and others, as well as improved illumination systems were developed. In 1851 German scientist and physician Hermann L. F. von Helmholtz (1821–1894) used a mirror with a tiny aperture (opening) to shine a beam of light into the inside of the eyeball. Helmholtz found that looking through the lens into the back of the eye only produced a red reflection. To improve on the image quality, he used a condenser lens that produced a 5× magnification Fig. 3.4. He called this combination of a mirror and condenser lens an *Augenspiegel* (eye mirror).

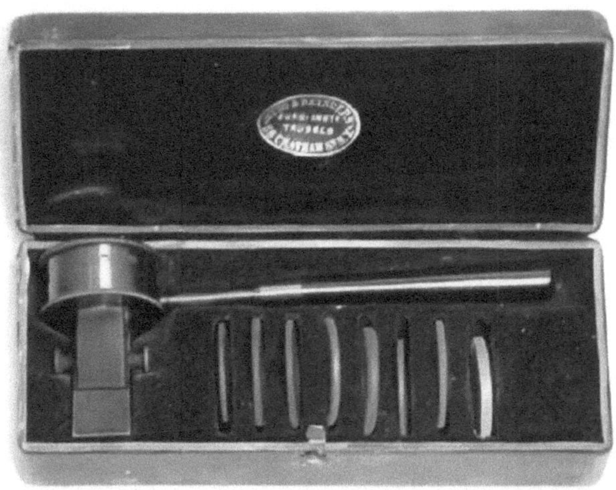

Figure 3.4: Helmholtz ophthalmoscope (c. 1851).

The term ophthalmoscope (eye-observer) did not come into common use until later. Helmholtz also invented the ophthalmometer, which was used to measure the curvature of the eye. In addition, Helmholtz studied color blindness and the speed of nervous impulses. He also wrote the classic Handbook of Physiological Optics.

In 1888 Prof. Reuss and Dr. Roth of Vienna used bent solid glass rods to illuminate body cavities for dentistry and surgery. This would be the earliest idea to use a precursor of an optical fiber for medical applications. Decades later, in 1926,

MEDICAL OPTICS

J. L. Baird of England and Clarence W. Hansell of the RCA Rocy Point Labs propose independently of each other fiber optic bundles as imaging devices. A few years later, German medical student Heinrich Lamm assembles the first bundles of transparent optical fibers to carry the image from a filament lamp but is denied a patent. Then in 1949, Danish researchers Holger M. Hansen and Abraham C. S. van Heel begin investigating image transmission using bundles of parallel glass fibers. Prof. Harold H. Hopkins from Imperial College in London begins work in 1952 to develop an endoscope based on bundles of glass fibers. University of Michigan Medical professor Basil Hirschowitz visits Imperial College in 1954 to discuss with Prof. Hopkins and graduate student, Narinder Kapany, about their ideas for imaging fiber bundles. Hirschowitz hired undergraduate student Larry Curtis to develop a fiber optic endoscope at the University of Michigan. Curtis fabricates the first clad optical fiber from a rod-in-tube glass drawing process. Prof. Hirschowitz tests first prototype fiber optic endoscope using clad fibers in February of 1957 and then introduces it to the American Gastroscopic Society in May of the same year.

The first solid-state laser was built in 1960 by Dr. T. H. Maiman at Hughes Aircraft Company. Within the year, Dr. Leon Goldman, chairman of the Department of Dermatology at the University of Cincinnati, began his research on the use of lasers for medical applications and later established a laser technology laboratory at the school's Medical Center. Dr. Goldman is known as the "father of laser medicine." He is also the founder of the American Society for Lasers in Medicine and Surgery. However, the first medical treatment using a laser on a human patient was performed in December 1961 by Dr. Charles J. Campbell of the Institute of Ophthalmology at Columbia–Presbyterian Medical Center, who used a ruby laser that is used to destroy a retinal tumor. Since then, lasers have become an integral part of modern medicine.

During the 1980s and 1990s, extensive research was conducted to develop fiber-optic-based chemical and biological sensors for diverse medical applications.

OCT is a newer optical medical imaging technique, first introduced in the early 1990s, that uses light to capture micrometer resolution, three-dimensional images from within biological tissue based on low-coherence, and optical interferometry. OCT is a technique that makes it possible to take sub-surface images of tissues with micrometer resolution. It can be thought of as the optical equivalent of an ultrasound scanning system. This is an active area of medical research at the moment.

3.4 FUTURE TRENDS

Optics and photonics, as mentioned earlier, are powerful, versatile, and enabling technologies for the development of present and future generations of medical devices, instruments, and techniques for diagnostic, therapy, and surgical applications.

Given the present R&D activity worldwide based on optical and photonic techniques it should be no surprise to expect a broader utilization of optically based solutions across the healthcare industry and medical profession. In the future, advances in the development of ever smaller and thinner medical probes and catheters should be expected, as well as broad utilization of OCT devices to become as common as ultrasound scanning devices are today. There will also be a proliferation of laser-based treatments and therapies. Endoscopy, for its part, will continue to evolve and more sophisticated and smaller devices will be developed that will combine more functions (from the standard illumination and visualization) with direct tissue analysis and laser treatment. Optical imaging techniques will continue to advance along with digital X-rays to make non-invasive examination and diagnosis safe, fast and with greater resolution and pinpoint accuracy.

Other future capabilities brought on by optics will be in the form of the so-called lab-on-a-fiber or LOF for short, where optical fibers are combined with micro- and nano-sized functionalized materials that react to specific physical, chemical, or biological external effects and can thus serve as elements to build multi-function, multi-parameter sensing devices. Light would remotely excite the functionalized materials which are embedded in the fiber's coating material. These materials in turn will react to specific biological or chemical substances (*analytes*) and induce an optical signal change proportional to the given analyte concentration.

Some future innovations can already be witnessed today in the form of optical devices used in combination with smart portable cell phones. For example, several new companies have now developed accessories for attachment to smartphones, which turn them into electronic video equivalents of conventional medical examination instruments such as otoscopes (to view inside ears), ophthalmoscopes (to view the inside of eyes), or even simple microscopes. Such devices are passive, optical elements that couple images from the patient to the video lens onto the smartphone's digital camera transform it into a fully functioning, network-connected medical instrument, capable of sending images and video remotely to a consulting doctor. Figure 3.5 depicts a cell phone otoscope in use, while Fig. 3.6 depicts a smartphone version of an ophthalmoscope and a dermal loupe.

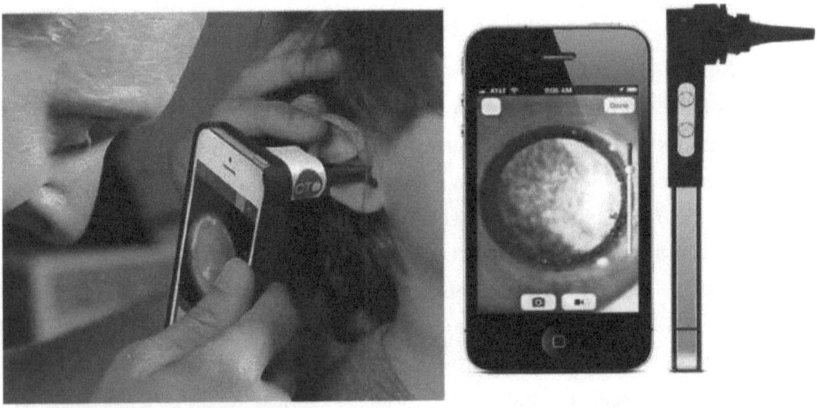

Figure 3.5: A smartphone otoscope.

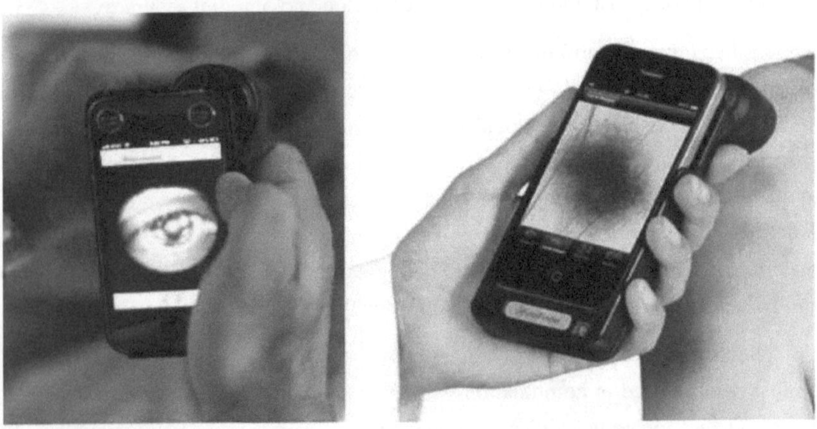

Figure 3.6: Examples of an ophthalmoscope and a dermal loupe attached to a smartphone.

Another such smartphone innovation is the so-called CellScope developed by researchers at the University of California at Berkeley. The CellScope is a microscope that attaches to a camera-equipped cell phone and produces two kinds of microscopy imaging: brightfield and fluorescence. The idea is that such device can then be used in the field (on remote locations or those where little medical infrastructure is available) and take magnified pictures of disease samples and transmit them to medical labs via mobile communication networks, and screen for hematologic and infectious diseases in areas that lack access to advanced analytical equipment.

3.5 EARLY AND TRADITIONAL MEDICAL OPTICAL INSTRUMENTS

As discussed earlier, optics has been used throughout the centuries as a technology to assist medical doctors perform examinations of patients. Many of the medical instruments in use today rely on optics and optical components to perform their intended function. In particular, there a set of very basic but very popular and common medical instruments that were developed in the nineteenth century and continue to be used in the medical profession of today. Among these optical instruments we have the *otoscope*, the *ophthalmoscope*, *retinoscope*, *laryngoscope*, and even basic devices such as the head mirror.

In general, many of the basic optical medical instruments have in common the goal to provide both a more direct illumination and optical magnification of the area under examination. Conceptually, these optical instruments are similar to a telescope or microscope, but their optical design is different. Typically, a medical instrument consists of a tubular structure fitted with an objective lens on the distal (patient) end, and an objective lens on the viewing (doctor) end, represented as (1) and (2) in Fig. 3.7.

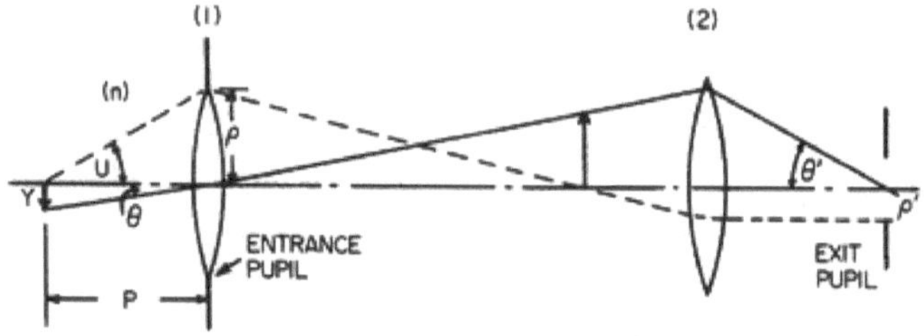

Figure 3.7 Schematic of a basic medical optical instrument.

This lens arrangement produces a magnification of the object under inspection on the objective side (distal end), which has a size Y, and is positioned a distance P from the entrance pupil of the objective lens. The visual magnification factor M_V is calculated as Eq. 3.1:

$$M_V = \theta' D/Y \quad (3.1)$$

where θ' is the angle of the light ray from the eyepiece, D is the viewing distance from the observer to the eyepiece. Hence, the magnification factor M is inversely proportional to the working distance P.

In the sections to follow, we shall describe the basic optical operating principles and uses of such devices. Our discussion of these devices is by no means exhaustive but is intended to provide the reader with an overall idea of the utilization of optics in medicine and brief introduction about medical optical instruments.

3.5.1 Head Mirror

The most basic optical medical instrument is the so-called head mirror see Fig. 3.8. A head mirror has historically been used by doctors since the eighteenth century for examination of the ear, nose, and throat. It consists of simple circular concave mirror—made of glass, plastic, or metal—with a small opening in the middle and mounted on an articulating joint to a head strap made of leather or fabric. The mirror is positioned over the physician's eye of choice, with the concave mirror surface facing outwards and the hole directly over the physician's eye.

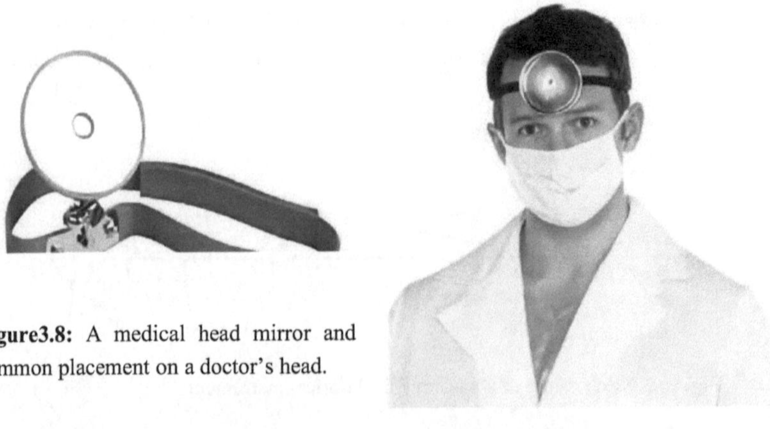

Figure3.8: A medical head mirror and common placement on a doctor's head.

In use, the patient sits and faces the physician. A bright lamp is positioned adjacent to the patient's head, pointing towards the physician's face and hence towards the head mirror. The lamp's light gets concentrated by the curvature of the mirror and reflected off it towards the area of examination, and along the line of sight of the doctor, thus providing shadow-free illumination. When used properly, the head mirror thus provides excellent shadow-free illumination.

A French obstetrician named Levert, who was fascinated with the intricacies of the larynx and dabbled with mirrors, is credited with conceiving the idea for the head mirror back in 1743. Today's head mirror has withstood the test of time and is still routinely used by ophthalmologists and otolaryngologists, particularly for examination and procedures involving the oral cavity.

3.5.2 Otoscope

An *otoscope* is a hand-held optical instrument with a small light and a funnel-shaped attachment called an ear speculum, which is used to examine the ear canal and eardrum (tympanic membrane). It is also called *auriscope*. The otoscope is one of the medical instruments most frequently used by primary care physicians. Health care providers use otoscopes to screen for illness during regular check-ups and also to investigate ear symptoms. Ear specialists—such as otolaryngologists and otologists—use otoscopes to diagnose infections of the middle and outer ear (otitis media and otitis externa).

The design of a modern otoscope is very simple. It consists of a handle and a head Fig. 3.9. The handle is long and texture for easy gripping and contains batteries to power an integrated light. The head houses a magnifying lens on the eyepiece with a typical magnification of 8 diopters; a cone-shaped disposable plastic speculum at the distal end; and an integrated light source (either lamp bulb, LED, or fiber optic). The doctor inserts a disposable speculum into the otoscope, straightens the patient's ear canal by pulling onto the ear, and inserts the otoscope to peer inside the ear canal. Some otoscope models (called pneumatic otoscopes) are provided with a manual bladder for pumping air through the speculum to test the mobility of the tympanic membrane.

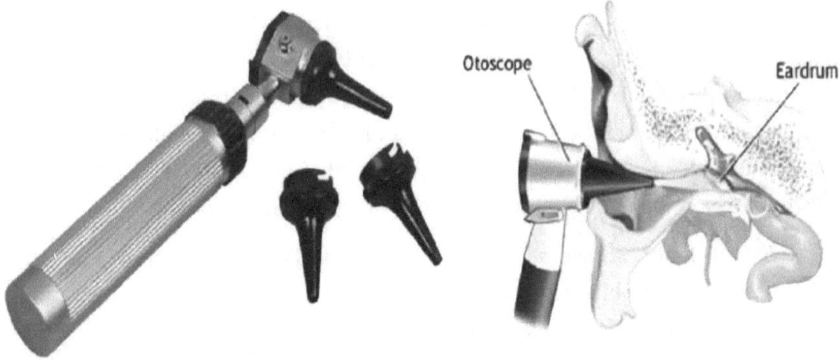

Figure 3.9: Otoscope for visual inspection inside the ear canal.

The most used otoscopes in emergency rooms and doctors' offices are monocular devices. They provide only a two-dimensional view of the ear canal. Another method of performing *otoscopy* (visualization of the ear) is use of a binocular microscope, in conjunction with a larger metal ear speculum, with the patient supine and the head tilted, which provides a much larger field of view and depth perception, thus affording a three-dimensional perception of the ear canal. The microscope has up to 40× power magnification, which allows for more detailed viewing of the entire ear canal and eardrum.

The otoscope is a valuable tool beyond its primary role as an examination tool for detecting ear problems. It can also be used for transillumination, dermatologic inspection, examination of the eye, nose, and throat and as an overall handy light source.

3.5.2.1 History of the Otoscope

Early ear examinations were performed by direct observation of the ear canal during daylight. Consequently, examinations were limited to times of the day and year when there was adequate bright daylight. Furthermore, a device was needed to gain more direct access to the ear canal and to keep it open and provide direct illumination inside. Hence, over the years, the use of a *speculum* (a conical shape device that can be safely inserted into the ear) was adopted. In 1363 Guy de Montpellier in France described the first aural and nasal specula. However, some means or direct illumination was needed to perform more effective ear examinations. The next major requirement was for an adequate method of directing concentrated natural daylight into the depths of the ear canal, which was accomplished by using a perforated mirror mounted either on a handle or on the head, which shone light directly into the ear canal. This allowed the doctor to look down the center of the beam of light, thus eliminating shadow effects and parallax (difference in the apparent position of an object viewed along two different lines of sight) Figs. 3.10 and 3.11.

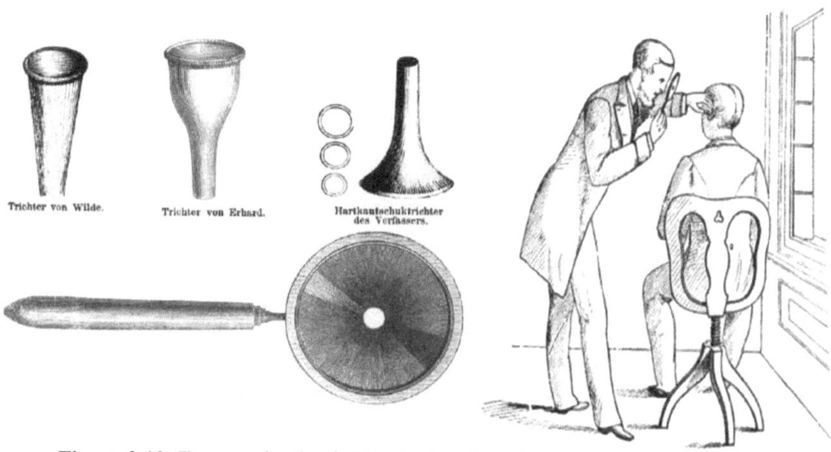

Figure 3.10: Ear examination in the nineteenth century.

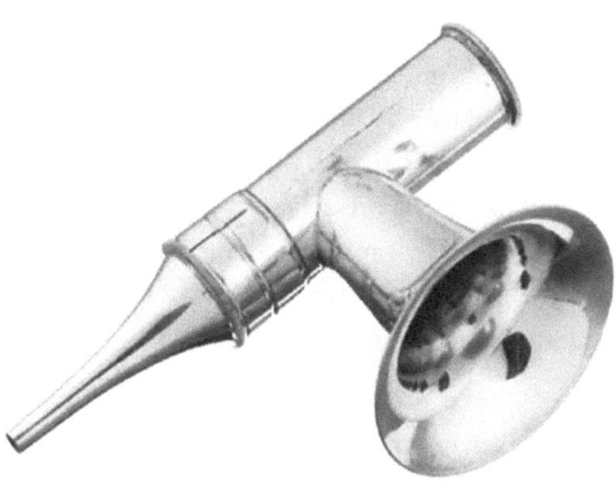

Figure 3.11: Bunton's Auriscope (c. 1880). It can be observed the metal tip speculum, the rear objective lens for viewing, as well as the middle horn used to direct light from a candle or lamp.

Von Troltsch is generally credited with popularizing the use of a mirror in *otoscopy* after he showed it in 1855 at a meeting of the Union of German Physicians in Paris. He ultimately fastened the mirror to his forehead as is still currently practiced by some doctors. The size and focal length of the mirror was not standardized for some time. To catch more light, used huge mirrors and only gradually was a diameter of 6–7 cm eventually adopted. A further improvement to Von Troltsch's early auriscope is Brunton's device which was first described in an 1865 Lancet article. This auriscope combined mirror and speculum into a single instrument and worked on the principle of a periscope: light from a candle or lamp was concentrated by a funnel and then reflected by a plane mirror set at an angle of 45° into the ear canal. The mirror had a central perforation through which the doctor could view the ear. Brunton's auriscope was fitted with a magnifying lens for the observer and could also be sealed with plain glass at the illuminating end. These were the first otoscopes to be electrically illuminated.

3.6 OPHTHALMOSCOPE

An *ophthalmoscope* is an optical instrument for examining the interior of the eyeball and its back structures (called the *fundus*) through the pupil by injecting a light beam into the eye and looking at its back-reflection. An ophthalmoscope is also referred to as a *funduscope*. The fundus consists of blood vessels, the optic nerve, and a lining of nerve cells (the retina) which detects images transmitted through the cornea, a clear lens-like layer covering of the eye. Ophthalmoscopes are used by doctors to exam the interior of eyes and help diagnose any possible conditions or detect any problems or diseases of the retina and vitreous humor. For instance, a doctor would look for changes in the color the fundamental body, the size, and shape of retinal blood vessels, or any abnormalities in the *macula lutea* (the portion of the retina that receives and analyzes light only from the very center of the visual field). Typically, special eyedrops are used to dilate the pupils and allow a wider field of view inside the eyeball.

A modern ophthalmoscope Fig. 3.12 consists essentially of two systems: one for illumination and another for viewing. The illuminating system is comprised of light source (a halogen or tungsten bulb), a condenser lens system, a reflector (a prism, mirror, or metallic plate) to illuminate the interior of the eye with a central hole through which the eye is examined. The viewing system is made of a sight hole and a focusing system, usually a rotating wheel with lenses of different powers. The lenses are selected to allow clear visualization of the structures of the eye at any depth and compensate for the combined errors of refraction between patient and examiner.

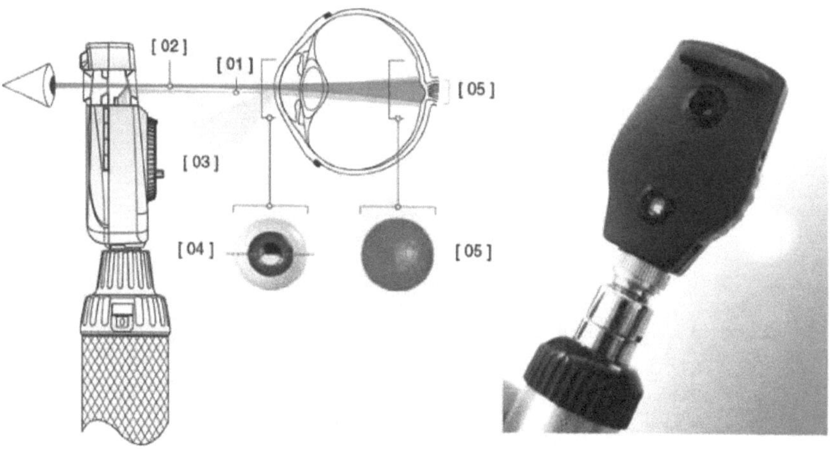

Figure 3.12: Aspect of a modern ophthalmoscope. A light beam is projected into the eye (*1*). The medical examiner has a direct line of sight into the back of the eye (fundus) (*2*). Path of light reflected the cornea and iris (*3*). Image observed at the pupil (*4*). Image observed at the back of the eye (*5*) (Images courtesy of Heine).

German physician Hermann von Helmholtz is credited with the invention of the ophthalmoscope back in 1851, which he based on an earlier version developed by Charles Babbage in 1847. Helmholtz original ophthalmoscope see Fig. 3.13 was very basic (made or cardboard, glue, and microscope glass plates) but it allowed him to place the eye of the observer in the path of the rays of light entering and leaving the patient's eye, thus allowing the patient's retina to be seen. In 1915, Francis A. Welch and William Noah Allyn invented the world's first hand-held direct illuminating ophthalmoscope and resulted in the formation of the Welch Allyn medical company, which is still in business today.

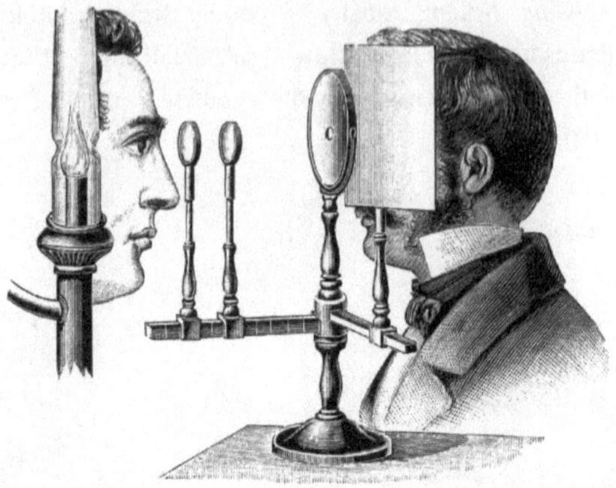

Figure 3.13: Nineteenth century illustration of Helmholtz original ophthalmoscope.

There are two types of ophthalmoscopes: *direct* and *indirect*. A *direct ophthalmoscope* produces an upright (unreversed) image with 15× magnification. The direct ophthalmoscope is used to inspect the funds of the eye, which is the back portion of the interior eyeball. Examination is best carried out in a darkened room. Macular degeneration and opacities of the lens can be seen through direct ophthalmoscopy. The instrument is held at close range to the patient's eye and the field of view is small (less than 10°) Fig. 3.14. The magnification M of a direct ophthalmoscope is equal to:

$$M = F_e/4 \qquad (3.2)$$

where F_e is the power of the eye.

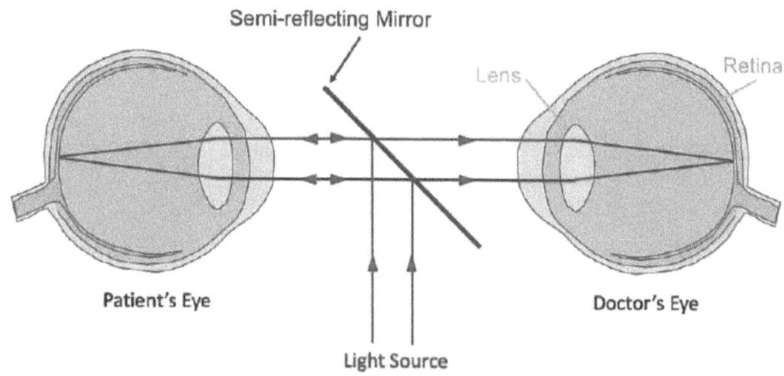

Figure 3.14: Optical raytracing for a direct ophthalmoscope. Light from the illuminating source is reflected into the eye and then back reflected by the fundus through a mirror (with either a hole through it or with partial reflectivity). O is the observer's eye, while P is the patient's eye; M, semi-silver mirror.

An *indirect ophthalmoscope* produces an inverted (reversed) image with a 2–5× magnification and formed. A small hand-held lens and either a slit lamp microscope or a light attached to a headband are used to form an image of the back of the eye in space, at approximately arm's length from the doctor. An indirect ophthalmoscope provides a stronger light source, a specially designed objective lens, and opportunity for stereoscopic inspection of the interior of the eyeball. It is invaluable for diagnosis and treatment of retinal tears, holes, and detachments.

This aerial image is usually produced by a strong positive lens ranging in power from +13 diopter to +30 diopter that is held in front of the patient's eye. The practitioner views this aerial image through a sight hole with a focusing lens to compensate for *ametropia* and accommodation. This instrument provides a large field of view (25–40°) and allows easier examination of the periphery of the retina. This instrument has been supplanted by the binocular indirect ophthalmoscope Fig. 3.15. The magnification of an indirect ophthalmoscope *M* is equal to:

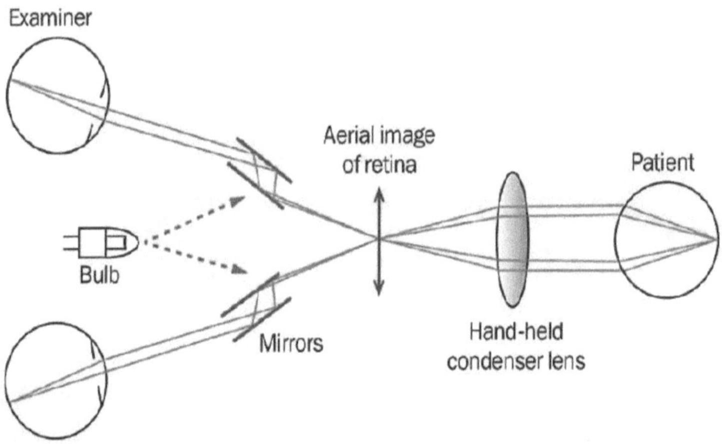

Figure 3.15: Optical raytracing for a binocular indirect ophthalmoscope. The light source mounted on the doctor's head illuminates a hand-held condenser lens which forms an inverted stereoscopic image of the retina in free space (aerial image).

$$M = F_e/F_c \quad (3.3)$$

where F_e and F_c are the powers of the eye and of the condensing lens, respectively.

3.7 RETINOSCOPE

A *retinoscope* is an optical hand-held device used by optometrists to measure the optical refractive power of the eyes and whether corrective glasses might be needed and the associated prescription value. As shown in Fig. 3.16, a person can have normal vision (*emmetropia*), *myopia* (nearsightedness), *hyperopia* (farsightedness), or astigmatism. The retinoscope is used to illuminate the internal eye (while the patient is looking for a far fixed object) and observe how the reflected light rays by the retina (called the *reflex*) align and move with respect to the light reflected directly off the pupil. If the input light beam focuses in front of or behind the retina, there is a "refractive error" of the eye. A high degree of refractive power indicates that the light focus remains in front of the retina, in which case the eye displays myopia. Conversely, if the focal spot happens behind the retina, there is little refractive power and the eye has hyperopia. The error of refraction is then corrected by using a *phoropter*, which introduces a series of lenses of various optical strengths until the retina focuses at the right position on the retina.

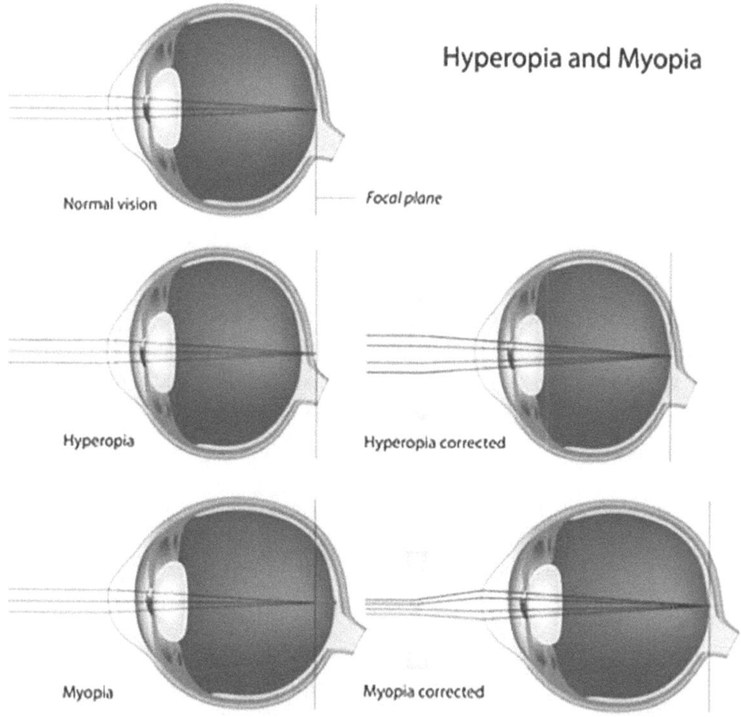

Figure 3.16: Types of human vision and associated corrective optical lenses.

The retinoscope consists of a light, a condensing lens, and a mirror Fig. 3.17. The mirror is either semi-transparent or has a hole through which the practitioner can view the patient's eye. During the procedure, the retinoscope shines a beam of light through the pupil. Then, the optometrist moves the light vertically and horizontally across the patient's eye and observes how the light reflects off the retina see pictures in Fig. 3.18. If the light reflex in the patient's pupil moves "with" or "against" motion. If the reflex moves in same direction, then the correction requires plus power (myopia) and motion against direction of the retinoscope, which means negative power correction (hyperopia).

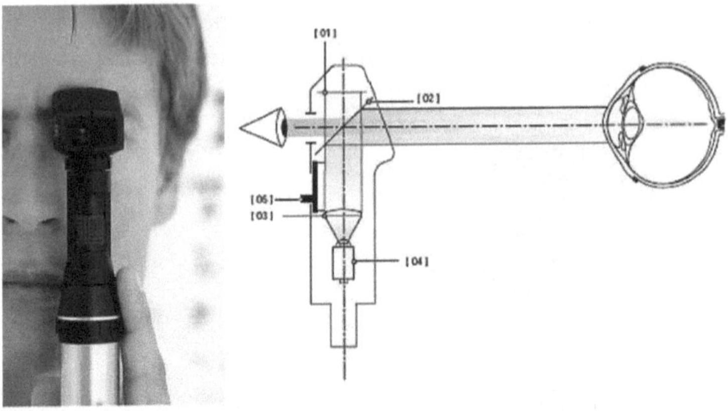

Figure 3.17: A modern retinoscope. An integrated lamp or LED light source (*4*) shines light through a collimating lens (*3*) onto a partially reflective mirror (*2*), which directs the light to the eye. The back-reflected light from the fundus and the cornea is examined by the doctor through the eyepiece (*1*) and focus adjusted using the lens dial (*5*) (Image courtesy of Heine).

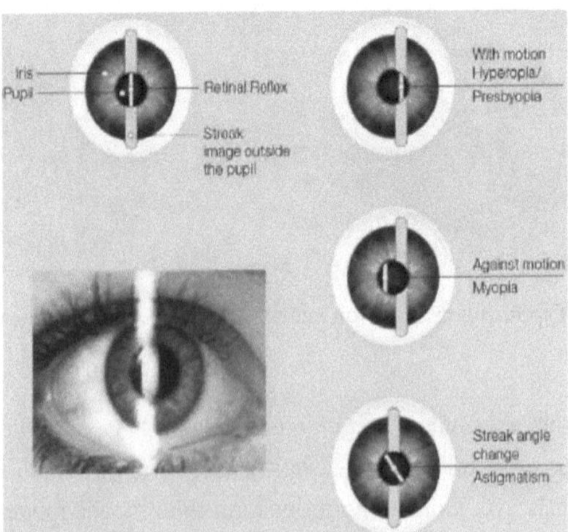

Figure 3.18: Aspect of reflex images from the human eye seen by a doctor using a retinoscope. If the reflex moves in same direction, then myopia is detected; if reflex is noted on motion against direction of the retinoscope, hyperopia is present. If the reflex line is oblique instead of vertical, then astigmatism is present. An aligned reflex means correct vision (*Source*: Heine).

To determine the corrective refractive lens power needed, lenses of increasing refractive power are placed in front of the eye and the change in the direction and pattern of the reflex is observed. The optometrist keeps changing the lenses until reaching a lens power that provides adequate focus on the retina, which manifests as alignment of the reflex with the streak light image outside of the pupil.

3.8 PHOROPTER

A *phoropter* is an ophthalmic binocular refracting testing device, also called a *refractor*. It is commonly used by ophthalmologists, optometrists, and eye care professionals during an eye examination to determine the corrective power needed for prescription glasses. It is commonly used in combination with a retinoscope.

Figure 3.19 shows a photograph of phoropter which consists in double sets (one for each eye) of rotating discs containing convex and concave spherical and cylindrical lenses, occludes, pinholes, colored filters, polarizers, prisms, and other optical elements. The patient sits in front of the device and the lenses within a phoropter refract light to focus images on the patient's retina at the right spot to compensate for each individual eye refractive errors. The optical power of these lenses is measured in 0.25 diopter increments. By changing these lenses, the examiner is able to determine the spherical and cylindrical power, and cylindrical axis necessary to correct a person's refractive error. These instruments were first devised in the early to mid-1910s.

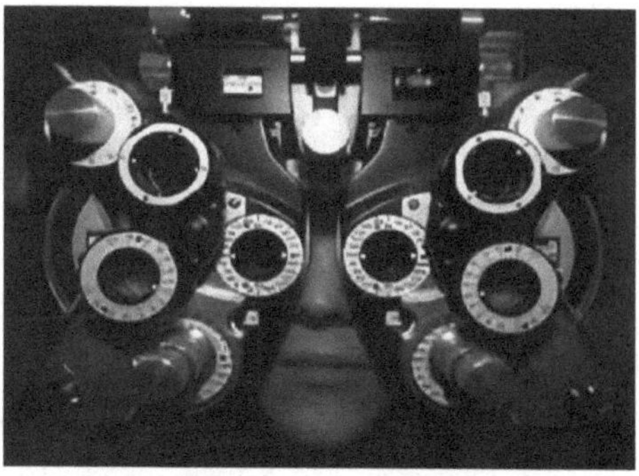

Figure 3.19: A phoropter is commonly used by optometrists to determine the necessary corrective lens prescription.

3.9 LARYNGOSCOPE

A *laryngoscope* is an optical instrument used for examining the interior of the larynx and structures around the throat. There are two types of laryngoscopes: *direct* and *indirect* laryngoscopes. A direct laryngoscope Fig. 3.20 consists of a handle containing batteries, an integrated light source, and a set of interchangeable blades for easy reach and placement into a patient's throat. Besides being used for visualization of the glottis and vocal cords, a direct laryngoscope may also be used during surgical procedures to remove foreign objects in the throat, collect tissue samples (biopsy), remove polyps from the vocal cords, perform laser treatments and, very commonly, as a tool aid to facilitate tracheal intubation during general anesthesia or in cardiopulmonary resuscitation.

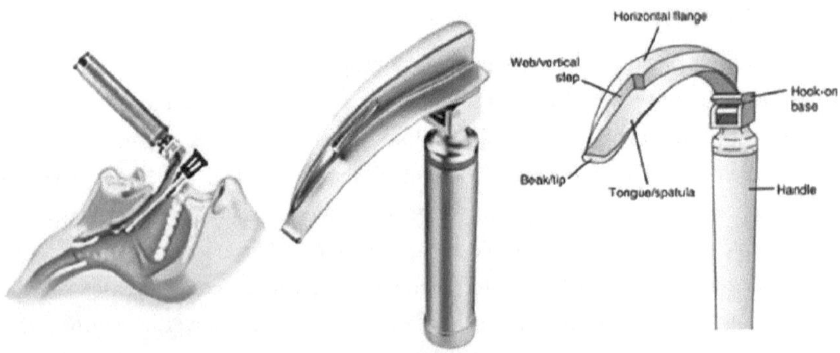

Figure 3.20: A direct laryngoscope and its insertion into a human throat for examination.

The blades in a laryngoscope help provide leverage to open wide the mouth and throat, as well as to keep the tongue in place and avoid a gag reflex. There are two basic styles of laryngoscope blades most used: curved and straight. The Macintosh blade is the most widely used of the curved laryngoscope blades, while the Miller blade is the most popular style of straight blade. Blades come in different sizes, to accommodate different patients.

An *indirect* laryngoscope consists of a combination of a small mirror mounted at an angle on a long stem and a light source. The mirror is usually circular in form and made in various sizes but is small enough to be placed in the throat behind the back of the tongue. The source of light is either a small bright lamp worn on the forehead of the observer, or a concave mirror, also worn on the forehead, for the purpose of concentrating light from some other source. Light is reflected to the back of the throat by the mirror and directed to illuminate up the interior of the larynx. The mirror also serves to reflect to the doctor an image of the throat, to appreciate the structure of the glottis and vocal cords.

Some historians credit Benjamin Guy Babington (1794–1866), with the invention of the laryngoscope back in 1829, who called his device the *glottiscope.* However, Manuel Garcia (1805–1906)—a Spanish tenor and singing maestro—experimented back in 1854 with a combination of throat mirror and light to observe the action of his own vocal cords and larynx when producing tones and sounds. His observations were published in the Royal Philosophical Magazine and Journal of Science in 1855, and they constitute the first physiological records of the human voice as based upon observations in the living subject. For this, he is also recognized as the original inventor of the laryngoscope. Figure 3.21 shows a photograph and illustration of his original laryngoscope device.

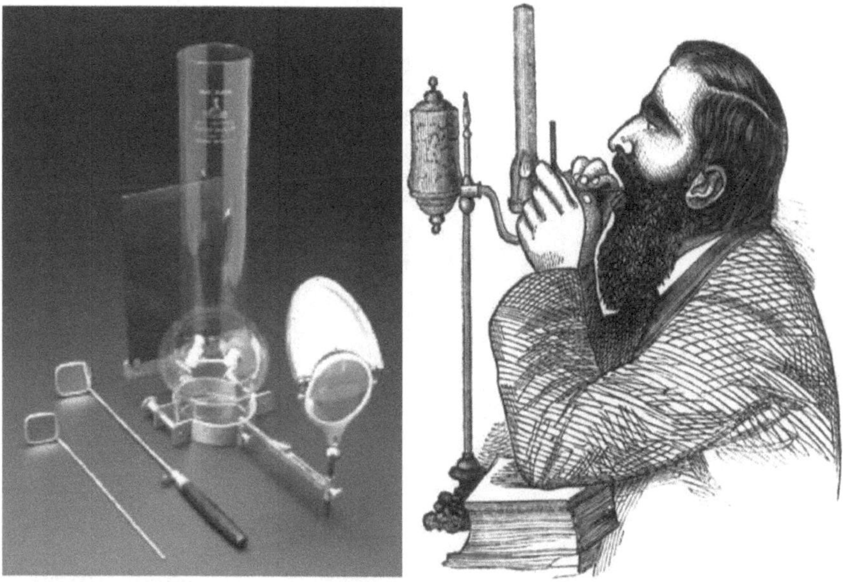

Figure 3.21: Original indirect laryngoscope developed by Manuel Garcia to view the movement of his own vocal cords (c. 1870).

MEDICAL OPTICS

Mirror-based laryngoscopy for the investigation of laryngeal pathology was pioneered back in 1858 by Johann Czermak, a professor of physiology at the University of Budapest. Czermak applied an external light source and a head-mounted mirror to improve visualization. During this period of time, a laryngoscopic examination was made as depicted in Fig. 3.22. The patient opens his mouth as widely as possible, protruding his tongue. The doctor, with a small napkin takes the protruded tongue between his thumb and forefinger and holds it in place, so as to enlarge opening of the mouth as much as possible. The laryngeal mirror is next inserted and dexterously positioned to the back of the mouth to direct the light from the external light source (mirror or lamp) into the back of the throat. An image of the lower throat is reflected back by the mirror for the doctor to view and assess the condition of the larynx.

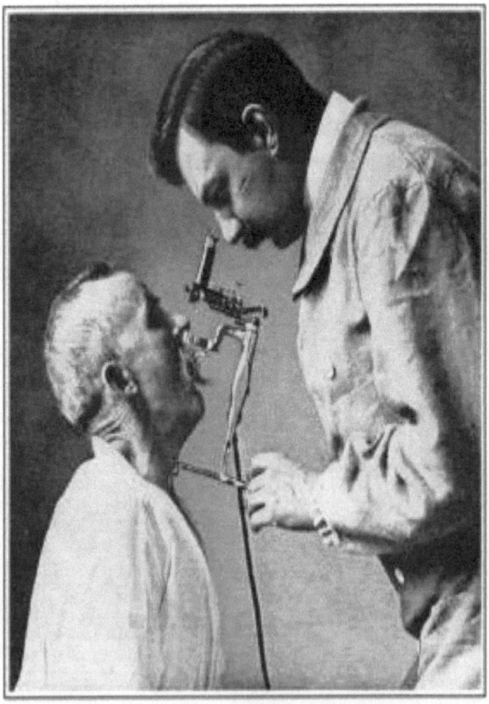

Figure 3.22: Nineteenth century illustration of a mirror-based laryngoscope examination of a patient's throat.

All previous observations of the glottis and larynx had been performed under indirect vision (using mirrors) until 1895, when Alfred Kirstein (1863–1922) of Germany performed the first direct laryngoscopy in Berlin, using an esophagoscope he had modified for this purpose, calling device an autoscope, and the modern, direct laryngoscope was born.

3.10 FIBER OPTIC MEDICAL DEVICES AND APPLICATIONS

The field of fiber optics has undergone tremendous growth and advancement over the last 50 years. Initially conceived as a medium to carry light and images for medical endoscopic applications, optical fibers were later proposed in the mid-1960s as an adequate information-carrying medium for telecommunication applications. Ever since, optical fiber technology has been the subject of considerable research and development to the point that today light wave communication systems have become the preferred method to transmit vast amounts of data and information from one point to another.

Given their EM immunity, intrinsic safety, small size and weight, autoclave compatibility and capability to perform multi-point and multi-parameter sensing remotely, optical fibers and fiberoptic-based devices are seeing increased acceptance and new uses for a variety of biomedical applications—from diverse endoscopes to laser-delivery systems, to disposable blood gas sensors, and to intra-aortic probes. This section illustrates—through several application and product examples—some of the benefits and uses of biomedical fiber sensors, and what makes them such an attractive, flexible, reliable, and unique technology.

3.11 OPTICAL FIBER FUNDAMENTALS

At the heart of this technology is the optical fiber itself. A hair-thin cylindrical filament made of glass (although sometimes they are also made of polymers) that can guide light through itself by confining it within regions having different optical indices of refraction. A typical fiber structure is depicted in Fig. 3.23. The central portion—where most of the light travel is called the core. Surrounding the core there is a region having a lower index of refraction, called the cladding. From a simple point of view, light trapped inside the core travels along the fiber by bouncing off the interfaces with the cladding, due to the effect of the total internal reflection occurring at these boundaries Fig. 3.24. Though, the optical energy propagates along the fiber in the form of waveguide modes that satisfy Maxwell's equations as well as the boundary conditions and the external perturbations present at the fiber.

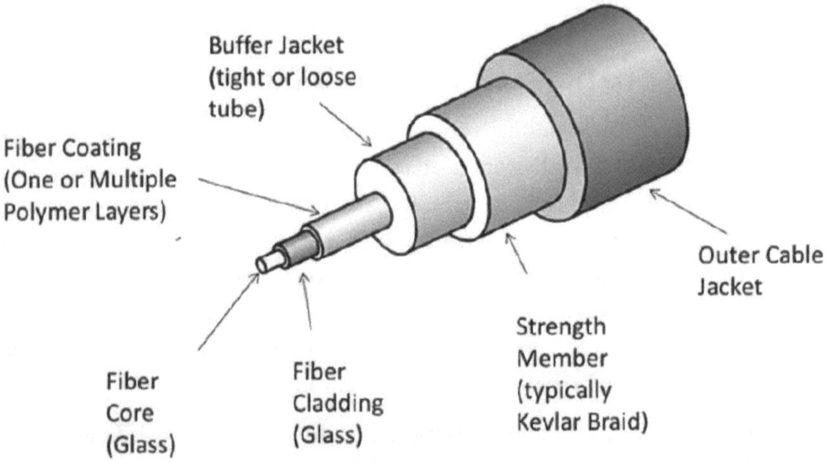

Figure 3.23 Schematic of an optical fiber.

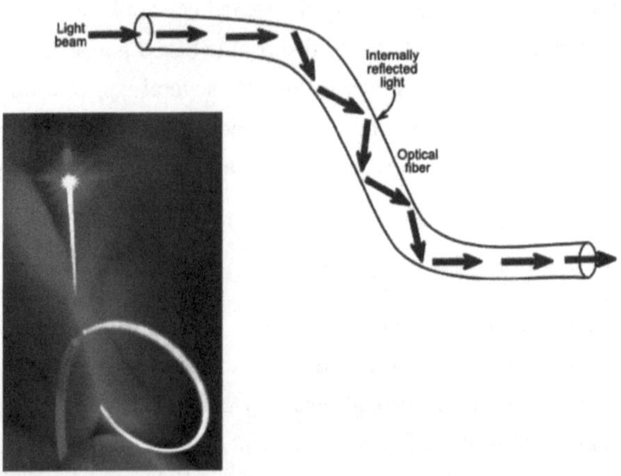

Figure 3.24: An optical fiber can guide light through the principle of total internal reflection. This allows the transmission of light energy (and signals) through any patch or shape taken by the optical fiber.

Refraction occurs when light passes from one homogeneous isotropic medium to another; the light ray will be bent at the interface between the two media. The mathematical expression Eq. 3.4 that describes the refraction phenomena is known as Snell's law,

$$n_0 \sin \phi_0 = n_1 \sin \phi_1 \qquad (3.4)$$

where n_o is the index of refraction of the medium in which the light is initially travelling, n_1 is the index of refraction of the second medium, Φ_o is the angle between the incident ray and the normal to the interface, and Φ_1 is the angle between the refracted ray and the normal to the interface.

Figure 3.25a shows the case of light passing from a high-index medium to a lower-index medium. Even though refraction is occurring, a certain portion of the incident ray is reflected. If the incident ray hits the boundary at ever-increasing angles, a value of $\phi_0 = \phi_C$ will be reached, at which no refraction will occur. The angle ϕ_c is called the critical angle. The refracted ray of light propagates along the interface, not penetrating into the lower-index medium, as shown in part Fig. 3.25b. At that point, $\sin \phi_c$ equals to unity. For angles ϕ_0 greater than ϕ_c, the ray is entirely reflected at the interface, and no refraction takes place see Fig. 3.25c. This phenomenon is known as *total internal reflection.*

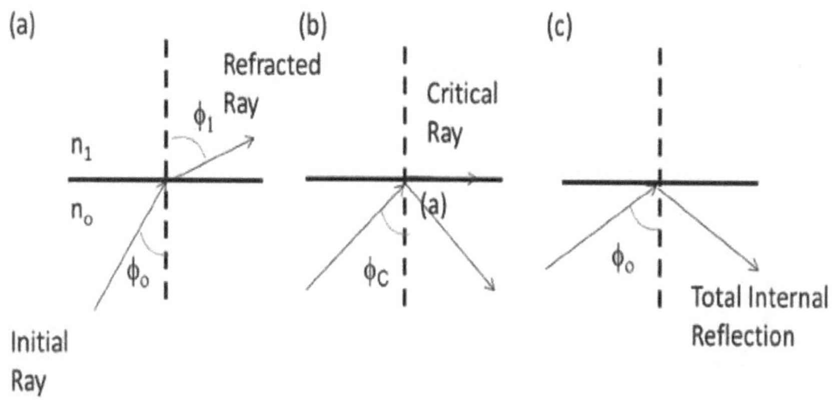

Figure 3.25: Light reflection and refraction between two media with different indices of refraction.

In Fig. 3.26, a ray of light incident upon the end of the optical fiber at an angle θ will be refracted as it passes into the core. If the ray travels through the high-index medium at an angle greater than Φ_c it will reflect off the cylinder wall, will have multiple reflections, and will emerge at the other end of the optical fiber. For a circular fiber, considering only meridional rays, the entrance and exit angles are equal. Considering Snell's law for the optical fiber, core index n_0, cladding index n_1, and the surrounding media index n,

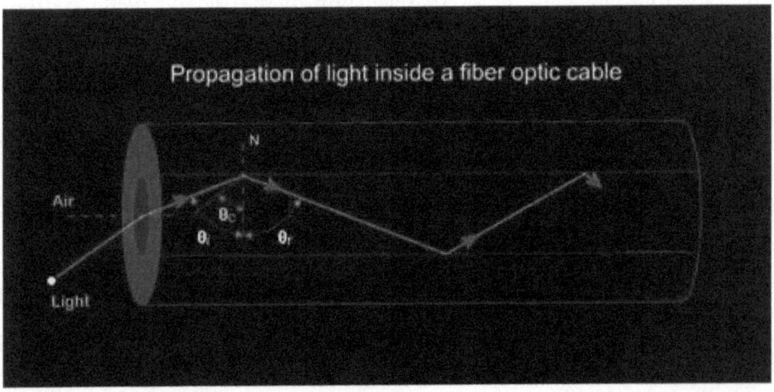

Figure 3.26: Light ray propagation along the core of an optical fiber. At the entrance to the fiber, a conical region is defined by the so-called acceptance angle, which is the region in space where light can be effectively collected and coupled into the fiber for guiding.

$$\begin{aligned} n\sin\theta &= n_0 \sin\theta_0 \\ &= n_0 \sin\left(\frac{\pi}{2} - \phi_c\right) \\ &= n_0\left[1 - (n_1 - n_0)^2\right]^{1/2} \\ &= \left(n_0^2 - n_1^2\right)^{1/2} = \text{Numerical Aperture.} \qquad (3.5) \end{aligned}$$

The term $n\sin\theta$ is defined as the *numerical aperture* or NA for short. The NA is determined by the difference between the refractive index of the core and that of the cladding. It is a measure of the light-acceptance capability of the optical fiber. As the NA increases, so does the ability of the fiber to couple light into the fiber, as shown in Fig. 3.27. The larger NA allows the fiber to couple in light from more severe grazing angles. Coupling efficiency also increases as the fiber diameter increases, since the large fiber can capture more light. Therefore, the maximum light-collection efficiency occurs for large-diameter-core fibers and large-NA fibers.

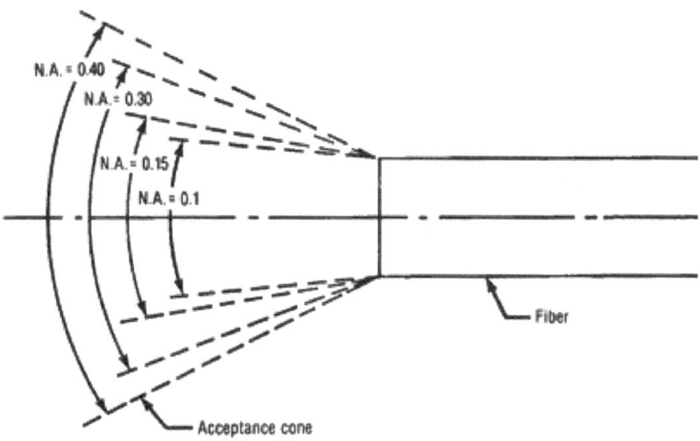

Figure 3.27: The greater the NA of an optical fiber, the bigger the acceptance cone, and broader the angle of capture of light by the fiber.

3.12 COHERENT AND INCOHERENT OPTICAL FIBER BUNDLES

In medicine, optical fibers have been considered for illuminating and imaging applications since the 1920s. Typically, a single glass optical fiber has a diameter ranging from 1 mm down to ~8 μm. However, a single optical fiber cannot transmit an image—only a bright light spot would be observed at its end. Hence, in order to carry a reasonable amount of light for illumination purposes, or to transmit and image, hundreds to thousands of optical fibers need to be assembled into bundles. Bundles of multiple single optical fibers of small diameter solid glass rods can thus be used to guide light or transmit images around bends and curved trajectories.

Glass optical fiber bundles are of two types: *incoherent* and *coherent*. An *incoherent* bundle consists of a collection of fibers randomly distributed in the bundle and is typically intended for illumination purposes only. In contrast, a *coherent* optical fiber bundle has an ordered array of fibers in which the relative position of each individual fiber at its input and output with respect to the bundle is maintained. That is to say, the position of individual fibers is at same locations over the cross section of both bundle ends as depicted in Fig. 3.28. In between the ends, the fibers need not have a fixed orientation and can move flexibly. Coherent bundles are used for conveying an image from one end to the other by the effect created by the grouping of the individual light conducted by each fiber which is perceived in the eye of the observer as a full image. To achieve better image quality and resolution, many small diameter fibers are needed for a given bundle diameter. Typically, fibers used in bundles have diameters on the order of 8–12 μm and their count can range from about 2000 up to 40,000. In the case of imaging bundles, larger diameter fibers are used of 30–50 μm in diameter.

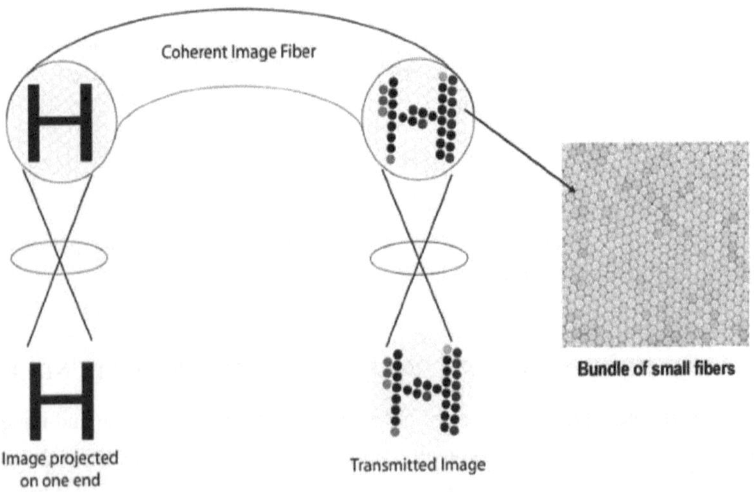

Figure 3.28: A coherent optical fiber bundle. Images are accurately transmitted by preserving the relative position of the fibers at each end of the bundle. The bundle consists of a multitude of individual glass fibers of a small diameter (~12 μm) that create a lattice effect.

Fabrication of illumination (non-coherent) and imaging (coherent) bundles is based on the same processes of drawing optical fibers or glass rods through heating furnaces and doing repeated draws of multi-stack sets, to achieve arrays with the desired quantity of fibers of the appropriate diameter. There are three common fabrication methods for coherent bundles: fused image bundles, wound image bundles, and leached image bundles. Figure 3.29 illustrates the three steps needed to fabricate fused as well as leached image fiber bundles.

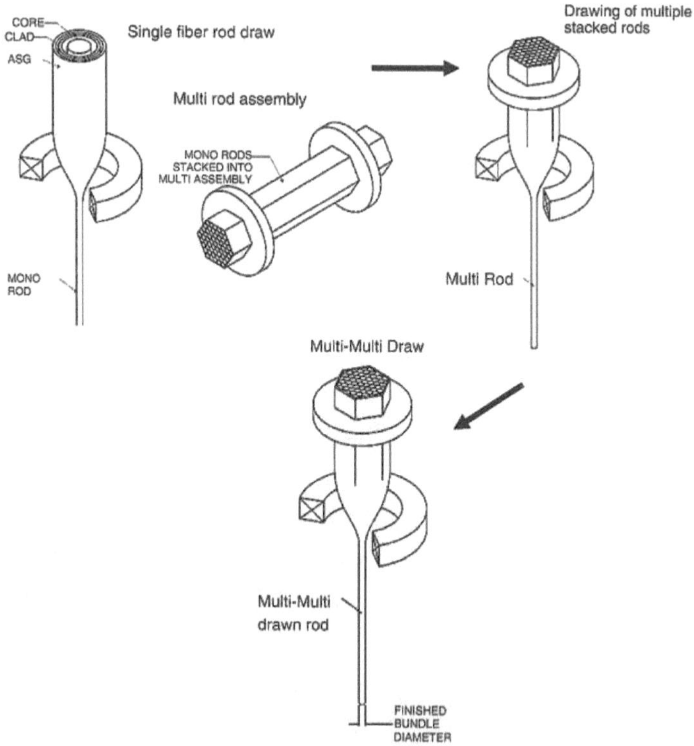

Figure 3.29 Fabrication process to make fiber bundles.

An individual fiber (or rod) is made by starting with a so-called perform made by the tube-in-rod technique where a single glass rod (which will become the fiber's core) is inserted into a tube made of glass with a lower refractive index (cladding). In the case of a leached bundle, an additional glass jacket made of a leachable glass is used. This glass perform is placed in an electric heating furnace that runs at a temperature close to the softening point of the glass. The heat causes the solid glass road to soften. Once soft, the glass is pulled down into a thin filament by a pulling mechanism. The final diameter of the filament is controlled by the ratio of the speeds between the advancing preform and the drawn fiber. Typically, the initial drawn fiber is more of a solid rod with a 2 mm diameter. In the next drawing stage, a multitude of mono fibers are stacked together and drawn in the furnace to produce a multi-fiber rod. The filament drawn from a multi-fiber preform consists of several 100 monofilament fibers. In the third stage, several multi-fiber rods are stacked together to perform the so-called multi-multi drawing process. The multi-multi stack assembly is fed through the furnace and drawn into a filament of rod of the desired diameter. Such filaments will be composed of thousands of individual glass fibers. As shown in Fig. 3.30, imaging multi-fiber arrays of square, circular, or hexagonal shape and in different sizes can be fabricated with this process.

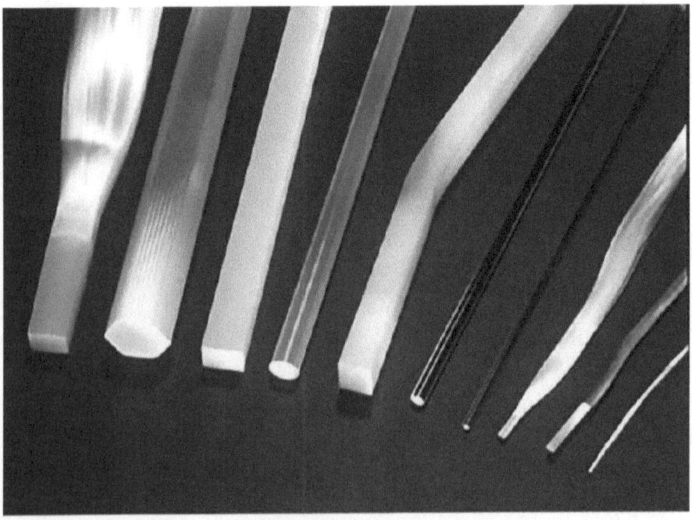

Fig. 3.30: Photograph of different styles and shapes of drawn coherent optical fiber bundles.

In the case of leached fiber bundles, each bundle end is properly secured and the entire bundle is soaked in an acid solution which will dissolve the leachable glass, allowing the fibers to move freely between the bundle ends.

Wound imaging bundles are made by winding a multi-fiber array as a single layer on a drum and then stacking the desired number of layers manually in a laminating operation.

3.13 ILLUMINATING GUIDES

Fiber optic illuminating guides are non-coherent and are used primarily to guide light to a desired point to provide illumination and enhance visual clarity. Imaging bundles are typically made of 30–50 μm diameter fibers, with NA values around 0.6. Most commonly, illuminating bundles are used as part of fiberscopes, endoscopes, and personal lights for surgeons. As seen in Fig. 3.31, when surgeons are operating on a patient, they need cool, bright light to help then see better tissues and organs—the closer the direct illumination to the operating field, the better. Rigid, light-guiding rods are also made (from single solid glass rods or from multi-core rods) for applications in dentistry and light therapy see Fig. 3.32.

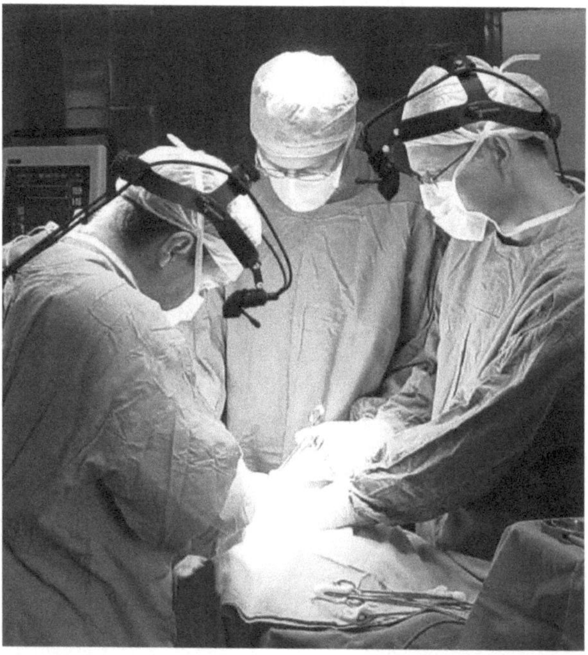

Figure 3.31: Fiber optic illuminators used in the operating room by surgeons.

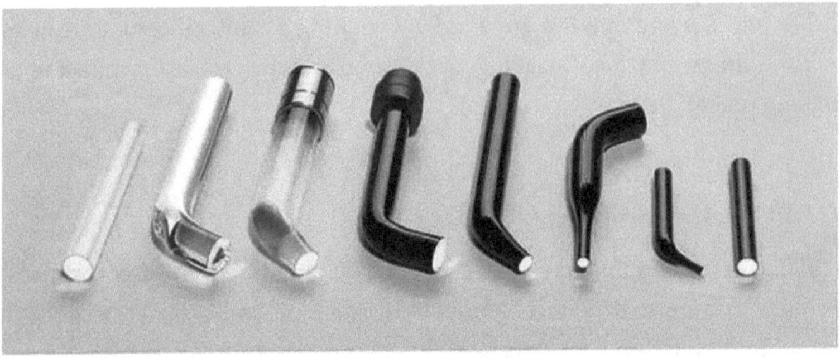

Figure3.32: Solid fiber optic illuminating rods.

3.14 FIBERSCOPES AND ENDOSCOPES

An endoscope is an optical instrument used for direct visual inspection of hollow organs or body cavities. Typically, an endoscope is generally introduced through a natural opening in the body Fig. 3.33, but it may also be inserted through an incision. Instruments for viewing specific areas of the body include the bronchoscope, colonoscope, cystoscope, gastroscope, laparoscope, proctoscope, and several others. Although the design may vary according to specific use, all endoscopes have similar construction and elements: an objective lens (distal end), illuminating fiber bundle, imaging coherent fiber bundle, fixed or articulating handle, and an eyepiece (proximal end). Accessories that might be used for diagnostic or therapeutic purposes include irrigation channels, suction tips, tubes, and suction pump; forceps for removal of biopsy tissue or a foreign body; biopsy brushes; an electrode tip for cauterization; as well as a video camera, video monitors, and image recorder. Many modern endoscopes have also articulating ends that are remotely controlled by the doctor using knobs on the handle that adjust pull wires inside the body of the endoscope. Figure 3.34 shows a modern, flexible, and fiber-optic endoscope.

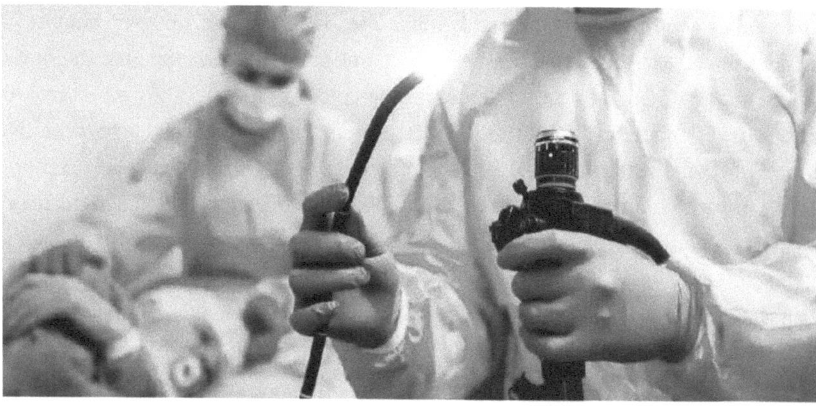

Figure 3.33: Endoscopes are commonly used by doctors to inspect patients' internal organs through body cavities, such as the nose or throat.

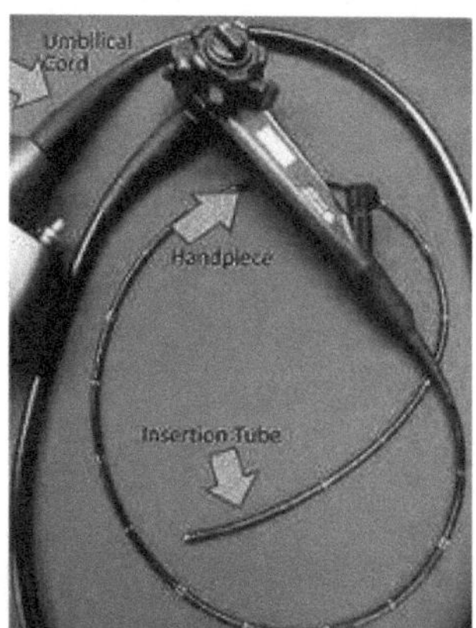

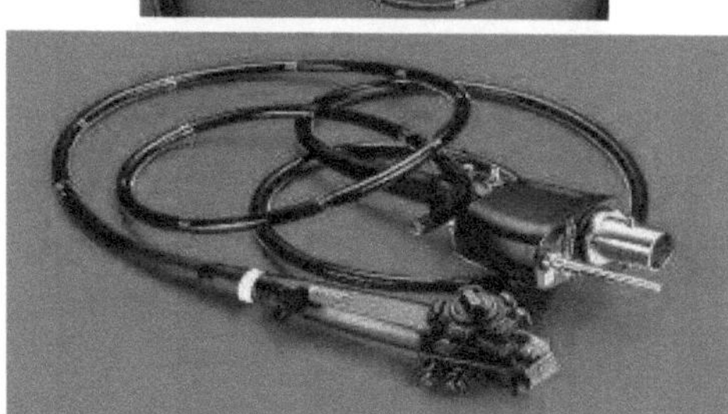

Figure 3.34: Aspect of a modern, flexible fiberscope fitted with articulating knobs, camera lens, and instrument port on the distal end.

Endoscopes can be rigid or flexible as depicted in Fig. 3.35. Modern endoscopes (both flexible and rigid) make use of fiber optic imaging bundles to achieve image transmission. However, earlier models relied on miniature flat or rod lenses to guide images from the objective end to the eyepiece as shown in Fig. 3.36. Hippocrates II (460–377 BC) reported using catheters and primitive forms of visualization tubes over two millennia ago. In the nineteenth century, endoscopy was very rudimentary and relied on the insertion of long, rigid metal tubes into body cavities. In 1910 Victor Elner used a gastroscope to view the stomach, while in 1912 the first semi-flexible gastroscope was developed. Then, Heinrich Lamm was the first person to transmit images through a bundle of optical fibers in 1930. In 1957, clad optical fibers were first proposed and developed by Lawrence Curtis as a graduate student at the University of Michigan, under the supervision of Dr. Basil Hirschowitz, who in 1957 demonstrated the first fiber optic endoscope. From then on, the devices became known as *fiberscopes*. The fiberoptic endoscope has great flexibility, reaching previously inaccessible areas and has become the norm in medicine.

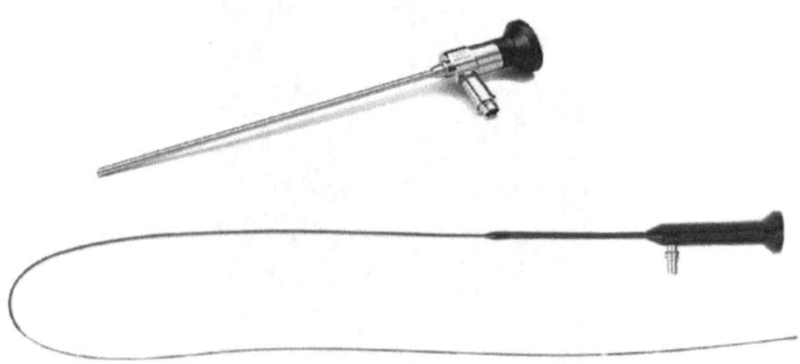

Figure 3.35: Examples of a rigid (*upper*) and flexible (*lower*) endoscopes.

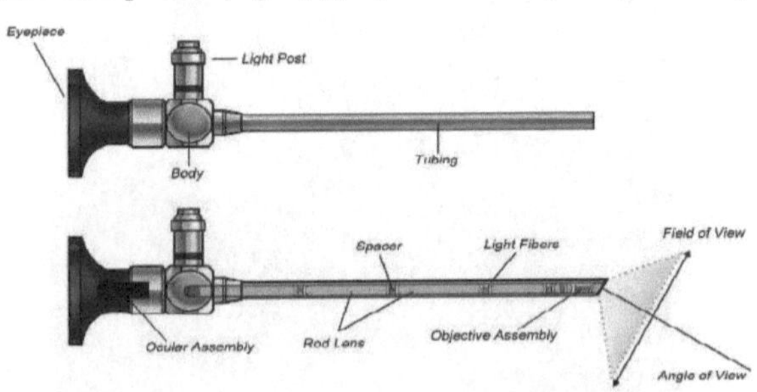

Figure 3.36: Early designs of rigid endoscopes using rod or glass lenses for image relaying.

3.15 FUSED FIBER FACEPLATES AND TAPERS FOR DIGITAL X-RAYS

Another type of coherent imaging conduit is the fiber optic fused faceplate (FOFP). FOFPs are made as pre-arranged blocks of multiple pre-drawn multi-fiber glass rods (known as boules), which are then fused together under elevated heat and pressure to form a solid piece Fig. 3.37. Typical individual fiber element sizes range from as small as 4 to 25 μm or larger. Thin plates are then sliced from the fused boule, ground and polished to the desired thickness—ranging from ~100 mm down to a practical limit of 50 μm. Typical shapes are round or rectangular. Depending on the intended application, the FOFP end faces can be coated with a specific spectral filtering, phosphorescent, or anti-reflective coating.

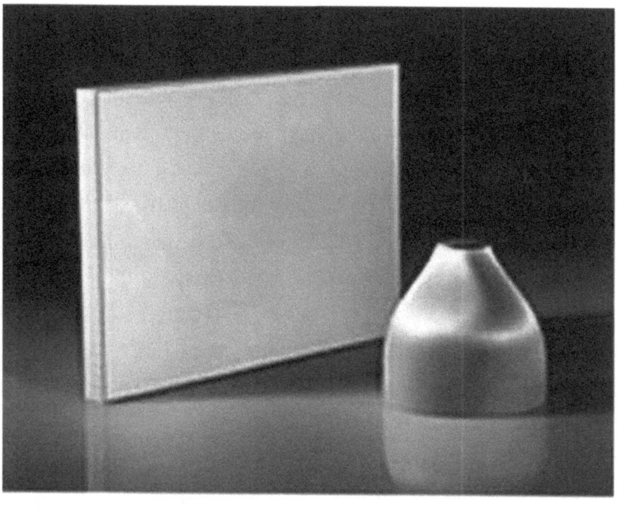

Figure 3.37: A fused fiberoptic faceplate (*back*) and taper (*front*). Photo courtesy of Schott glass.

Optically, an FOFP behaves as zero-thickness optical window transferring an image, fiber by fiber, from one face of the plate to the other. Image magnification or reduction can be achieved by tapering the cross section of the bulk plate during the manufacturing process. In this case, the boule is drawn down, and a neck region is formed with an hour-glass shape piece. The piece is cut into two pieces, machined and the ends polished resulting in a fused fiber optic taper.

Faceplates and tapers also function as dielectric barriers and mechanical interface and are optically used as a two-dimensional image conduit for energy conversion, field-flattening, distortion correction, and contrast enhancement. They are typically used for imaging applications bonded to cathode ray tubes (CRT) and LCD displays, image intensifiers, charged coupled device (CCD) or complementary metal-oxide semiconductor (CMOS) detectors, image plane transfer devices, X-ray digital detectors, among others.

In the medical area, fiber optic tapers and faceplates have found widespread use for both dental and medical digital radiography (such as mammography, fluoroscopy, intra-oral, panoramic, or cephalometric) where instead of using conventional film to obtain the X-ray images, an electronic photosensitive device such as a CCD or CMOS detector chip is used to convert the X-ray energy into electronic pixel signals via the use of an intermediate faceplate. Digital radiography offers high-resolution images while greatly reducing patient and sensor exposure to harmful X-rays by using low-dose X-ray sources. In addition, digital X-ray imaging speeds the availability of images for diagnostic, while also making the viewing, sharing, transmitting, and storing of X-ray patient data so much easy and compatible with modern electronic record systems. Furthermore, faceplates also provide a critical X-ray absorbing barrier between the X-ray emitter and the semiconductor detector device, prolonging their service life and reducing background noise.

As shown in Fig. 3.38, when an X-ray source emits radiation energy (that would pass through the patient) the transmitted energy impinges on a scintillator plate which converts the radiation rays into visible photons. The scintillating coating—e.g., cesium iodide (CSI) or gadolinium oxysulfide (Gadox) doped with Tl or Eu—is deposited directly on the large end of a fused fiber-optic taper. The light is then transferred and reduced through the taper and coupled to a digital CCD chip where a black and white image is formed which can then be viewed on a computer screen or monitor and readily archived as an electronic image file.

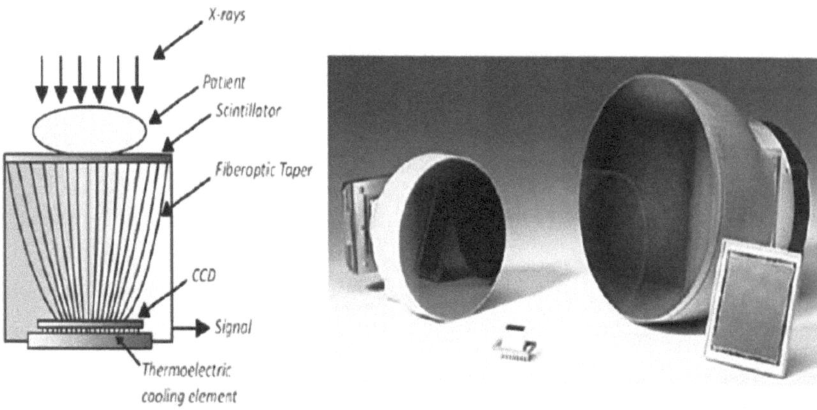

Figure 3.38: In digital X-rays, a fused fiberoptic taper is used to guide the light image from a scintillator an electronic CDD detector array for processing and visualization.

3.16 CONCLUSIONS

As discussed in this section, optics is a useful, practical, versatile, and powerful technology that, throughout history, has helped humankind perform visual examination, diagnostics, and therapeutics on both the sick and healthy. Optics technology and optical components are at the core in a variety of modern-day optical devices and instruments such as endoscopes, patient monitoring probes, and sensors, as well as in advanced robotic assisted surgery systems.

The harnessing power of light, and its interaction with living matter, is extremely useful and beneficial for a variety of medical purposes and treatments ranging from laser procedures for tattoo removal, to eye surgery to vessel and tissue ablation and coagulation, up to modern photodynamic therapy treatments. We have seen how the field of optics is a subset of a more complex and interdisciplinary area of research known as Biophotonics.

New advancements in optics and photonics are driving the development of a new generation of imaging tools—such as optical coherence and photo-acoustic tomography—that can readily provide two and three-dimensional images of diverse human body tissues and organs.

MEDICAL OPTICS

Optics has, and will continue to be, an *enabling technology* for the advancement of medicine promoting unimaginable new devices, techniques, and applications to happen in the not-too-distant future.

4

CHAPTER

ENDOSCOPY DEVICE

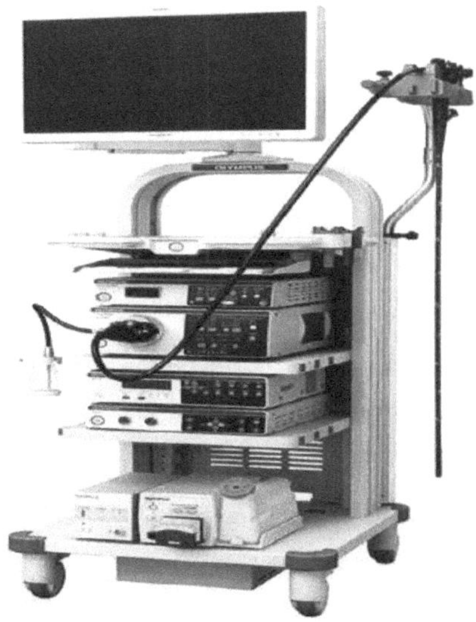

4.1 COMPONENTS OF ENDOSCOPY DEVICE

1- A thin, long flexible tube.

2- A lens or lens system.

3- A light transmitting system (Optical Fiber).

4- The eyepiece.

5- Control system.

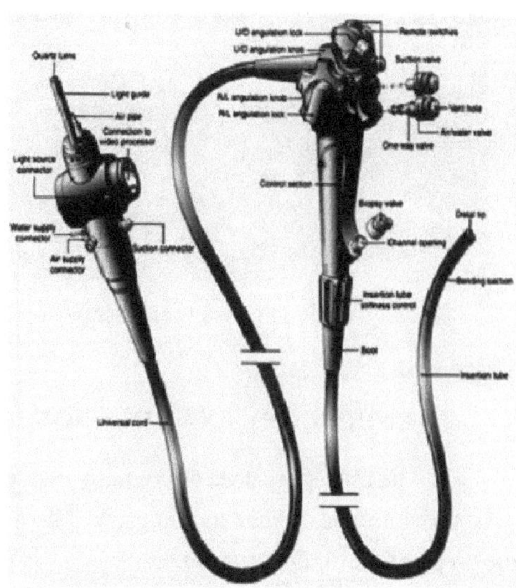

Figure 4.1: Component of endoscopy device.

4.2 HOW DOSE ENDOSCOPY DEVICE WORK

Basically, a typical endoscope uses fiber optics, which allow for effective transmitting of light. In this technique (fiber optics) light is transmitted through a flexible fiber of glass (transparent) known as optical fiber.

The optical fiber allows for light to travel through curved paths, whichmakes one of the best systems to view spaces that would normally be difficult to reach.

Here, total internal reflection makes it possible for light to travel along the fibers with the light rays hitting the fiber walls at an angle (minimumangle of 82 degree).

Given that individual fibers can be thinner than human hair, fiber optics isone of the best techniques to enter and view different areas of the body.

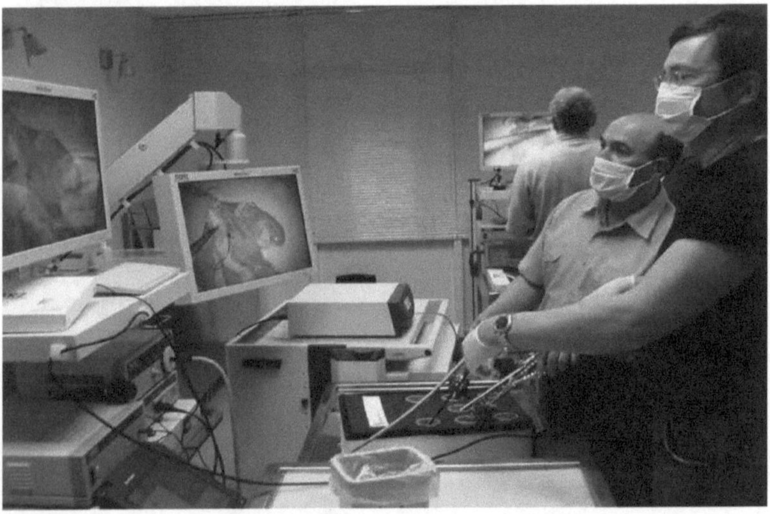

Figure 4.2: Monitor results endoscopy device

4.3 ENDOSCOPY EXAMINATION PREPARATIONS

1- The procedure does not require an overnight stay in the hospital andusually only takes around 1 hour to complete. The doctor will provide instructions about the preparation for the procedure.

2- For many types of endoscopies, the individual needs to fast for around 12 hours, though this varies based on the type.

3- For procedures investigating the gut, laxatives may be taken the night before to clear the system.

4- A doctor will carry out an examination before the endoscopy. It is important to mention all current medications (including supplements) and any previous procedures.

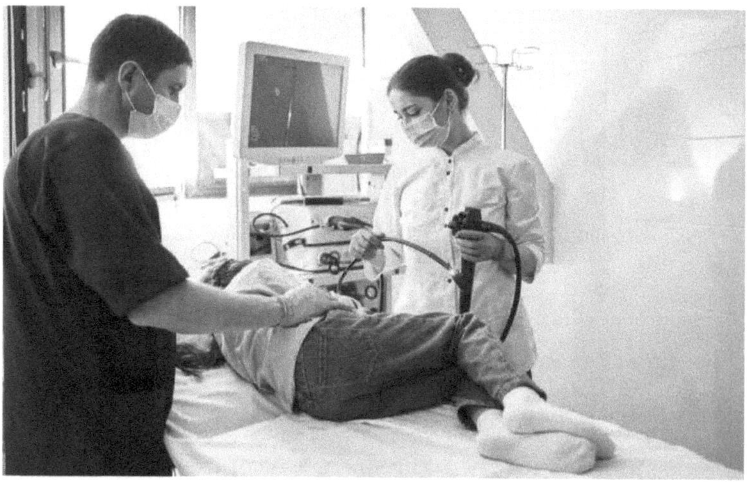

Figure 4.3: Examining the patient with a endoscopy device.

4.4 MAIN REASONS FOR CARRYING OUT AN ENDOSCOPY

Investigation: If an individual is experiencing vomiting, abdominal pain, breathing disorders, stomach ulcers, difficulty swallowing, or gastrointestinal bleeding, for example an endoscope can be used to searchfor a cause.

Confirmation of a diagnosis: Endoscopy can be used to carry out abiopsy to confirm a diagnosis of cancer or other diseases.

Treatment: An endoscope can be used to treat an illness directly; for instance, endoscopy can be used to cauterize (seal using heat) a bleedingvessel or remove a polyp.

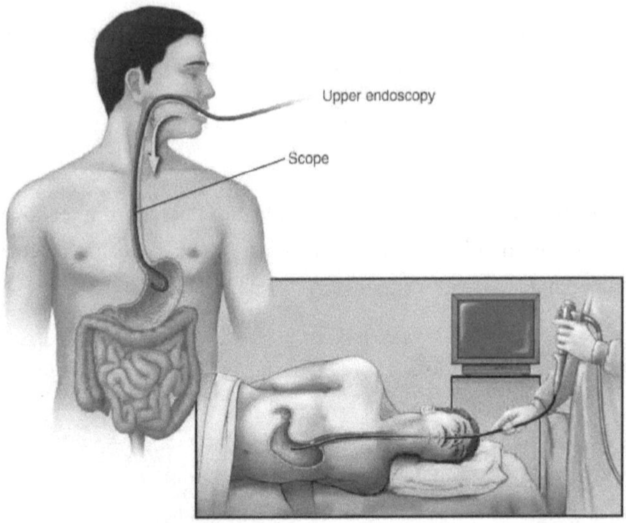

Figure 4.4: Illustration showing the endoscopy device inserted into the patient's stomach.

Benefits of Endoscopy:

1- No prior preparations are required of patients.

2- Laparoscopic surgery requires only a small incision through which a diagnosis or surgery can be made.

3- Using this technique, patients lose less blood during and after surgery and can recover much faster compared with standard surgical procedures.

Risks of Endoscopy:

1- Over-sedation, although sedation is not always necessary.

2- Feeling bloated for a short time after the procedure.

3- Mild cramping.

4- A numb throat for a few hours due to the use of local anesthetic.

5- Persistent pain around the endoscopy.

4.5 CAPSULE ENDOSCOPY DEVICE

It is the most important type of endoscopy; Capsule endoscopy was developed in the mid-1990s and involves a wireless camera. The camera is small enough to fit into a capsule (roughly the size of a vitamin tablet)and can, therefore, be swallowed.

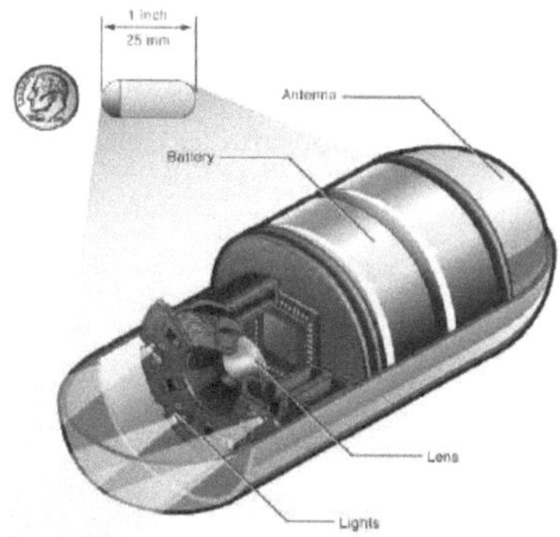

Figure 4.5: Illustration showing the endoscopy capsule.

As the capsule travels through the digestive tract, it takes thousands of pictures, which are transmitted to a device attached to a wearable belt.

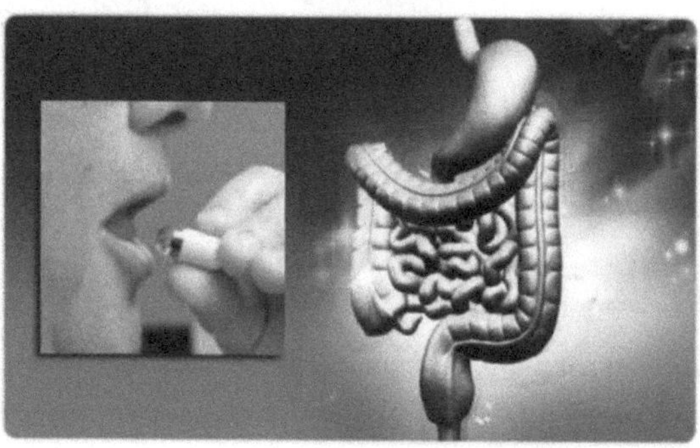

Figure 4.6: Illustration showing the as the capsule travels through the digestive tract.

Capsule endoscopy is used to image the small intestine, a region that is difficult to image using standard endoscopy. It is also very useful for examining the small intestinal mucosa and diagnosing Crohn's disease.The capsule usually passes through the digestive system within 24-48 hours.

While capsule endoscopy has been deemed a sufficient alternative to an esophagogastroduodenoscopy, limitations Trusted Source are observed, including clear visualization and active movements that need controlling. To remedy this issue, magnetic manipulation is used.

This is a relatively new technique and was given FDA approval for use inthe United States in 2001. To date, more than 500,000 capsule endoscopyprocedures have been carried out, and nearly 1,000 articles have been published covering its clinical use.

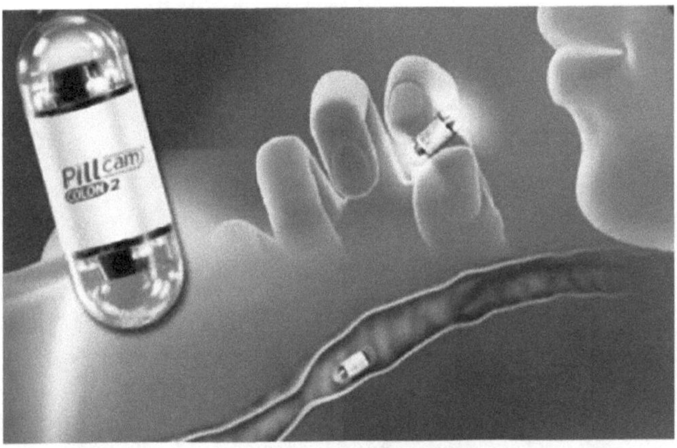

Figure 4.7: Illustration showing them as the endoscopy capsule march.

4.6 PREPARING FOR AN ENDOSCOPY

An endoscopy does not require an overnight stay in the hospital and usually only takes around 1 hour to complete. The doctor will provide instructions about the preparation for the procedure.

For many types of endoscopies, the individual needs to fast for around 12 hours, though this varies based on the type.

For procedures investigating the gut, laxatives may be taken the night before to clear the system.

A doctor will conduct an examination before the endoscopy. It is important to mention all current medications (including supplements) and any previous procedures.

4.7 ENDOSCOPY PROCEDURE

The procedure will depend to some extent on the reason for the endoscopy.

There are three main reasons for carrying out an endoscopy:

- **Investigation:** If an individual is experiencing vomiting, abdominal pain, breathing disorders, stomach ulcers, difficulty swallowing, or gastrointestinal bleeding, for example, an endoscope can be used to search for a cause.

- **Confirmation of a diagnosis:** An endoscopy can carry out a biopsy to confirm a diagnosis of cancer or other diseases.

- **Treatment:** An endoscope can treat an illness directly; for instance, endoscopy can be used to cauterize (seal using heat) a bleeding vessel or remove a polyp.

Sometimes, an endoscopy will be combined with another procedure such as an ultrasound scan. It can be used to place the ultrasound probe close to organs that can be difficult to image, such as the pancreas.

Modern endoscopes sometimes come with sensitive lights that use narrow-band imaging. This type of imaging uses specific blue and green wavelengths that allow the doctor to spot precancerous conditions more easily.

An endoscopy typically happens while the person is conscious, although sometimes the person receives local anesthetic (commonly an anesthetic spray to the back of the throat). Often, the person is sedated.

For endoscopy procedures involving entry through the mouth, a mouth guard will protect the teeth and lips as the tube is inserted.

4.8 ENDOSCOPE USE IN SURGERY

Endoscopy has advanced in recent years, enabling some forms of surgery using a modified endoscope. This makes the surgery less invasive.

Procedures such as the removal of the gallbladder, sealing and tying the fallopian tubes, and the removal of small tumors from the digestive system or lungs are now commonplace.

A laparoscope is a modified endoscope used for keyhole surgery (also referred to as laparoscopic surgery).

Laparoscopic surgery requires only a small incision and can be used for appendectomies (removal of the appendix), hysterectomies (removal of the uterus), and prostatectomies (removal of prostate tissue).

Using this technique, people lose less blood during and after surgery and can recover much faster compared with standard surgical procedures.

4.9 RISKS AND SIDE EFFECTS OF ENDOSCOPY

An endoscopy is a relatively safe procedure. However, there are certain risks involved. Risks depend on the area that is being examined.

Risks of endoscopy may include:

- over-sedation, although sedation is not always necessary
- feeling bloated for a short time after the procedure
- mild cramping
- a numb throat for a few hours due to the use of local anesthetic
- infection of the area of investigation, which most commonly occurs when additional procedures are carried out at the same time (the infections are normally minor and treatable with a course of antibiotics)
- persistent pain around the endoscopy
- perforation or tear of the lining of the stomach or esophagus, a rare but serious complication
- internal bleeding, usually minor and sometimes treatable by endoscopic cauterization
- complications related to preexisting conditions

Any of the following symptoms should be reported to a doctor:

- dark-colored stool
- shortness of breath
- severe and persistent abdominal pain
- chest pain
- Vomiting Blood

4.10 RECOVERING FROM AN ENDOSCOPY

Recovery will depend on the type of procedure. For an upper endoscopy, which lets a doctor examine the upper gastrointestinal tract, the person will undergo observation after the procedure. This usually lasts around 1 hour while any sedative medication wears off.

The person should not usually work or drive for the rest of the day because of the sedative effect of the medication used to prevent the pain. Any cognitive effects Trusted Source should be reported to a doctor prior to leaving the procedure area or after.

There may be some soreness. With this type of endoscopy, there may be bloating and a sore throat. However, these usually resolve quickly.

Takeaway

Endoscopic procedures are typically minimally invasive and can be done through the mouth, anus, or in small incisions. These procedures may be used to investigate, diagnose, or treat various conditions.

These procedures have low complication rates, and a person is typically discharged within a few hours. Some side effects may occur, such as a sore throat or bloating. However, they will typically resolve quickly. A person should speak with their doctor if lingering effects occur.

Optical Fiber Structure:

A typical optical fiber consists of a core, a cladding, and a polymer jacket (buffer coating).

The polymer coating is the first line of mechanical protection The coating also reduces the internal reflection at the cladding, so light is only guided by the core.

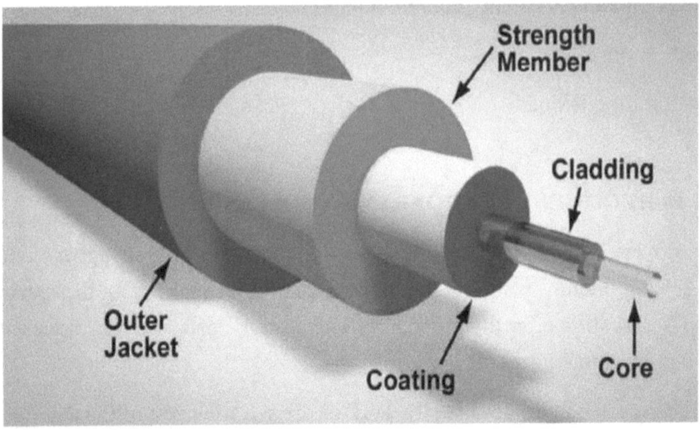

Figure 4.8: Fiber optic components.

Principle of operation:

1- An optical fiber is a cylindrical dielectric waveguide (no conducting waveguide) .

2- Optical fiber transmits light along its axis through the process of total internal reflection.

3- The fiber consists of a core surrounded by a cladding layer, both of which are made of dielectric materials, to confine the optical signal in the core.

4- The refractive index of the core must be greater than that of the cladding.

5- Light can be fed into optical fibers using lasers or LEDs.

5

CHAPTER

OPTICS AND HUMAN VISION

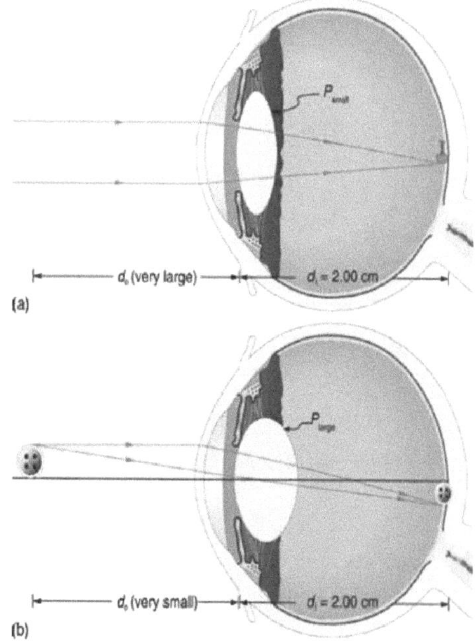

5.1 LIGHT

Light

1-Particles known as photons

2-Act as 'waves'

Two fundamental properties

1- Amplitude

2-Wavelength

a- Frequency is the inverse of wavelength

b- Relationship between wavelength (λ: lambda) and frequency (f), as illustrated in Figure 5.1.

$$\lambda = c / f$$

Where c = speed of light = 299,792,458 m / s

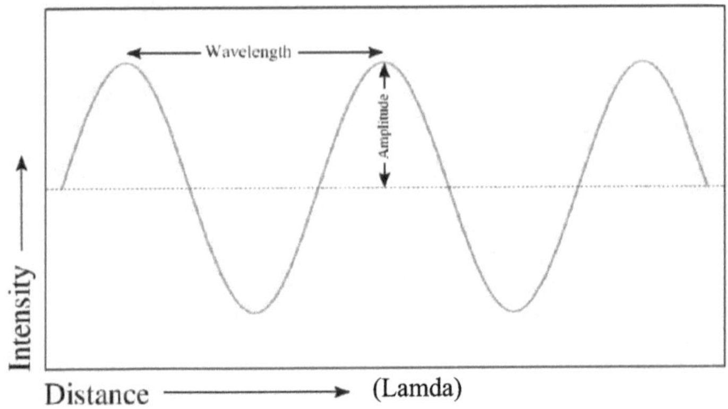

Figure 5.1: Diagram of a light wave.

Wavelength can be measured between any two points with the same phase, such as between crests.

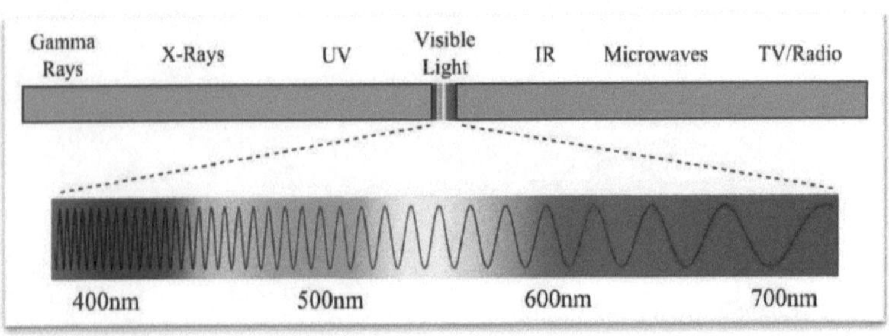

Figure 5.2: Electromagnetic Spectrum, showing the visible light range.

5.2 ELECTROMAGNETIC SPECTRUM

1- Microwave hyperthermia therapy is a type of medical treatment in which body tissue is exposed to slightly higher temperatures to damage and kill cancer cell or to make cancer cell more sensitive to the effects of radiation and certain anti- cancer drugs.

2- Infrared radiation is emitted by all objects above absolute zero, Infrared is used in locating tumors.

3- Visible Typically optical fibers are used to transfer light to the end of the endoscope and a miniature video records the image and viewed on a video screen.

4- Ultraviolet light in treatment of psoriasis and ultraviolet light against germs.

5- X-ray photons have much more energy (1-100 kev) Soft tissue does not absorb X-ray radiation well but it is still possible, that is why you don't only see bones.

Figures 5.3 and 5.4 show different types of machines producing images of the body.

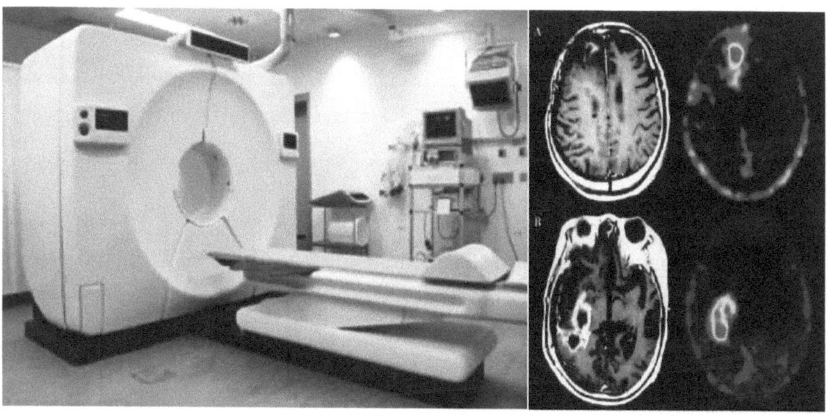

Figure 5.3: CT-Scan machine producing X- ray slices of the body.

Gamma ray Positron Emission Tomography (PET):

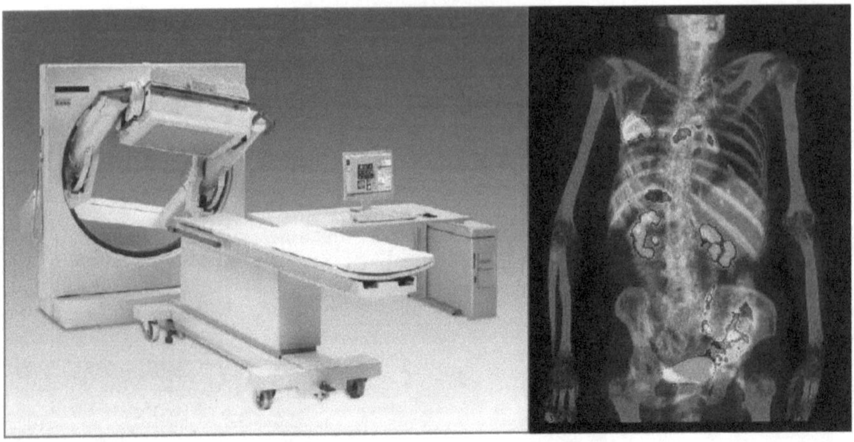

Figure 5.4: Nuclear medical imaging, 3D images, taken by Gamma ray machine.

Example 5.1:

To reach tumors deep within a patient's body so-called hard X- ray is used. An X-ray tube generator operating at 500 KV is used.

a- What is the energy of the operating generator?

b- What is the wavelength of the X- ray?

Solution:

a- $E = eV$ (e = electron charge = 1.6×10^{-19} C)

$E = 1.6 \times 10^{-19} \times 500 \times 1000$

$E = 8 \times 10^{-14}$ J

b- $E = hf$ (h = planks constant = 6.6×10^{-34} J.s)

(f = the frequency of the X- ray)

$E = h \times c/\lambda$

$\lambda = h \times c/E$

$\lambda = 6.6 \times 10^{-34}$ J.s $\times 3 \times 10^{8}$ m.s^{-1}/8×10^{-14} J

$\lambda = 2.4 \times 10^{-12}$ m

$\lambda = 2.48 \times 10^{-3}$ nm.

Example 5.2:

The frequency is associated with a certain diagnostic X-ray photon 1.7 x10^{19} Hz.

a- Find the energy of X-ray.

b- At what voltage X-ray tube was operating?

Solution:

a- E = hf

$E = 6.6\text{x } 10^{-34}\text{ J.s x } 1.7\text{ x}10^{19}\text{ Hz}$

$E = 11.22\text{ x } 10^{-15}\text{ J}$

b- E = ev

v = E / e

$v = 11.22\text{ x } 10^{-15}\text{ J} / 1.6\text{ x } 10^{-19}\text{ C}$

$v = 7.0125\text{ x } 10^{-34}\text{ V}$

5.3 THIN LENSES

A lens is a transparent device that allow light to pass through and refracts A is an optical device with perfect or approximate axial symmetry. Thin lenses are those whose thickness is small compared to their radius of curvature, as shown in Figures 5.5 and 5.6.

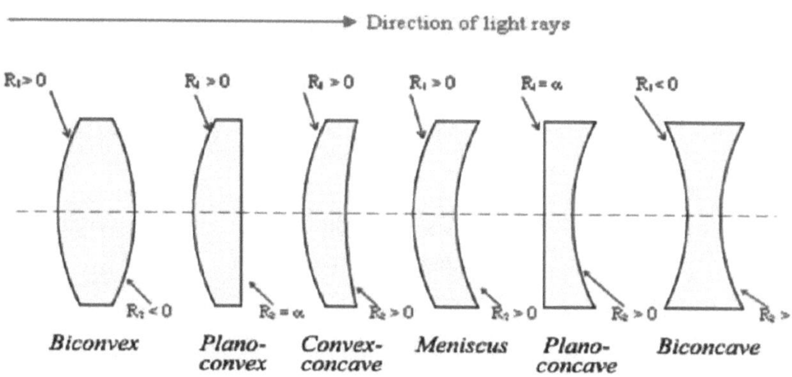

a- Converging lenses b- Diverging lenses

Figure 5.5: Different types of converging and diverging lenses.

(a)

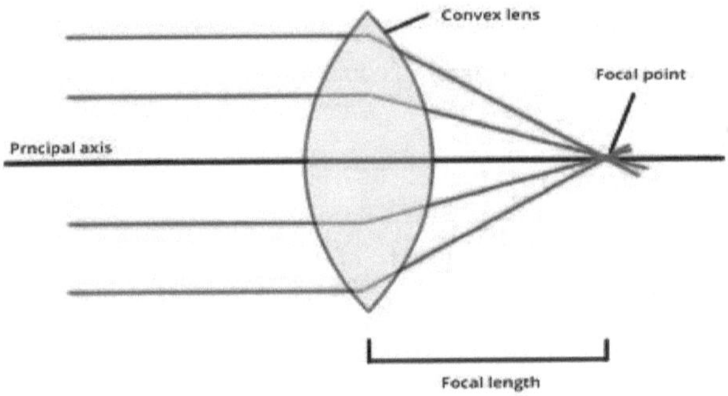

(b)

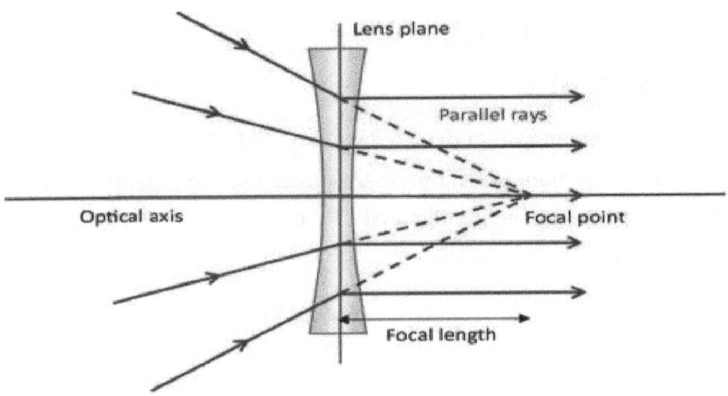

Figure 5.6: Converging lens (a) or diverging lens (b).

In converging, Parallel rays are brought to a focus by a converging lens. The property of image is really inverted and virtual upright.

A diverging lens makes parallel light diverge; the focal point is that point where the diverging rays would converge if projected back. The properties of image virtually upright.

Example 5.3:

If F_1 is 25 cm, and F_2 is 1m, what is F total?

Solution:

$$\frac{1}{F_T} = \frac{1}{F_1} + \frac{1}{F_1}$$

$$\frac{1}{F_T} = \frac{1}{25} + \frac{1}{100} = \frac{5}{100}$$

$\therefore$ FT = 20 cm

5.4 THIN LENS EQUATION

- A lens is a transparent device that allows light to pass through while causing it to either converge or diverge.
- Assume that a camera is focused on a target object using a single converging lens:
  - Let S_1 be the distance from the lens to the target.
  - Let S_2 be the distance from the lens to the film.
  - The focal length, f, is a measure of how strongly a lens converges light
  - The magnification factor, m, is another measure.
  - The optical zoom of a digital camera is usually larger than 1
  - The magnification factor of a single lens is usually less than 1, as shown in Figure 5.7.

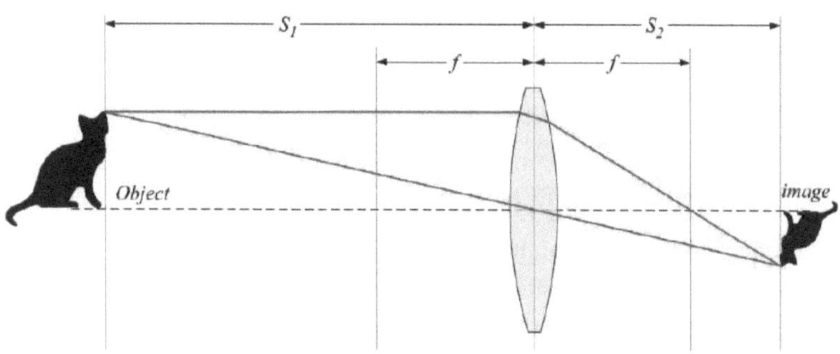

Figure 5.7: Distances S_1 and S_2 for the calculation of magnification factors.

$$m = \frac{image\ size}{object\ size} = \frac{S_2}{S_1} \qquad (5.1)$$

$$\frac{1}{S_1} + \frac{1}{S_2} = \frac{1}{f}$$

5.4.1 Optics and f-stop

- F-number is the ratio of focal length to the diameter of the aperture (lens opening)
- F-stops are pre-defined aperture settings that are typically factors of 2 with respect to amount of light allowed into the camera.
- Doubling "area" of a circle implies scaling the aperture diameter by square (2) or 1.4.
- F-stops are geometric sequences involving powers of the square-root of 2.

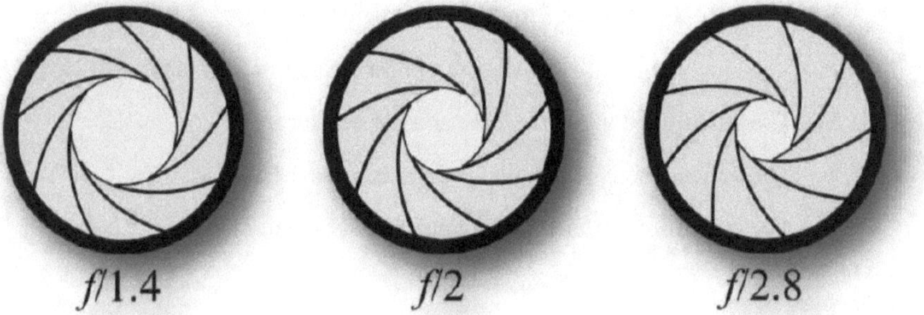

Figure 5.8: Different f-stop ratio of focal length to the diameter of the lens opening (aperture).

5.5 THE HUMAN EYE

The human eye is one of the most valuable and sensitive organs. It enables us to see the wonderful world and the colors around us. On closing our eyes, we can identify objects to some extent by their smell, taste, sound they make or by touch. It is, however, impossible to identify colors while closing the eyes. Thus, of all sense organs, the human eye is the most significant one as it enables us to see the beautiful, colorful world around us.

The human eye is like a camera. Its lens system forms an image on a light-sensitive screen called the retina. Light enters the eye through a thin membrane called the cornea. It forms the transparent bulge on the front surface of the eyeball as shown in Fig. 5.9. The eyeball is approximately spherical in shape with a diameter of about 2.3 cm. Most of the refractions for the light rays entering the eye occurs at the outer surface of the cornea. The crystalline lens merely provides the finer adjustment of focal length required to focus objects at different distances on the retina. We find a structure called iris behind the cornea. Iris is a dark muscular diaphragm that controls the size of the pupil. The pupil regulates and controls the amount of light entering the eye. The eye lens forms an inverted real image of the object on the retina. The retina is a delicate membrane having enormous number of light-sensitive cells. The light-sensitive cells get activated upon illumination and generate electrical signals. These signals are sent to the brain via the optic nerves. The brain interprets these signals, and finally, processes the information so that we perceive objects as they are.

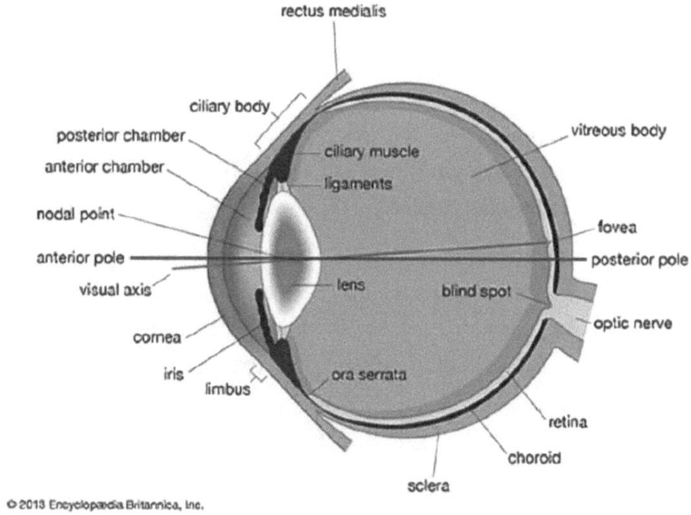

Figure 5.9 The human eye.

Damage to or malfunction of any part of the visual system can lead to significant loss of visual functioning. For example, if any of the structures involved in the transmission of light, like the cornea, pupil, eye lens, aqueous humor and vitreous humor or those responsible for conversion of light to electrical impulse, like the retina or even the optic nerve that transmits these impulses to the brain, is damaged, it will result in visual impairment. You might have experienced that you are not able to see objects clearly for some time when you enter from bright light to a room with dim light. After some time, however, you may be able to see things in the dim-lit room. The pupil of an eye acts like a variable aperture whose size can be varied with the help of the iris. When the light is very bright, the iris contracts the pupil to allow less light to enter the eye. However, in dim light the iris expands the pupil to allow more light to enter the eye. Thus, the pupil opens completely through the relaxation of the iris.

Cornea: The transparent part of the eye. It is the clear transparent bump on the front of the eye that does about two- thirds of focusing of light.

Visual axis: A straight line that passes through the center of the colored part of the front eye. The function of iris is adaptation of vision from light to dark and vice.

Versa. It is believed that the iris aids the eye by increasing or decreasing incident light on the retina until the retina adapts to the new lighting condition. In addition, under bright light conditions it plays an important role in reducing lens defects.

The pupil: It is the small opening in the center of iris where light enters the lens. It appears black because essential all of the light that enters is absorbed inside the eye. (Under average light conditions, the opening is about ≅ 4mm). It can change from ≅ 3mm in diameter in bright light to 8mm in dim light. The physiology reason for this change in size is not clear.

Aqueous humor (It fills the space between the lens and the cornea. This fluid, mostly water, $n \cong 1.33$.

The Lens is variable in shape and could focus objects at various distances at both its front and back surfaces. It is more curved in the back than in the front.

The focusing power of lens is smaller than that of the cornea (1/3), because it is surrounded by substances that have indexes of refraction close to its own. The lens it's made up of layers somewhat like anion and all layers do not have the same n.

The lens act as a fine adjustment for focusing different distance, so called accommodation on Retina, optic nerve to the visual cortex, as shown in Figures 5.10 and 5.11.

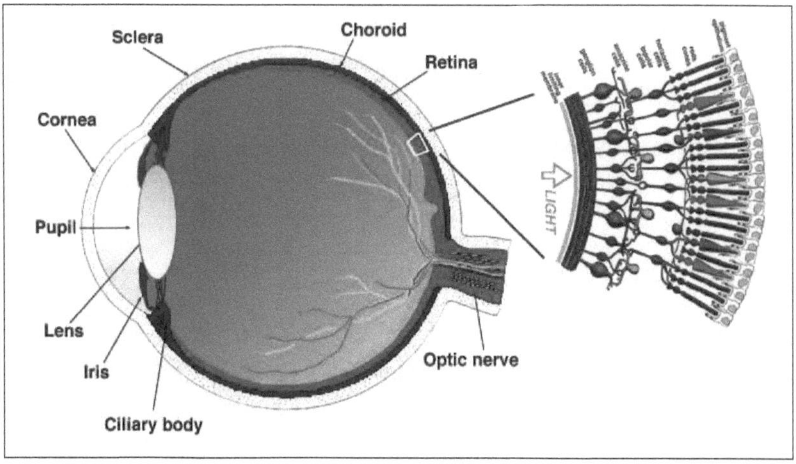

Figure 5.10: Anatomy of eye showed all parts concerning image formation.

5.5.1 Power of Accommodation

The eye lens is composed of a fibrous, jelly-like material. Its curvature can be modified to some extent by the ciliary muscles. The change in the curvature of the eye lens can thus change its focal length. When the muscles are relaxed, the lens becomes thin. Thus, its focal length increases. This enables us to see distant objects clearly. When you are looking at objects closer to the eye, the ciliary muscles contract. This increases the curvature of the eye lens. The eye lens then becomes thicker. Consequently, the focal length of the eye lens decreases. This enables us to see nearby objects clearly.

MEDICAL OPTICS

The ability of the eye lens to adjust its focal length is called accommodation. However, the focal length of the eye lens cannot be decreased below a certain minimum limit. Try to read a printed page by holding it very close to your eyes. You may see the image being blurred or feel strain in the eye. To see an object comfortably and distinctly, you must hold it at about 25 cm from the eyes. The minimum distance, at which objects can be seen most distinctly without strain, is called the least distance of distinct vision. It is also called the near point of the eye. For a young adult with normal vision, the near point is about 25 cm. The farthest point up to which the eye can see objects clearly is called the far point of the eye. It is infinite for a normal eye. You may note here that a normal eye can see objects clearly that are between 25 cm and infinite.

Sometimes, the crystalline lens of people at old age becomes milky and cloudy. This condition is called cataract. This causes partial or complete loss of vision. It is possible to restore vision through cataract surgery.

Why do we have two eyes for vision and not just one?

There are several advantages of our having two eyes instead of one. It gives a wider field of view. A human being has a horizontal field of view of about 150° with one eye and of about 180° with two eyes. The ability to detect faint objects is, of course, enhanced with two detectors instead of one.

Some animals, usually prey animals, have their two eyes positioned on opposite sides of their heads to give the widest possible field of view. But our two eyes are positioned on the front of our heads, and it thus reduces our field of view in favor of what is called stereopsis. Shut one eye and the world looks flat – two-dimensional. Keep both eyes open and the world take on the third dimension of depth. Because our eyes are separated by a few centimeters, each eye sees a slightly different image. Our brain combines the two images into one, using the extra information to tell us how close or far away things are.

5.5.2 Specifications of the Optical System

1. Observation of events over **~180°** angle when looking intently at an object directly ahead of it.

2. Blinking to clean and lubricate the lens.

3. Clear distance viewing between. ~ **25cm to infinity ∞.**

4. Operating effectively between the daylight and dark night (**$\sim 10^{10}$:1 intensity**). Brilliant day light to a very dark night.

5. The eye has an automatic aperture adjustment (**iris**).

6. Cornea (**has no blood supply**) made of living cells and can repair **the** local damage.

7. The eye has a self-regulating pressure system that maintains the internal pressure of **~20mm Hg** and thus **keeps the eye in shape.**

8. Mountain in a well-protected casing.

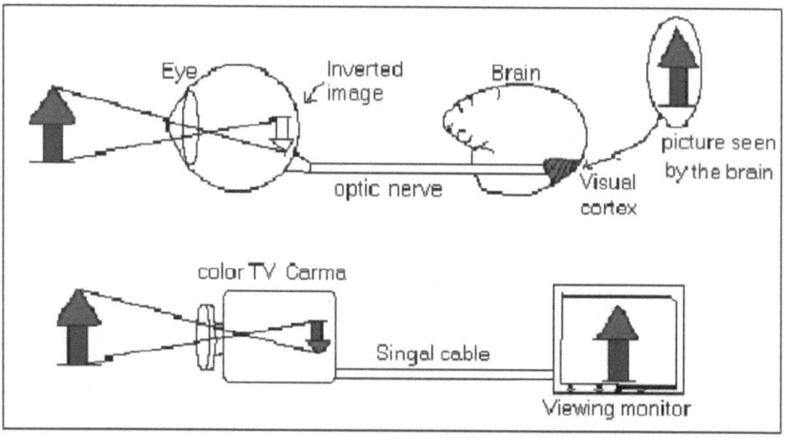

Figure 5.11: Schematic diagram, showing object, lens and image system of the eye.

9. The image appears upside down on the light sensitive retain at the **back** of the eyeball, but **the brain automatically corrects for this.**

10. The brain blends the images from both eyes giving good depth **perception** and **the 3D viewing**.

11. The muscles of the eye (**six muscles**, the muscles work in pair) **permit** flexible movement up, down, side-ways and diagonally.

All six muscles are attached to the skull.

One pair controls up and down movement.

One pair control left and right movement.

One pair controls rotation.

After a little practice, the eye can even be made to go in circle.

5.5.3 The amount of Bending depends on

The curvatures of its surfaces: Human eye is convex lens crystalline, the focal length of this lens is changed by special muscle around the lens, and the focal length depend on the radius of the curvature (R).

$$F = \frac{1}{2} R \qquad (5.2)$$

5.5.4 Light detector of the eye

Light incident on retina through the lens of eye. Retina is the light sensitive part of the eye that converts the images into electrical nerve impulses that are sent to the brain.

5.5.5 The physical aspects of the retina

The absorption of visible light with energy > 1 ev causes a photochemical reaction in the photoreceptor and initiates the action potential then the light image convert into electrical signal sent to the brain through the optic nerve.

- Retina covers the back half of the eyeball.
- Most vision is restricted to a small area called yellow spot (~ 0.3 mm).

The image on the retina, real, is very small due to short image distance about (2cm) ≅ 20mm.

- Simple relation between the object and image size and object and image distance from the ratio of the lengths of sides of similar triangles, as shown in Figure 5.12.

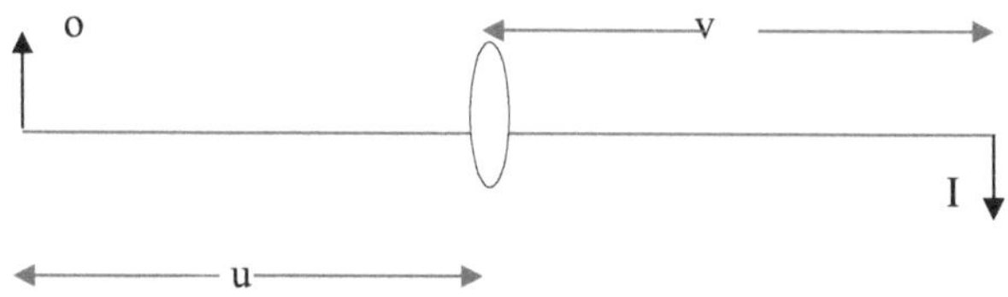

Figure 5.12: The relation between U, V, O and I of a lens.

$$\left[\frac{\text{Object size}}{\text{Image size}} = \frac{\text{object distance}}{\text{Image distance}}\right] = \left[\frac{O}{I} = \frac{u}{v}\right] \qquad (5.3)$$

Also the relation between U, V and f is given by:

$$\frac{1}{f} = \frac{1}{u} + \frac{1}{v}$$

In connection with equation (5,1), we have:

$U = S_1$ and $V = S_2$

Example 5.4:

How big is the image on the retina of a fly on a wall 3.0 m away? Assume the fly is 3mm in diameter and v = 0.02 m.

Solution:

We have:

U = object distance = 3.0 m

O = Object size = 3mm = 0.03m

V = Image distance = 0.02 m

I = Image size = ?

$$\therefore \quad \left[\frac{O}{I} = \frac{u}{v}\right] \longrightarrow \therefore I = \left(\frac{v}{u}\right) O$$

$$I = \left(\frac{0.02}{3.0}\right) 0.03 = 0.0002 \text{ m} = 0.02 \text{ cm}$$

5.6 DEFECTS OF VISION AND THEIR CORRECTION

Sometimes, the eye may gradually lose its power of accommodation. In such conditions, the person cannot see the objects distinctly and comfortably. The vision becomes blurred due to the refractive defects of the eye.

There are mainly three common refractive defects of vision. These are (i) myopia or near-sightedness, (ii) Hypermetropia or far-sightedness, and (iii) Presbyopia. These defects can be corrected using suitable spherical lenses. We discuss below these defects and their corrections.

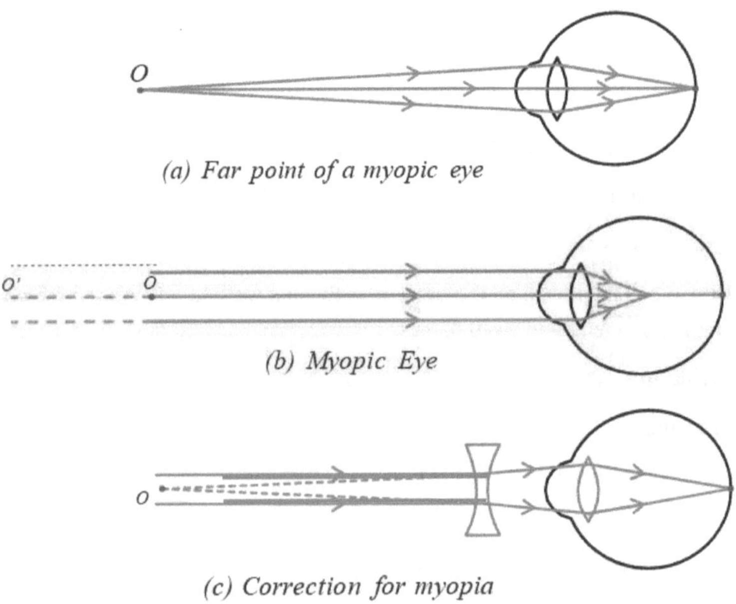

Figure 5.13 (a), (b) The myopic eye, and (c) correction for myopia with a concave lens.

(a) **Myopia**

Myopia is also known as near-sightedness. A person with myopia can see nearby objects clearly but cannot see distant objects distinctly. A person with this defect has a far point nearer than infinity. Such a person may see clearly up to a distance of a few meters. In a myopic eye, the image of a distant object is formed in front of the retina Fig. 5.13 (b) and not at the retina itself. This defect may arise due to

(i) excessive curvature of the eye lens, or (ii) elongation of the eyeball. This defect can be corrected by using a concave lens of suitable power. This is illustrated in Fig. 5.13 (c). A concave lens of suitable power will bring the image back on to the retina and thus the defect is corrected.

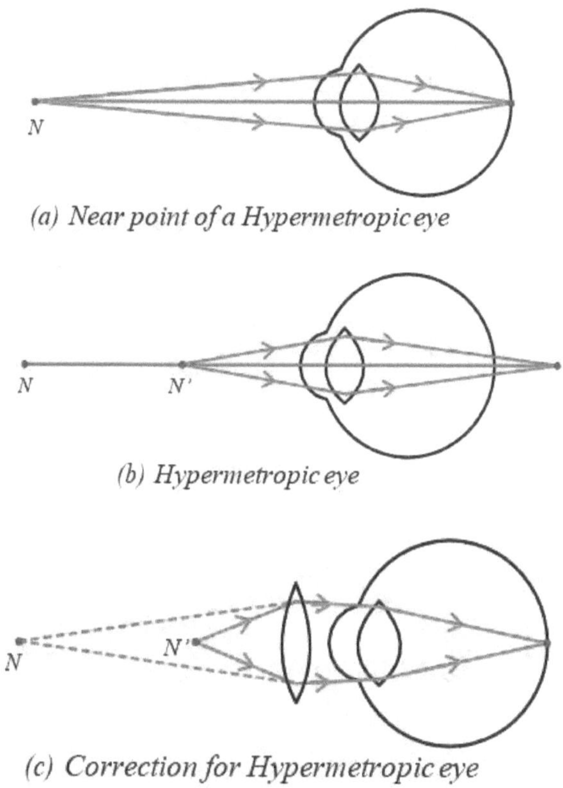

(a) Near point of a Hypermetropic eye

(b) Hypermetropic eye

(c) Correction for Hypermetropic eye

Figure 5.14 (a), (b) The hypermetropic eye, and (c) correction for hypermetropia

(b) Hypermetropia

Hypermetropia is also known as far-sightedness. A person with hypermetropia can see distant objects clearly but cannot see nearby objects distinctly. The near point, for the person, is farther away from the normal near point (25 cm). Such a person must keep reading material much beyond 25 cm from the eye for comfortable reading. This is because the light rays from a close by object are focused at a point behind the retina as shown in Fig. 5.14 (b). This defect arises either because (i) the focal length of the eye lens is too long, or (ii) the eyeball has become too small. This defect can be corrected by using a convex lens of appropriate power. This is illustrated in Fig. 5.14 (c). Eyeglasses with converging lenses provide the additional focusing power required for forming the image on the retina.

(c) Presbyopia

The power of accommodation of the eye usually decreases with ageing. For most people, the near point gradually recedes away. They find it difficult to see nearby objects comfortably and distinctly without corrective eyeglasses. This defect is called Presbyopia. It arises due to the gradual weakening of the ciliary muscles and diminishing flexibility of the eye lens. Sometimes, a person may suffer from both myopia and hypermetropia. Such people often require bi- focal lenses. A common type of bi-focal lenses consists of both concave and convex lenses. The upper portion consists of a concave lens. It facilitates distant vision. The lower part is a convex lens. It facilitates nearvision.

These days, it is possible to correct the refractive defects with

contact lenses or through surgical interventions.

5.7 RODS AND CONES SENSITIVITY

The Rods and Cons are distributed symmetrically in all directions from the visual axis except in one region the blind spot.

A. Cones: The Cones **(~ 6.5 million in each eye)**, their properties are:

1. Are primarily used for **daylight** or **photonic vision**. With the cones, we can see fine details and recognize different colors.

2. The cones are primarily found in the **fovea centralize** although some are scattered **throughout the retina.**

3. Each of the cones in the fovea has **its own telephone lines for the brain.** In the rest of the Retina several cones share one nerve fiber.

4. The cones are not uniformly sensitive to all colors but have a maximum sensitivity at about **550mv in the yellow-green region.**

5. The cones adapted most rapidly (**dark adaptation**) at the ~ **5**min in the fovea centralize has reached its best sensitivity.

Rods and cones are illustrated in Figure 5.15.

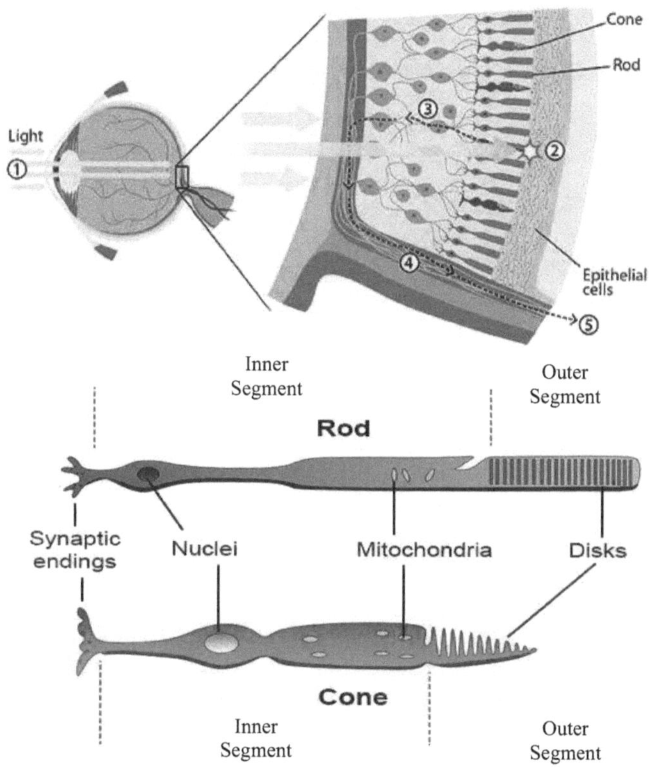

Figure 5.15: The light must pass through various cell layers to reach the rods and cones, in the Retina.

B. Rods: The rods **(~120 million in each eye and covered most of the retina), their properties are:**

1. Are they used for **night** or **scotopic vision** and for peripheral vision.

2. They are **not uniformly distributed over the retina** but have a maximum density at an **angle of about 20°.**

3. Hundreds of roads send their information to **same nerve fiber.**

4. The rods are most sensitive to the **blue-green light (~510-nm)** which has a wavelength shorter than the optimum for the cones (~ 550 nm).

5. The rods continue to **dark adapt** for **30-60 min** although their adaptation occurs in the **first 15min**.

Cone (LMS) and Rod (R) responses, as shown in Figure 5.16.

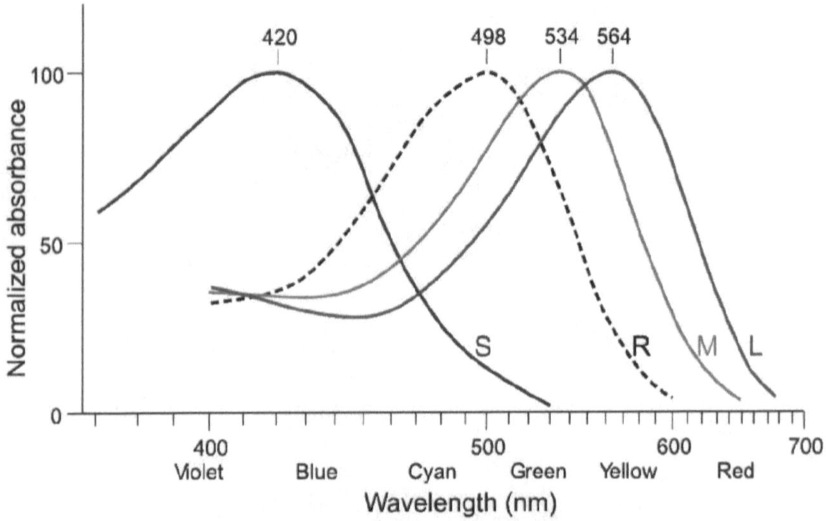

Figure 5.16: The rod is much more sensitive than the cones.

Table 5.1: Comparison between rods and cones.

Rods	Cones
Used for night vision	Used for day vision
Loss causes night blindness	Loss causes legal blindness
Low spatial resolution with higher noise	High spatial resolution with lower noise
Not present in fovea	Concentrated in fovea
Slower time response to light	Quicker time response to light
One type of photosensitive pigment	Three types of photosensitive pigment
Emphasis on motion detection	Emphasis on detecting fine detail

5.8 DIFFRACTION EFFECTS ON THE EYE

The iris produces a diffraction pattern on the retina like the diffraction of light pass through a small opening (slit). A when mono chromatic light (λ = 555 nm) from a distant source is brought to a focus retina.

From the relation $\mathbf{d\sin\theta = n\lambda}$ (5. 4)

Where:

d = diameter of the pupil of the iris.

θ = angle of the diffraction of the light

n = order of the diffraction

λ = Wavelength of the light

Example 5.5: A slit of width 0.5 mm is illuminated with 633 nm light. At what angle is the first minimum observed in the single slit diffraction pattern on a distant screen?

Solution:

$$\mathbf{d \sin\theta = n\,\lambda}$$

$$0.5 \times 10^{-3} \times \sin\theta = 1 \times 633 \times 10^{-9}$$

$$\sin\theta = \frac{633 \times 10^{-9}}{0.5 \times 10^{-3}} = 1266 \times 10^{-6}$$

$$\theta = \sin^{-1}(1266 \times 10^{-6}) = 0.07253$$

Example 5.6: the pupil of a cat`s eye narrows to a vertical slit of width o.5 mm in daylight. What is the angular resolution for horizontally separated mice? Assume that the average wavelength of the light is 500nm.

Solution:

$$\mathbf{d \sin\theta = n\,\lambda}$$

$$0.5 \times 10^{-3} \sin\theta = 1 \times 500 \times 10^{-9}$$

$$\sin\theta = \frac{500 \times 10^{-9}}{0.5 \times 10^{-3}} = 1000 \times 10^{-6} = 0.001$$

5.9 THE RESOLUTION OF THE EYE

The minimum angular separation of the two equidistance points of light which can just be resolved by the eye.

5.9.1 The test of vision

The property of our eyes to determine whether we need corrective lenses test by using eye charts. Snellen chart to test vision is usually viewed from 20 ft [6 meters], as shown in Figure 5.17.

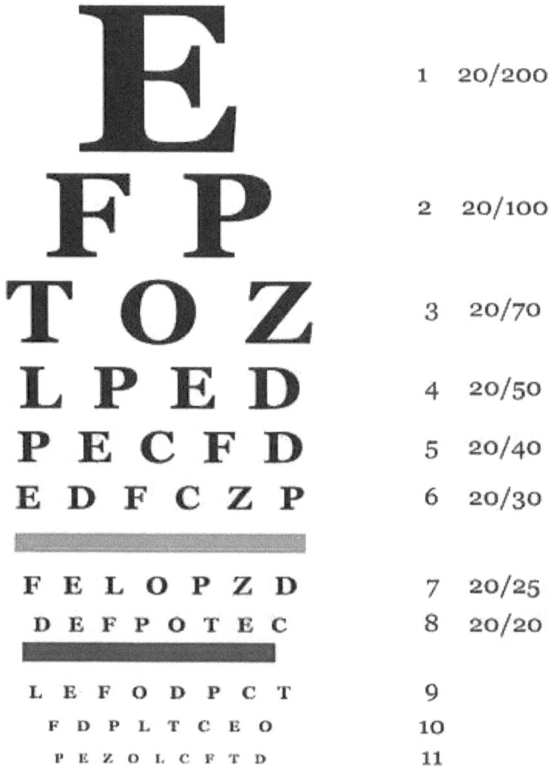

Figure 5.17: Snellen Chart.

5.9.2 The kind of test

1- $\frac{20}{20} = \frac{6}{6}$ It means that you can read detail from 20 ft. that a person with good vision can read from 20 ft.

2- $\frac{20}{20} = \frac{6}{12}$, you can read from 20 ft., that a person with good vision can read from 40 ft.

3- $\frac{20}{20} = \frac{6}{18}$ You can read from 20 ft. that a person with good vision can read from 60 ft.

Meter = 3.333 ft.

5.10 THE STRENGTH (POWER) OF OPTIC SYSTEM

The strength (power) [refractive power]:

Is the reciprocal length of the focal length of this system in meter.

∴ The power

$$\mathbf{P} = \frac{1}{f\ (meter)} \qquad (5.5)$$

f = the focal length in (m)

P = the power of eye (D)

Where D is unit of strength of this system when F in meter.

$$\therefore \text{D} = \text{diopter} = \frac{1}{f\ (M)} \qquad (5.6)$$

Diverging lens with negative focal length (-f)

5.10.1 The power of human eye

a- **Far – point:** The point at which distant objects are focused when the focusing muscle is relaxed.

Normal eye far – point (∞).

b- **Near – point:** The closest point at which object can be focused when the lens is its thickest.

Normal eye near – point (25 cm).

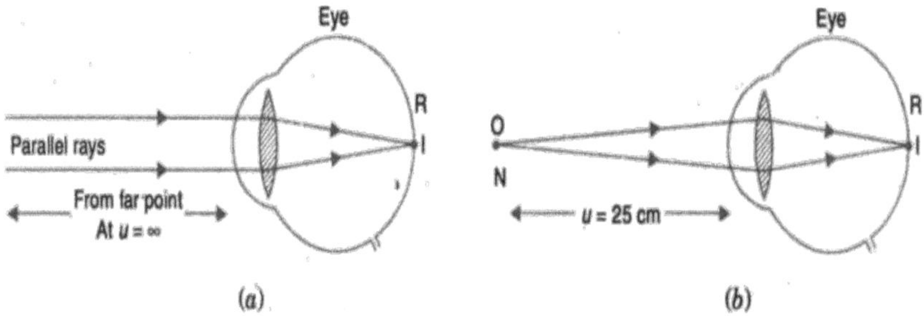

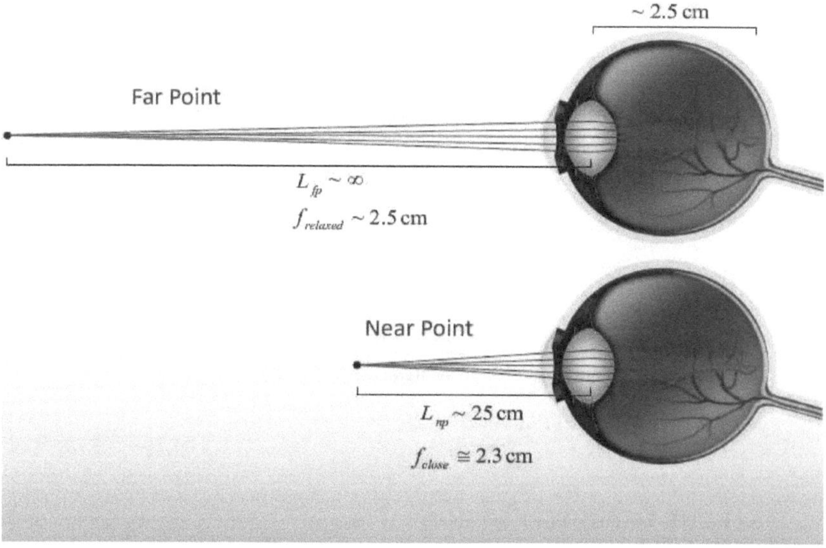

Figure 5.18: Far and Near point for the human eye.

Example 5.7:

A-What is the power of a normal human eye in diopter when focusing on an object at the far point of the eye? Assume the lens to retina distance is 2 cm.

Solution:

∴ The power of eye at far points $p\infty$

$$P\infty = \frac{1}{+f\,(\infty)} \Longrightarrow \frac{1}{f} = \frac{1}{u} + \frac{1}{v} = \frac{1}{\infty} + \frac{1}{v}$$

$\therefore \frac{1}{f} = \frac{1}{v}$

$P_\infty = \frac{1}{v} = \frac{1}{0.02\ m} = \mathbf{50\ D}$

B- What is the power of a normal eye in diopter when focusing on an object at near point of the eye? Assume the lens to retina distance is 2 cm.

Solution:

p_N = power at near point $= \frac{1}{f_N}$

$P_N = \frac{1}{v} + \frac{1}{u} = \frac{1}{v} + \frac{1}{0.25}$ u= 25 cm near point

$P_N = \frac{1}{0.02} + \frac{1}{0.25} = 50 + 4 = 54D$

C- What`s power of accommodation of the normal human eye lens.

Solution:

$\therefore P_{acc} = P_N - P_f$

$P_{acc} = 54D - 50D = 4D$

The normal eye with good vision, near point (N. P) = 0.25m,

Far point (F.P) = and $P_{acc} = 4D$

5.11 THE DEFECTIVE VISION

The types of emmetropia:

5.11.1 Myopia (near – sightedness) short sight

The causes:

a- Cornea is too curved (focal length too short) or eyeball

D > 0.02 m.

b- Image of distant object forms in front of retina.

c- Image on retina is blurred.

The eye point:

(f.p) far point of this eye < f.p of normal (∞)

N.P $\cong$ 0.25 m or little value than 0.25 m.

The correction of this defect by using diverging lens with focal length in magnitude is equal to the f.p of myopic eye.

The prescribed lens must produce a virtual image at the f.p of the eye of an object at (∞) infinity so that the relaxed eye can focus on the retain of the rays coming from the lens and striking it.

In the myopic eye, the parallel rays are focused by the relaxed eye to a position in front of the retina only near object see clearly, as shown in Figure 8.15 (upper).

5.11.2 Hyperopia (far – sightedness), long sight

The causes:

a- Cornea is not curved enough (focal length too long or eyeball too short).

b- Image of distant object from behind retina.

c- Image on retia is blurred.

The eye point:

N.P near point > N.P of normal eye (0.25m).

F.P $\cong \infty$

The correction:

By using converging lens. The parallel rays are focused to a point behind the retina, using the corrective lens which will bring the eye`s near point back to the normal value by produce virtual image of an object placed at new near point (25m) which will appear to the eye to lie at the old near point, as shown in Figure 8.16 (lower).

5.11.3 Astigmatism

In this case the cornea curvature is asymmetric (curvature different in one direction than in another). A cylindrical lens is used for correction.

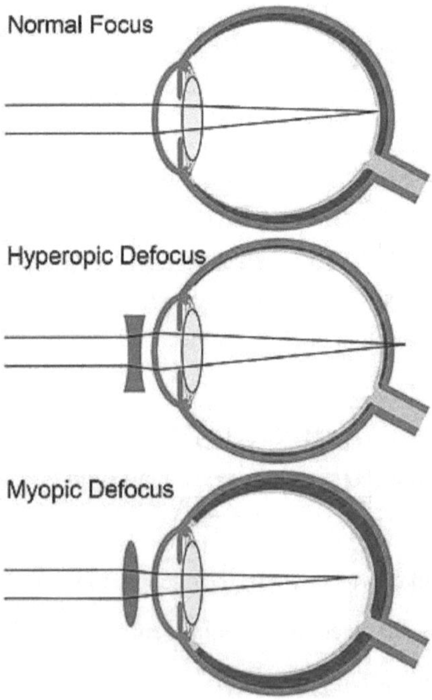

Figure 5.19: Normal eye focus, and the correction of hyperopic and myopic defocusing, using diverging and converging lenses respectively.

5.12 INSTRUMENT USED IN OPHTHALMOLOGY

1- Ophthalmoscope to examine the interior of the eye.

2- Retinoscopy: to determine the prescription of a corrective lens

3- Keratometer: to measure the curvature of the cornea.

4- Lensometer: to measure the focal length of a lens

5- Tonometer: to measure eye pressure, application tonometer.

Example 5.8:

The near point of eye is 100 cm in front of the eye. What lens should be used to see clearly an object 25 cm in front of the eye.

Solution:

Defect: hyperopia

Correction: using converging lens

Object at near point (25 cm) U = 25 cm⟶ Virtual image at the old new point v = -1m

Lens:

$$\therefore \frac{1}{f} = \frac{1}{u} + \frac{1}{v} = \frac{1}{25} - \frac{1}{1oo} = \frac{4-1}{100} = \frac{3}{100}$$

f = 33 cm. That's a converging lens of focal length 33 cm.

Examples 5.9:

A man has a near point at 50 cm and far point at ∞.

1. What is his useful accommodating power?
2. What spectacle lens are used?

The solution:

1. When eye focused at ∞.

$$p_\infty = \frac{1}{f_\infty} = \frac{1}{\infty} + \frac{1}{D}$$

and when eye is accommodating to it max.

$$P_N = \frac{1}{F_N} = \frac{1}{0.5\,M} + \frac{1}{D}$$

∴ useful accommodating power:

$P_N - P_\infty = 2$ D

2. The man has long sight (hyperopia)

+ Ve lens (converging) is used to bring his near point back to normal value (25 cm), This spectacle produces a virtual image of an object placed at the new point (25 cm)which will appear to the man to lie at old near point.

∴The eye is fully accommodated.

Example 5.10: A myopic male has near and far point of 20 and 250 cm.

1- What spectacle lens is used.

2- What is his near point.

Solution:

1- The defect is myopia. The correction by using –Ve lens diverging concave lens.

5.13 THE CORRECTION LENS

This lens produces a virtual image at the far point of the eye of an object at ∞. The relaxed eye can focus on the retina, the rays coming from the lens and striking it.

The lens has focal length F, u = ∞ from the law of the lens, v = -250.

$$\frac{1}{f} = \frac{1}{u} + \frac{1}{v} = \frac{1}{\infty} - \frac{1}{250\ cm}$$

∴ f = -250 cm ⟶ power = - 0.4 D

∴ the correction lens has strength of – 0.4 D.

The kind of the lens is diverging.

2- The nearest point when wearing the lens will be at distance (d) from the eyes. The virtual image produced by the lens must be at the near point of the eye in order that the fully accommodating ⟶ v = - 20 cm and u = d

$$\frac{1}{F} = \frac{1}{u} + \frac{1}{v}$$

$$-\frac{1}{250\ cm} = \frac{1}{d} - \frac{1}{20}$$

d = 21.7 cm

5.14 QUESTIONS

1. A man can see distinctly only object which lie between 25cm-400cm from his eye:

a) What is the useful power of accommodation of his eyes?

b) What spectacles should be prescribed for the man?

c) What is the minimum distance from his eyes at which he can hold the book?

d) Write the required prescription for his eyes.

2. A near – sighted person wants to see to infinity but does not see clearly beyond 2 meters. What kind and strength of eyeglasses do they need?

3. A near – sighted person wants to see to infinity but does not see clearly beyond 1 meter. What kind and strength of eyeglasses do they need?

4. A far – sighted person sees no closer than 1 meter. They want to read at the normal 25 cm distance. What kind and strength of eyeglasses do they need?

5. A far – sighted person sees no closer than 0.75 meter. They want to read at the normal 25 cm distance. What kind and strength of eyeglasses do they need?

6. A person is nearsighted with a far point of 17 cm and needs glasses to correct for this. What power lenses should be used if the lenses are 2 cm from the eye?

7. A person is farsighted with a near point of 50 cm. What power lens will correct this problem?

8. What is the power of accommodation of the eye, when object viewed from 20- 500cm from his eye?

9. Bifocal lenses are prescribed for a patient, the components having focal length of 40cm & -300cm.

What are the new and far points of the patient's eye?

MEDICAL OPTICS

10. 45-year-old man can see with his left eye between 25 → 300 cm and in his right eye between 15cm→ ∞. A man has astigmatism at his left eye which requires a lens of focal length + 0.5m at axis 120°. The patient requires magnification glasses of focal length 0.25m. Write the required prescription for this patient.

11. What is meant by power of accommodation of the eye?

12. A person with a myopic eye cannot see objects beyond 1.2 m distinctly. What should be the type of corrective lens used to restore proper vision?

13. What is the far point and near point of the human eye with normal vision?

14. A student has difficulty reading the blackboard while sitting in the last row. What could be the defect the child is suffering from? How can it be corrected?

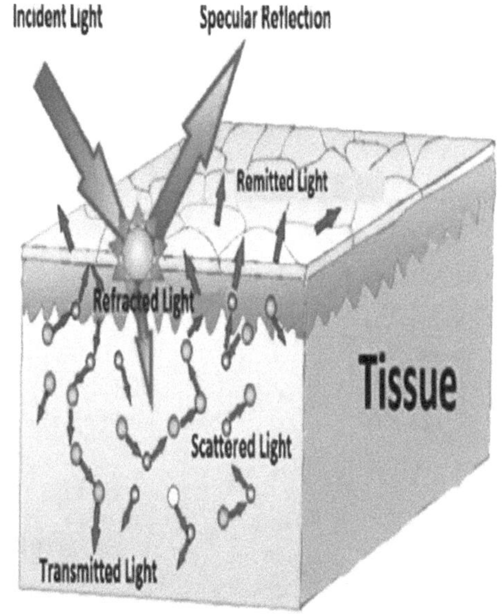

6

CHAPTER

OPTICAL PROPERTIES OF TISSUES

6.1 NATURE OF LIGHT

Light is electromagnetic wave seen by humans. Light has the properties of a wave and a particle. Visible light wavelengths between about 400 nm-700 nm. Wavelength is the distance that light travels in one oscillation. The intensity of the light varies depending on the number of particles.

6.1.1 Light Interaction

Reflection Refraction Absorption Fluorescence Scattering these interactions depends on constituents of tissue, Optical properties of tissue and Propagation of light.

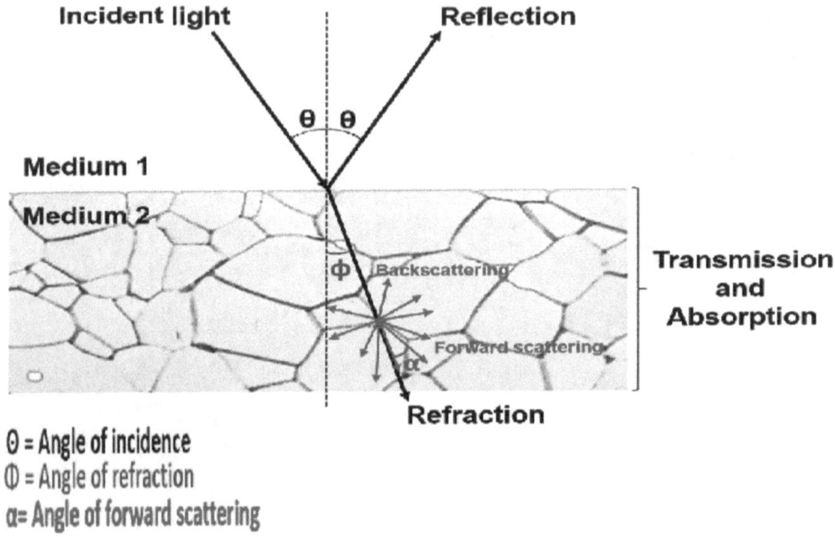

Figure 6.1 Light interaction in medium.

6.1.2 Overview

The transmittance T of a medium is de ned as the ratio of the transmitted intensity of light I_T to the incident intensity of light I_0, on that medium, i.e.

$$T = \frac{I_T}{I_0} \quad (6.1)$$

Similarly, the absorbance A of a medium is the ratio of the absorbed intensity (or radiant ux) I_A to the incident intensity,

$$A = \frac{I_A}{I_0} \quad (6.2)$$

The reactance R of a medium is the ratio of the re ected intensity I_R to the incident intensity:

$$R = \frac{I_R}{I_0} \quad (6.3)$$

For a material that absorbs a fraction of incident light whilst transmitting the rest, or vice versa

$$I_0 = I_T + I_A + I_R, \qquad (6.4)$$

where I_A, I_T and I_R are wavelength dependent. Hence

$$T(\lambda) + R(\lambda) + A(\lambda) = 1. \qquad (6.5)$$

6.2 REFRACTION

When light travels from one material to another it usually changes direction. The bending of light that occurs at the borderline of two materials is called refraction. Refraction is caused by the change in speed experienced by a wave when it changes medium. The amount of bending depends on the optical properties of the two materials- characterized by their index of refraction:

n. The refractive index n, determines the speed of light. The refractive index of tissue is 1.35- 1.55.

The relationship between the angles of incidence and refraction and the indices of refraction of the two media is known as Snell's Law. The law of refraction predicts the amount of bend.

θ_1 is the angle of incidence, θ_2 is the angle of refraction and n_1 and n_2 are the speeds of light in the media

Formula for Snell's Law:

$$n_1 \sin\theta_1 = n_2 \sin\theta_2$$

$$n_1 = index\ of\ refraction\ of\ first\ medium$$
$$\theta_1 = angle\ of\ incidence$$
$$n_2 = index\ of\ refraction\ of\ second\ medium$$
$$\theta_2 = angle\ of\ refraction$$

6.3 SCATTERING

Change of direction of propagation of energy of light. It is a physical process where light interacts with matter and changes direction.

Light scattering in tissue depends upon the size of the scattering particle, the wavelength of the light and the variation of the refractive indices of the various tissue components, such as cell membranes and organelles. Light scattering arises from the presence of heterogeneities within a bulk medium.

Types of Scattering

Elastic scattering: no energy change

Frequency of the scattered wave = frequency of incident wave

Gives insight into the static structure of material. The light scattered by a system has interacted with the inhomogeneity's of the system. Photons are mostly scattered by the structure whose size matches the wavelength

Types are Rayleigh and Mie scattering

(a) Rayleigh Scattering

• Scattering from very small particles i.e., $\leq \lambda/10$

• Rayleigh scattering is inversely related to fourth power of the wavelength of the incident light

(b) Mie Scattering

• For scattering particles comparable or larger than the wavelength, Mie scattering predominates. Because of the relative particle size, Mie scattering is not strongly wavelength dependent. Forward directional scattering.

Inelastic scattering: energy change

• Frequency of the scattered wave ≠ frequency of incident wave. Internal energy levels of atoms and molecules are exciting. It gives information about vibrational bonds of the molecule.

Types are Raman and Brillouin scattering

Applications

Diagnostic applications: Scattering depends on the size, morphology, and structure of the components in tissues (e.g. lipid membrane, collagen fibers, nuclei).

Variations in these components due to disease would affect scattering properties, thus providing a means for diagnostic purpose

Therapeutic applications: Scattering signals can be used to determine optimal light dosimeter and provide useful feedback during therapy

6.3.1 Scattering Cross-section

Similarly, for scattering we take the same considerations into account and we have

$$I = I_0 e^{-\mu_s L}, \quad (6.6)$$

where L is again the photon path length.

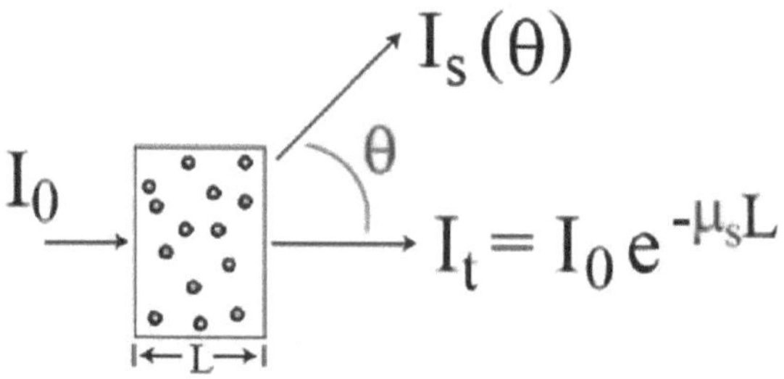

Figure 6.2: Transmission of light through a homogeneous scattering medium.

Analogously, the scattering coincidence Figure 6.2 can also be expressed as:

$$\mu_s = \rho_s \sigma_s, \quad (6.7)$$

where σ_s is the scattering cross section (cm^2) and ρ_s is the particle number density of the stutterers in the medium. By dentition

$$\sigma_a = Q_a A, \quad (6.8)$$

and Q_s is the scattering exigency with A being the geometrical area of the scattering particle, as illustrated in Figure 6.3.

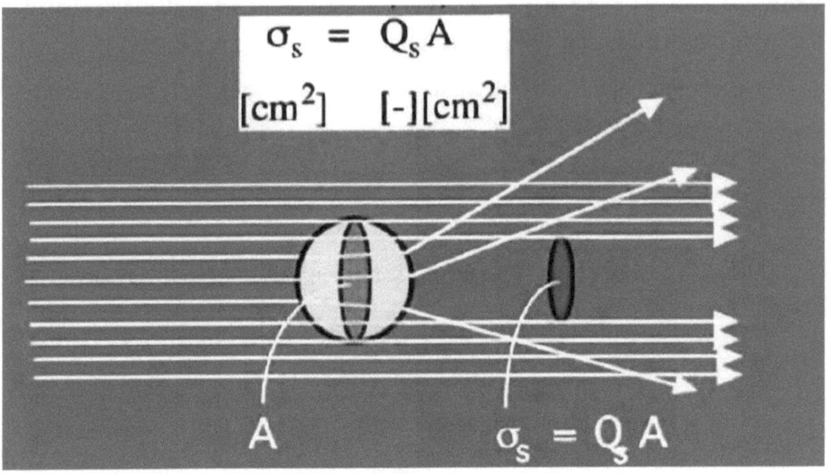

Figure 6.3: The scattering cross-section of a spherical particle.

6.3.2 Multiple Scattering

In nature, it is far more likely for electromagnetic waves to be scattered by many particles when incidents are upon a surface, rather than a single scattered. Waves that pass-through media which contain a large amount of discrete stutterers will undergo many scattering events, which makes the wave equation di cult to solve. Various techniques can be applied to account for these multiple scattering events.

A medium can be considered as a random distribution of single spheres, in which the attenuation due to scattering is negligible, provided the incident wavelength is much larger than the size of the scattering particles and the mean separation between stutterers. A frequency-dependent dielectric constant can, in this situation, describe the medium.

T-matrices and Green's functions can be used to approximate multiple scat- tiring processes, but in cases for large ensembles of scattering particles probe- ability density functions are used to determine the locations of individual scattering centers. Integral equations can also be set up to describe the led as it actuates through multiple scattering events. This actuating led can be expressed in terms of the average led $\mathbf{E}_j$ at the position of some arbitrary particle j by:

$$(\mathbf{E}) = \mathbf{E}^0 + S_j\,(\mathbf{E}_j)\,G\,(\mathbf{r}_j)\,d\mathbf{r}_j. \qquad (6.9)$$

This approximation and method of averaging is limited however and works well only in media with a small fractional volume of stutterers.

6.4 ABSORPTION

A process by which light is absorbed and converted into energy. Absorption depends on the electromagnetic frequency of the light and object's nature of atoms. Absorption of light is therefore directly proportional to the frequency. Most objects selectively absorb, transmit or reflect the light. When light is absorbed, heat is generated. Absorption occurs when the photon frequency matches the frequency associated with the molecule's energy transition. Electrons absorb the energy of light and transform it into vibrational motion.

The absorption of a photon results in: quantized change in charge separation, quantized excitation of vibrational modes. Electrons interact with neighboring atoms to convert vibrational energy into thermal energy.

6.4.1 Absorption Cross-section

Absorption by tissue can have either a therapeutic act or a destructive one. Energy from incident waves is transferred to the tissue at each absorption event, and if no absorption occurs then there is no energy transfer between the incident radiation and the tissue. Absorption of light by tissue also plays a diagnostic role in tissue spectroscopy and medical imaging, amongst others. Absorption can only occur if the energy of the incoming photon hv is identical to the difference in energy between energy levels ΔE in the molecule onto which radiation is incident, i.e.

$$\Delta E = hv. \qquad (6.10)$$

As a result of the absorption, the molecule undergoes a quantized change in charge separation and a quantized change in its vibrational state.

Classically we can adopt the following formalism for absorption. Consider a collimated beam of light with wavelength λ and intensity I_0 passing through a homogeneous medium with absorption coefficient μ_a (cm^{-1}). The light intensity I transmitted through the medium of width L is given by:

$$I = I_0 e^{-\mu_a L}, \tag{6.11}$$

where L is also known as the photon path length. Figure 6.4 illustrates this concept.

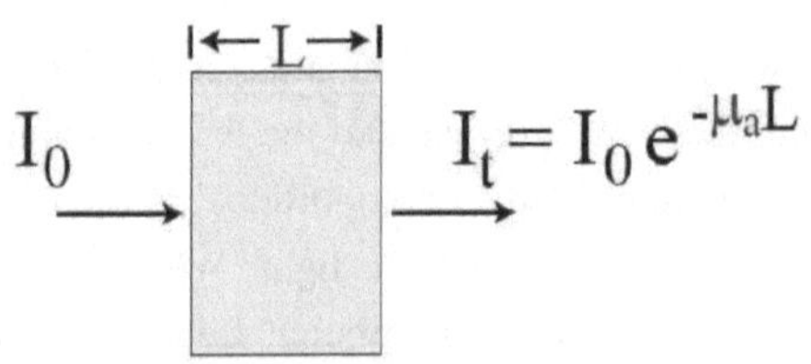

Figure 6.4: Transmission of light through a homogeneous absorbing medium.

The absorption coefficient can also be expressed as

$$\mu_a = \rho_a \sigma_a, \tag{6.12}$$

in which σ_a is known as the absorption cross section (cm^2) and ρ_a is the particle number density of the absorbers in the medium. By dentition:

$$\sigma_a = Q_a A, \tag{6.13}$$

where Q_a is the absorption exigency and A is the geometrical area of the absorbing particle. We can approximate the absorbing particle to ideally be a sphere, as shown in Figure 6.5.

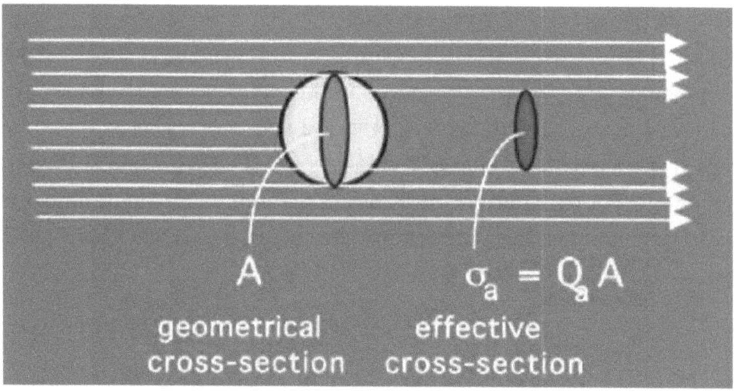

Figure 6.5: The absorption cross-section of a spherical particle.

6.4.1.1 Propagation of Light in Tissue

The characteristics of tissue and the propagation of photons, which include scattering and absorption events within tissue, and reaction and transmission at boundaries, determine the number of photons that will reach the epidermis or dermis before being absorbed by a chromosphere. Experimental evidence suggests that many scattering events occur for each photon propagating through tissue, especially at visible and near infrared (IR) wavelengths. The mean distance travelled by a photon between scattering events is between 0.01 and 0.2 mm. At these wavelengths incident photons are more often scattered in the forward direction rather than the backward direction. Most incident photos are never absorbed by the melanocyte, and besides being scattered, these photons can be absorbed by other chromospheres in the tissue, totally internally reacted at the interface between air and tissue or even reacted out of the tissue. To exactly understand the propagation of light in tissue then it would require modeling of the size and spatial distribution of the structures (absorbing and scattering) within the tissue, as well as their absorption and scattering properties. Tissue same lotion is clearly a di cult task and a simple way to represent tissue is to assume its base material to be largely absorbing, with a random distribution of stutterers within the volume of the sample. This sample would be isotropic and homogeneous over much of its volume, even though tissues are not.

One of the main objectives of tissue optics is the formulation of methods to determine the absorbing and scattering characteristics of tissue. The optical properties to be discussed are all wavelength dependent and considered in the relevant human tissue. These properties are ideally determined non- invasively, which can be achieved with laser light, however, many of these properties are not known accurately yet in the end of tissue optics. This is due to the result of changes that occur dynamically in tissues at die rent temperatures and water or oxygen concentrations, i.e. changes in the scattering and absorbing pro les of tissues.

Transport Cosecants

Tissue is considered as a turbid medium, i.e. An incident photon is likely to undergo both scattering, in all directions, and absorption when incident upon a tissue. When a photon travels over an in intestinal distance *ds* in tissue, the probability for scattering to occur over this in intestinal distance is given by $\mu_s ds$, and similarly the probability of absorption occurring is $\mu_a ds$, where μ_s and μ_a are the conceits of scattering and absorption respectively.

The mean free path for an absorption event is $\frac{1}{a}$ and for a scattering event is

$\frac{1}{s}$. In a turbid medium it is conventional to describe the sum of the absorption and scattering conceits, and this is known as the total attenuation

coincident or the transport coincident μ_t:

$$\mu_t = \mu_a + \mu_s. \tag{6.14}$$

Penetration Depth

The penetration depth δ of a collimated beam is de need as the mean free path for an absorption or scattering event, i.e. the mean distance into the tissue that a photon from the incident beam will travel before it undergoes scattering or absorption. It is hence the reciprocal of the attenuation coe cient

$$\delta = \frac{1}{\mu_t}. \tag{6.15}$$

Optical Depth

The optical depth OD, not to be confused with the physical depth d, is the product

$$OD = \mu_t d, \qquad (6.16)$$

i.e. a greater optical depth means the photons travel a greater distance, on average, into the tissue.

Albedo

The albedo a is dined as the ratio of the scattering coincident to the trans- port coincident

$$a = \frac{\mu_s}{\mu_t} \qquad (6.17)$$

For an optical albedo a = 0, the attenuation caused is by absorption only and for an albedo a = 1, only scattering occurs. Figure 6.6 depicts the albedo as a function of the scattering coincident, with the absorb

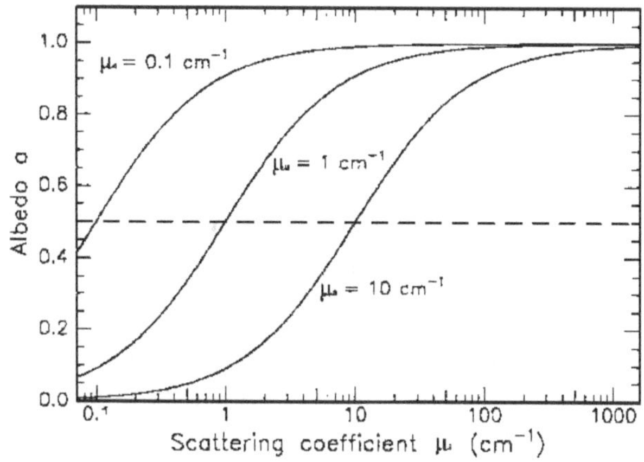

Figure 6.6: A graph of the optical albedo as a function of the scattering coincident.

Anisotropy

Light scattering in tissue is not isotropic, and collimated light is scattered strongly in the forward direction. Measurements of the angular dispersion after scattering can be made using tissue samples thin enough to ensure that only a single scattering event will occur. The anisotropy factor g is the measure of the degree of anisotropy in a tissue, and represents the average scattering angle by that tissue, i.e.

$$g = <\cos\theta> . \quad (6.18)$$

Total forward scattering means $g = 1$, total backscattering corresponds to $g = 1$ and isotrōpic scattering implies that $g = 0$. The converse is not true for isotropic scattering however, $g = 0$ does not necessarily indicate isotropic scattering. Mie theory can be used to nd analytical solutions for the phase function of plane electromagnetic waves by isotropic spherical particles of any size. The anisotropy factor can then be expressed as

$$g = <\cos\theta> = -1 \qquad \cos\theta f(\cos\theta) d\cos\theta \quad (6.19)$$

Biological tissues generally scatter visible and near infrared light strongly in the forward direction with anisotropy factors in the range 0.69 g 0.99 [15].

The reduced scattering coincident μ_s' [cm^{-1}] is dined as

$$\mu'_S = \mu_s(1 - g), \quad (6.20)$$

where $1/\mu_s$' is the mean path travelled by a collimated beam of light before it becomes isotropic [15]. Finally, the total transport coe cient μ_t can be found from

$$\mu_t = \mu'_S + \mu_a = \mu_s(1 - g) + \mu_a. \quad (6.21)$$

6.4.1.2 Attenuation of Light

It is di cult to accurately measure the transmission of collimated light, in theory, as measurements of transmission are likely to include scattered light. Light that is transmitted through the air-tissue interface will undergo scattering or absorption at some point in the tissue. The absorption coincidence of melanin in tissue decreases as the wavelength of the incident light in- creases, whereas the absorption by blood depends on the wavelength and the oxygenation of the blood. At certain wavelengths (known as isopiestic points) the absorption of oxygenated and deoxygenated blood is equal, as shown by the points of intersection of Figure 6.7.

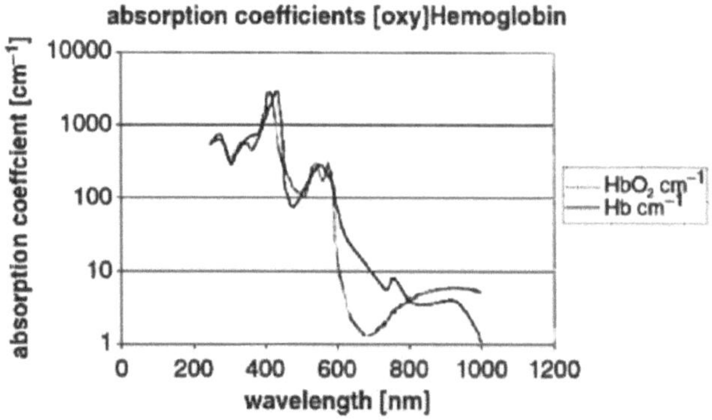

Figure 6.7: Absorption coincidence of oxy- and deoxyhemoglobin as a function of wavelength.

Proteins and amino acids become the primary absorbers at wavelengths in the UV spectral range and water is the most highly absorbing of the chromospheres at IR wavelengths. At wavelengths above that of 1.4 *μm*, the scattering in tissue becomes insignia ant as compared to the absorption. This wavelength is in the infrared range of the spectrum and hence the primary cause for attenuation in this range is water. The absorption coincident (and hence the transport coincident) of the tissue may then be estimated by the absorption coincident of water, considering the concentration of water in that tissue. Changes in the temperature of water can also act in its absorption characteristics.

Applications

Diagnostic applications: Absorption data can serve as spectral fingerprint of the molecule. Various types of Chromospheres (light absorbers) in Tissue Tumor detection and other physiological assessments (pulse oximetry)

Therapeutic applications: Absorption of energy is the primary mechanism that allows light from a source (laser) to produce physical effects on tissue for treatment purposes: Lasik Eye Surgery, Tattoo Removal.

6.5 LIGHT TRANSPORT INSIDE THE TISSUE

Tissue is a self-supporting bulk medium to transport light. Scattering and absorption occur simultaneously and are wavelength dependent. Reflection and refraction also occur. Maximum light will be delivered or penetrates the tissue when it is incident on the tissue at 90°. Scattering monotonically decreases *with* wavelength. Absorption is large in UV, near visible, and IR. Absorption is low in red and NIR. Modeling of light transport in tissues is often governed by the relative magnitudes of optical absorption and scattering.

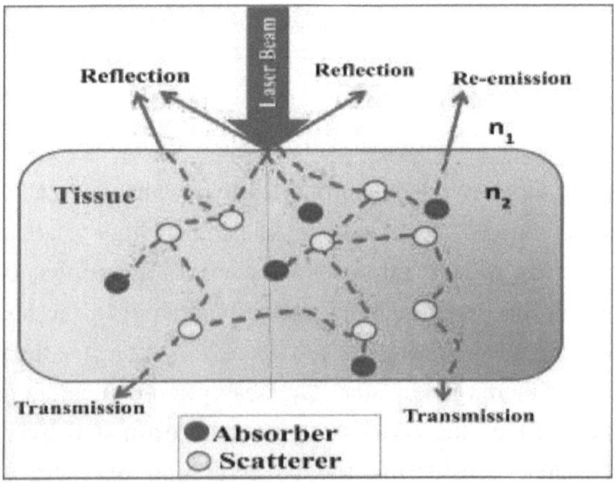

Figure 6.8: Light transport inside the tissue.

6.6 LASER CHARACTERISTICS AS APPLIED TO MEDICINE AND BIOLOGY

- *Laser* is a narrow beam of light of a single wavelength (monochromatic) in which each wave is in phase (coherent) with other near it.

- To generate laser beam three processes must be satisfied:

- Population inversion.
- Stimulated emission.
- Pumping source Optical and Electric **Types of Lasers**
- Solid

- Liquid
- Gas

Laser characteristics include reflection, refraction, absorption and scattering.

- Monochromaticity of laser light is responsible for its selective effect on biological tissues.
- The optical effects of lasers can be applied for different medical applications like diagnosis, therapy and surgery.
- Photocoagulation of retina
- Tissue welding
- Coagulation
- Tattoo Removal
- Lithotripsy
- Dermatology

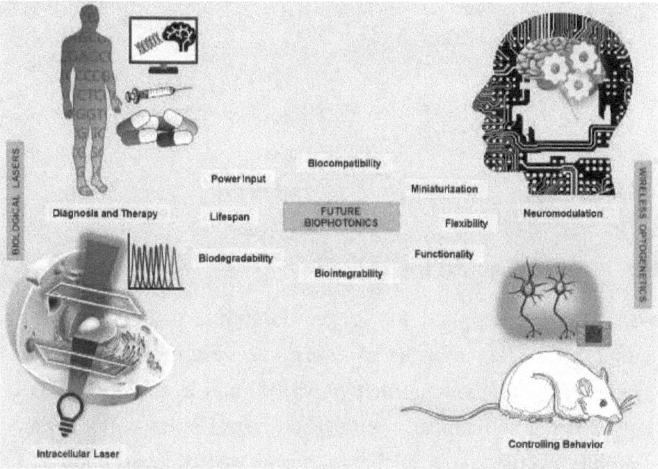

Figure 6.9: Laser characteristics as applied to medicine and biology.

6.7 LASER TISSUE INTERACTION

Types

1. Photochemical interactions
2. Thermal interactions
3. Photoablation
4. Plasma-induced ablation
5. Photodisruption.

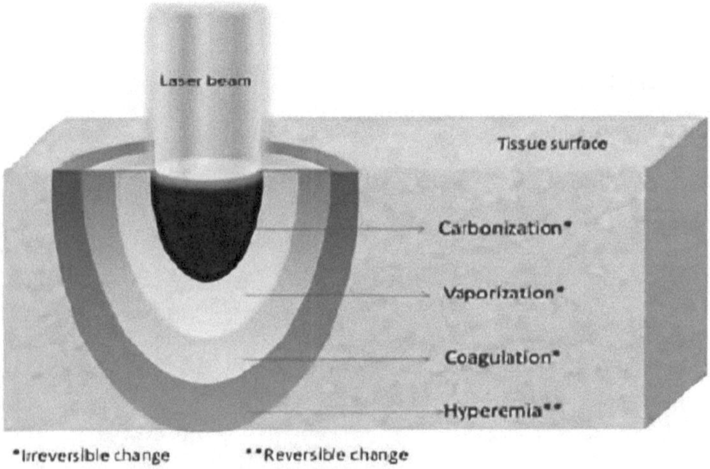

6.7.1 Photochemical Interactions

Lower intensities applied for longer durations. It causes a photochemical change- either by a slow transfer of energy as heat or by a specific chemical reaction as used in photodynamic therapy (PDT) and in LASIK vision correction. Laser energy can react chemically with specific molecules within tissue. Excimer lasers for modifying the shape of the cornea in LASIK procedures is based on - (UV) laser's ability to break covalent bonds in protein.

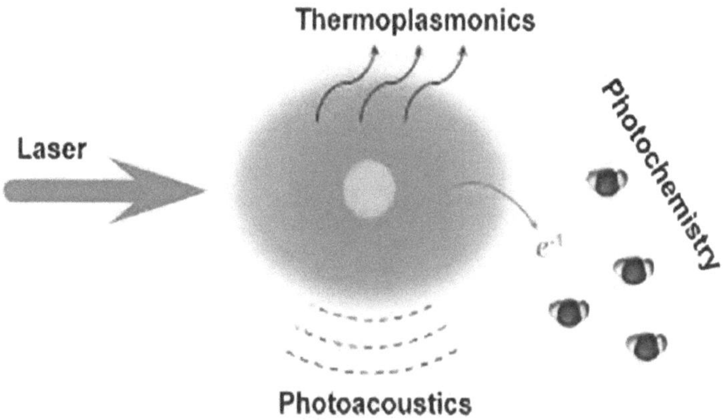

Figure 6.11: Laser energy reacts chemically with specific molecules within tissue.

6.7.2 Photothermal Interactions

A less intense- longer pulse will cause a rapid heating- photo thermal effect. When laser energy is absorbed by a chromosphere - and transformed into heat which is dissipated in the target- leading to denaturation of proteins at 42-65 C. Depending on the exposure time, tissue vaporization, or coagulation, or both will take place. An example of a photo thermal laser is the CO_2 laser- used to cut and vaporize tissue - which mostly consists of water. Water and thus soft tissue- vaporizes at 100 degrees C. When the laser hits soft tissue- rapid heating causes the water in the tissue to flash into steam- ablating the tissue. To minimize thermal damage- maximize the ablation- a short exposure time is necessary. This can be done by pulsed laser beam in such a way that the time it dwells over the tissue is less than its thermal relaxation time.

The thermal relaxation time- defined as the time taken by target structure to dissipate 50% of the energy absorbed- to surrounding tissue. This time is roughly equal to the square of the diameter of the target structure.

The thermal containment time- in which no heat (no thermal effect) is dissipated to surrounding tissue- and is roughly one-quarter of the thermal relaxation time.

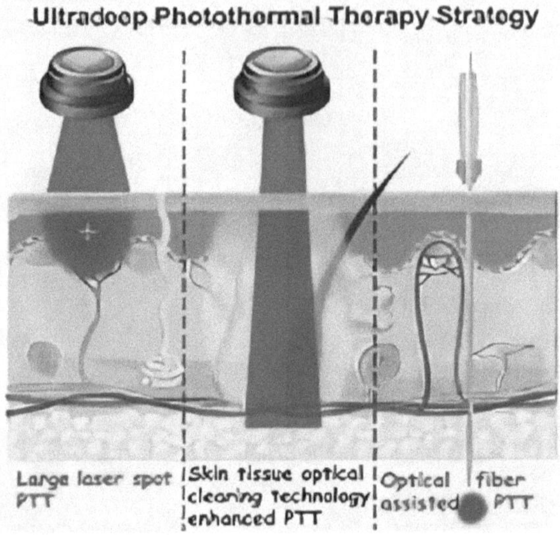

Figure 6.12: Photothermal Interaction.

6.7.3 Photoelectromechanical Interaction

Extremely intense- short pulse of laser light will usually cause an explosive expansion of tissue photoelectromechanical reaction. Photo disruptive. High energy- ultra short pulses of laser light cause extremely rapid heating of the target- with formation of a rapidly expanding thermal plasma. As the plasma collapses- the shock wave causes mechanical disruption of the target. This photomechanical disruption is utilized to treat tattoos- disruption of stones and certain pigmented skin lesions. When the laser fluence is very high, the electric field may attain the order of magnitude of the electric field present within the molecules. This electric field is in the range 107 to 1012 Vm^{-1}. Breaking of chemical bonds and ionization take place, leading to the well-known electric breakdown of the medium. It Produces shock wave. This is the origin of the sound emitted during air or gas breakdown. In biological (and other) materials, the plasma (ionized gas) expands rapidly, giving rise to an electroacoustic shock wave. This can destroy solid grains. The plasma absorbs the incoming laser beam, hence diminishing the treated volume. This is used in ophthalmology, when one destroys some opaque elements of the vitreous humor without damaging the retina.

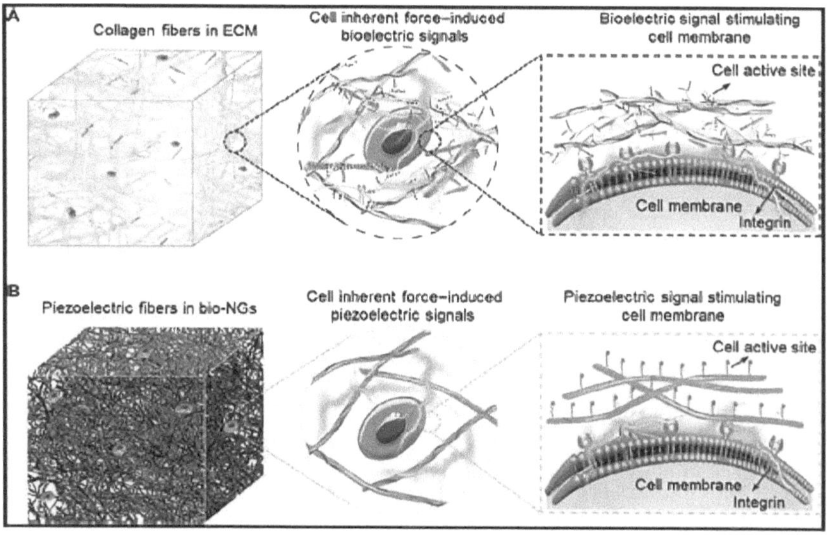

Figure 6.13: Cell activity modulation and its specific function maintenance by bio inspired electromechanical.

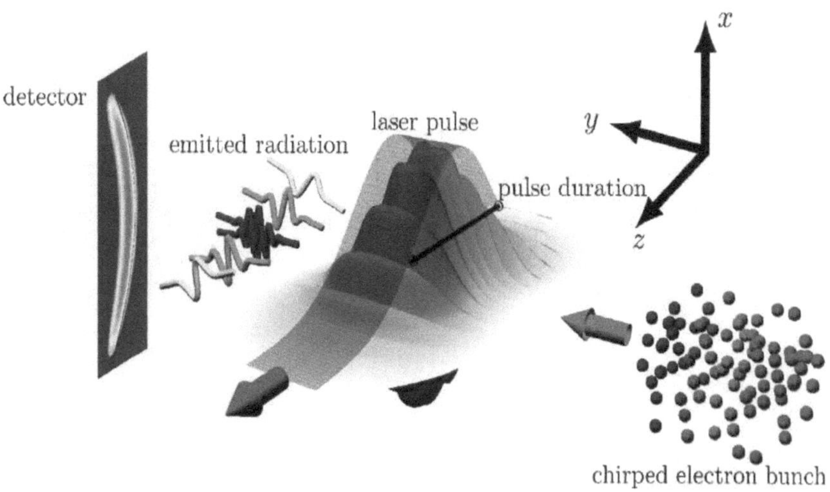

Figure 6.14: Determining the duration of an ultra-intense laser pulse directly in its focus Scientific Reports.

6.7.4 Photo Ablation

Visible and Ultraviolet laser beams are absorbed by electronic excitation. Property used to break chemical bonds without heating the material: photoablation. Condition for breaking a chemical bond by electronic excitation is that the photon energy, is equal to or larger than the bond energy. Photoablation is performed by lasers emitting ultraviolet light, i.e. excimer lasers. Along with bond breaking, there exists light energy in the form of thermal energy. This causes rapid detachment of the molecules into the gas phase, giving rise to the ablation of the material.

Advantage -Emit very short pulses (around 10^{-8} s), so that heat doesn't diffuse away from the irradiated zone. Photoablation is well localized to the irradiated regions. No thermal damage such as coagulation or vaporization. Another advantage is precision etching. Highly intense laser irradiation.

Photoablation is a two-step process:

1. excitation
2. dissociation

Interaction mechanism of photoablation is limited to the application of UV light. Pure photoablation is observed for the 193nm wavelength of the ArF excimer laser.

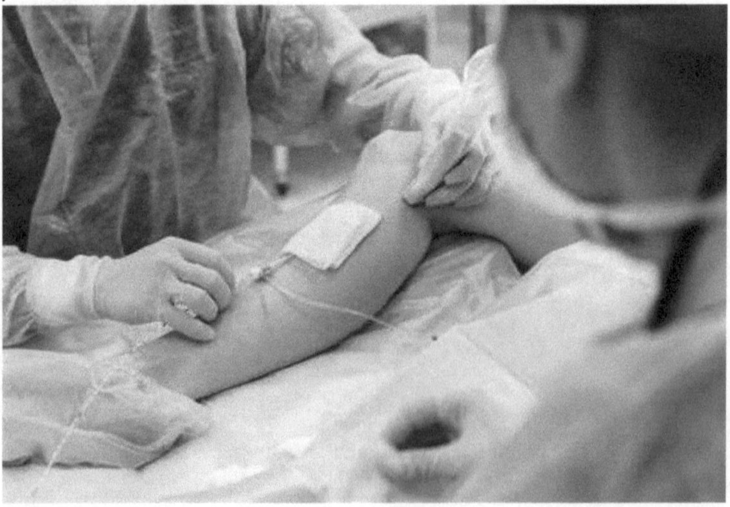

Figure 6.15: Laser Vein Ablation for Varicose Veins.

7

CHAPTER

INSTRUMENTATION IN PHOTONICS

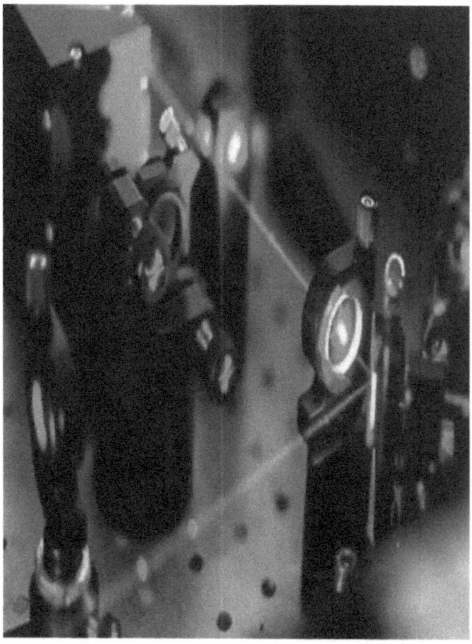

7.1 INSTRUMENTS FOR ABSORPTION, SCATTERING AND EMISSION MEASUREMENTS

Spectrophotometers measure spectroscopic properties related to the molecular composition and structure of biochemical species in the sample of interest. There are several types of spectroscopic measurements: absorption, scattering (elastic and inelastic), and emission.

Light at a certain wavelength is used to irradiate a sample of interest. This process is called "excitation." Properties of the light that emerges from the sample are measured and analyzed. One can measure the light emitted and scattered by the sample, processes that occur at wavelengths different from the excitation wavelength; the techniques involved are fluorescence, phosphorescence, and inelastic scattering (Raman scattering).

A basic spectrophotometer generally consists of the following components:

1. An excitation light source
2. Dispersive devices (optical filters, monochromators, or polychromators)
3. A sample (usually in a compartment with a sample holder)
4. A photometric detector (equipped with a read-out device)

7.1.1 Instrument for Absorption Measurements

The collimated output of a light source is focused on the entrance slit of an excitation monochromatorfor wavelength scanning. The output of the excitation monochromatic is directed to the sample inside the sample compartment. The light transmitted by the sample is collected through appropriate optics and focused onto a detector. This simple instrumental setup is often used in a single-beam absorption spectrometer.

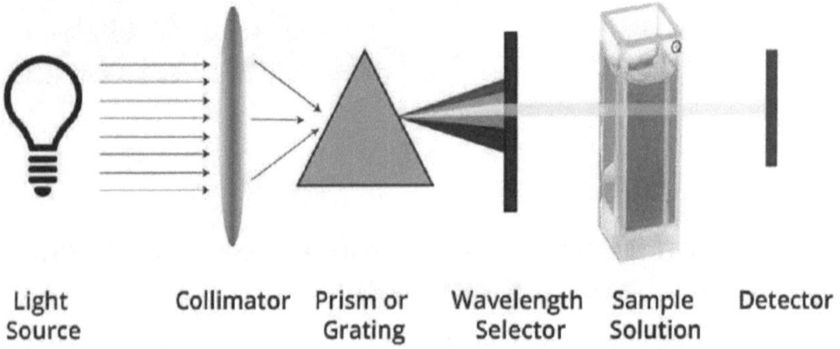

Figure 7.1 Absorption Measurement.

7.1.2 Instrument for Scattering Measurements

The elastic scattering (ES) technique involves detection of the backscattering of a broadband light source irradiating the sample of interest. A spectrometer records the backscattered light at various wavelengths and produces a spectrum that is dependent on sample structure, as well as chromosphere constituents. In general, the sample is illuminated with the excitation light, which is selected with a dispersive element and then directed to a specific point location (e.g., via an optical fiber) of the sample. The scattered light is measured at the same wavelength as the excitation wavelength. With inelastic scattering measurements, one measures the scattered light from the sample in a spectral region different from the excitation wavelength. In this case, the basic setup is like the ES setup but has an additional dispersive element to analyze the scattering emission from the samples.

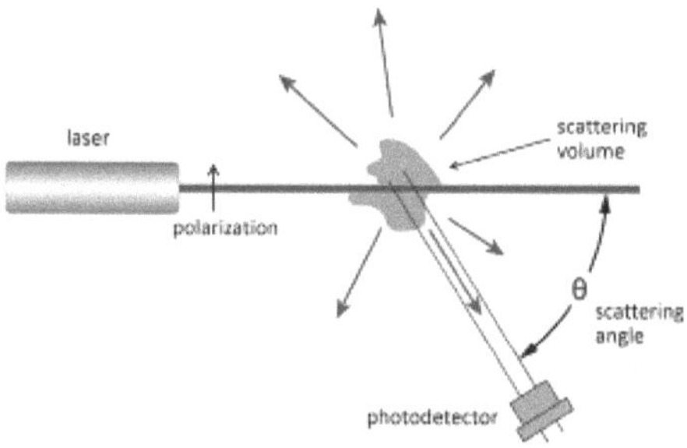

Figure 7.2 Scattering Measurement.

7.1.3 Instrument for Emission Measurements

The excitation light source is usually a laser or high-intensity xenon arc lamp. The collimated output of the light source is focused on the entrance slit of an excitation monochromatic output whose output is directed to the sample. When a laser is used as the excitation source, the excitation monochromatic is not required. The emission from the sample is collected through appropriate optics and focused on the entrance slit of an emission monochromatic. The excitation beam and the emission beam are usually focused at right angles for minimum interference from scattered light.

There are three basic classes of spectrophotometers: filter instruments, monochromatic instruments, and multichannel devices. The first type of device uses optical filters, whereas the latter two systems use prisms or gratings as dispersive elements. The three major features to consider are the intensity of the excitation light source, the resolution and throughput of the monochromators, and the sensitivity of the detector.

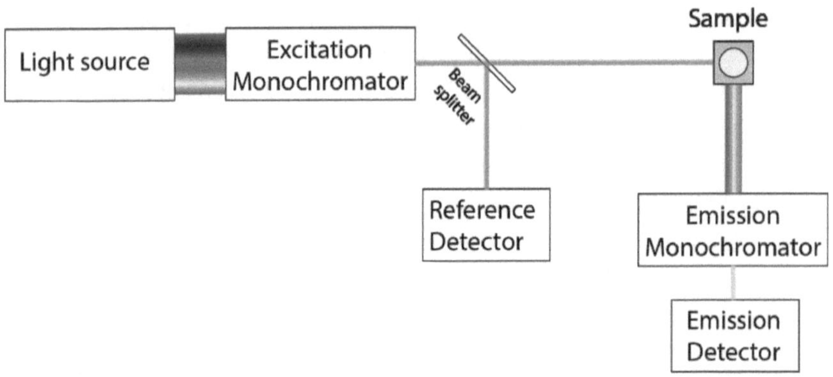

Figure 7.3 Emission Measurement.

7.2 EXCITATION LIGHT SOURCES

Light sources utilized in laser optics are high pressure mercury and sodium lamps, Lasers and LEDs.

7.2.1 High-Pressure Arc Lamps

High-pressure arc lamps are the most used radiation sources. These lamps produce intense quasi-continuum radiation ranging from the UV (<200 nm) to the near infrared (NIR) (>1000 nm) with only a few broad bands at approximately 450 to 500 nm. The lamps consist of two tungsten electrodes in a quartz envelope containing gases under high pressure, for example, xenon (Xe), mercury, an Xe–mercury mixture. Lamps of this type are commercially available in a wide range of input power from a few watts to several kilowatts. If excitation can be carried out at only one wavelength or a few fixed wavelengths of the mercury emission lines, the mercury lamp is probably the most effective radiation source. The Xe lamp, however, is more commonly used because it provides a smoother spectral profile more suitable for conducting excitation spectra measurements.

The Xe arc lamp is the most versatile light source for steady-state spectrometers. Xenon arc lamps typically have a lifetime between 400 and 600 hours. Three categories: continuous-output xenon short-arc lamps, continuous-

output xenon long-arc lamps, and xenon flash lamps. Xenon arc lamps of smaller sizes, down to 10 watts, are used in optics and in precision illumination for
] ·

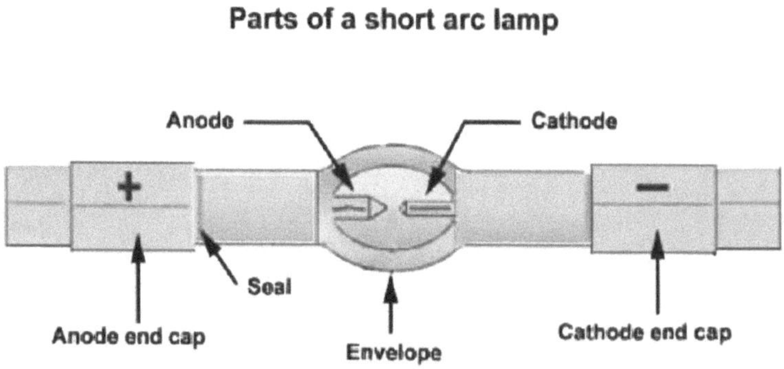

Figure 7.4 High Pressure Arc Lamp.

7.2.2 Light-emitting diodes

Light-emitting diodes (LEDs) are solid-state light sources that provide output over a wide range of wavelengths. These devices require little power and generate little heat. PN junction opto- semiconductor that emits a monochromatic (single color) light when operated in a forward biased direction. Emits light when activated by a suitable voltage is applied to the leads.

When a suitable voltage is applied to the leads, electrons recombine with electron holes within the device, releasing energy in the form of photons. exotic semiconductor compounds such as Gallium Arsenide (GaAs), Gallium Phosphide (GaP), Gallium Arsenide Phosphide (GaAsP), Silicon Carbide (SiC) or Gallium Indium Nitride (GaInN) all mixed at different ratios to produce a distinct wavelength of color.

Table 7.1 LED Materials and Colors.

Typical LED Characteristics			
Semiconductor Material	Wavelength	Colour	V_F @ 20mA
GaAs	850-940nm	Infra-Red	1.2v
GaAsP	630-660nm	Red	1.8v
GaAsP	605-620nm	Amber	2.0v
GaAsP:N	585-595nm	Yellow	2.2v
AlGaP	550-570nm	Green	3.5v
SiC	430-505nm	Blue	3.6v
GaInN	450nm	White	4.0v

7.3 TYPES OF LIGHT-EMITTING DIODES (LED)

1. Surface Emitting Diode

SLED is a five layered double hetrojunction on device consisting of a GaAs and GaAlAs layers. A massive electron injection into a thin active layer for recombination of electron and holes and enhanced focus of emitted light into the optical fiber. Plane of the active light emitting region is oriented perpendicularly to the axis of the fiber. From the substrate of the device, a well is etched. Fibers are connected in the well to accept the emitted light. The circular active area in practical surface emitters in normally 50μm in diameter and up to 2.5μm thick SLED. Only active region near the surface will emit significant amounts of light while absorbing from the other parts. Hence it is known as surface emitting LED.

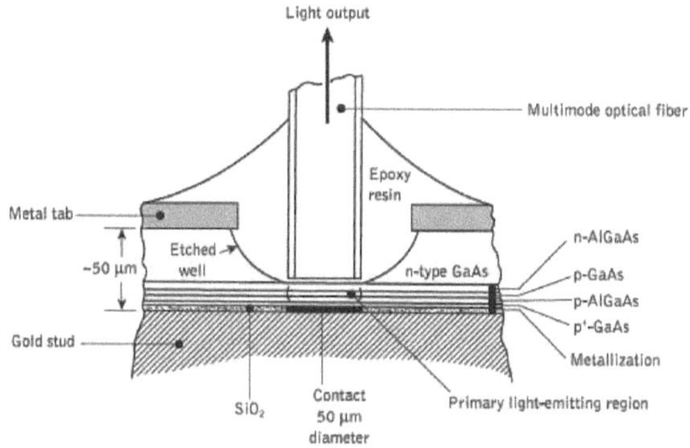

Figure 7.5: The structure of an AlGaAs DH surface – emitting LED (Burrus type).

2. Edge Emitting Diode

Primary active region of the ELED is a narrow stripe, which lies below the surface of the semiconductor substrate. The semiconductor substrate is cut or polished (facets) so that the stripe runs between the front and back of the device. Rear facet is highly reflective, and the front facet is antireflection coated. The rear facet reflects the light propagating toward the rear end-face back toward the front facet. By coating the front facet with antireflection material, the front facet reduces optical feedback and allows light emission. ELEDs emit light only through the front facet.

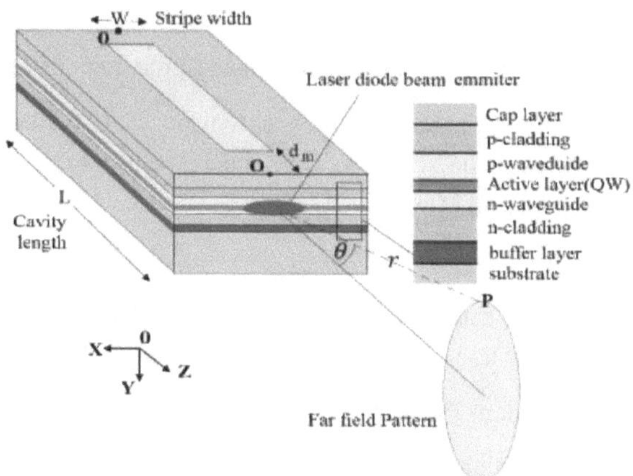

Figure 7.6: ELED emit light .

3. **Superluminiscent Diode**

A semiconductor device that emits low-coherence light of a broad spectrum like LED but high brightness like Laser Diode. Emission occurs by flowing forward current to a p-n junction. When a power supply is connected to the positive p-layer and the n-layer negative, electrons enter from the n-side and holes from the p-side. When the two meet at the junction, an electron drops into a hole and light is emitted. Light is reflected at the end surface of the active layer.

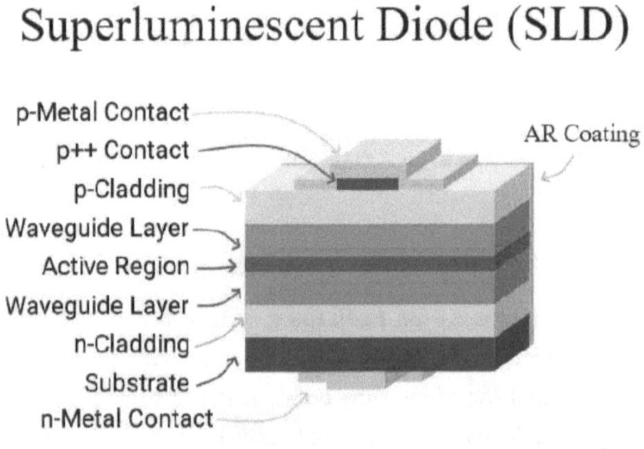

Figure 7.7 Super Luminiscent LED.

7.3.1 Laser/Laser Diode

LASER — Light Amplification by Stimulated Emission of Radiation

A Source of highly directional, monochromatic, coherent light. It Operates under a "stimulated emission" process. The semiconductor laser differs from other lasers (solid, gas, and liquid lasers)

Principle

The principle of laser is based on the stimulated emission of light. Components of a typical laser are:

1. Gain Medium for Population energy
2. Laser Pumping energy

3. Cavity 4. Reflector 5. Laser Beam

Semiconductor Laser

A semiconductor laser diode is a device capable of producing a lasing action by applying a potential difference across a modified p-n junction. This modified pn-junction is heavily doped and contained within a cavity thus providing the gain medium for the laser. A feedback circuit is also implemented in order to control the amount of current sent to the laser dialogue.

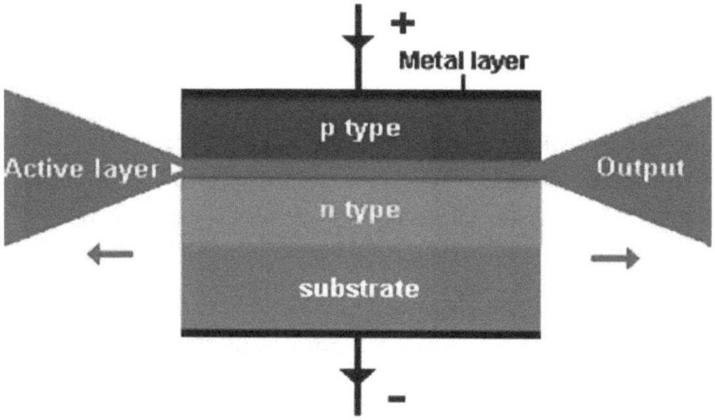

Figure 7.8 Semiconductor Laser Diode.

Components of laser diode- Metal contact, P-type material, Active region (n-type material), N- type material, Metal contact Materials include: GaAlAs,AlGaInP, InGaAsP

Semiconductor laser diodes are cheap and easy to use compared to other types of lasers. Precisely controlled current source is needed to regulate the amount of current to the laser diode.

7.4 OPTICAL FILTERS

Filters transmit only the desired wavelengths and either absorb or reflect light of unwanted wavelengths. It utilized to select a portion of the incoming light for use as an input for an optical system. It is used to select a portion of the light to be used as an output. It is used to split light into multiple components with differing wavelengths. Filter out background noise from the rest of the optical spectrum Properties

- Long pass filters transmit wavelengths above a cut-on wavelength.
- Short pass filters transmit wavelengths below a cut-off wavelength.
- Band pass filters transmit wavelengths in a narrow range around a specified wavelength.

7.4.1 Types

Absorbance filters -Color glass filters -absorb the unwanted wavelengths\ Light is blocked based on the absorption properties of the glass substrate used. Light that is blocked does not reflect off the filter; rather, it is absorbed and contained within the filter. Consist of dye molecules uniformly suspended in glass or plastic. Will often fluoresces.

Interference filters -Dichroic, Dielectric, reflective filters - Reflect the unwanted wavelengths. Composed of transparent glass or quartz substrate on which multiple thin layers of dielectric material, sometimes separated by spacer layers. They are wavelength selective.

Dichroic Filters- They used to direct light in different spectral region to different detectors. They are interference filters, long pass or short pass. Angle Sensitive. Reflects unwanted wavelengths and transmits the desired portion of the spectrum.

7.5 OPTICAL DETECTORS

An optical detector converts the optical signal into an electrical signal, which can then be further processed. Generates an electrical current proportional to the intensity of incident optical radiation.

7.5.1 Classification Diodes

PN-diodes - The photo- generated electron hole pairs in the depletion region of the diode contribute to the overall photocurrent. Operated under short circuit conditions or under reverse bias voltage.

PIN diodes - The depletion region is extended across the intrinsic or lightly doped layer and therefore more photo-generated carriers contribute to the photocurrent. All three layers (p-,i- and n-region) have the same optical band gap. The thicker the i-layer the further the sensitivity.

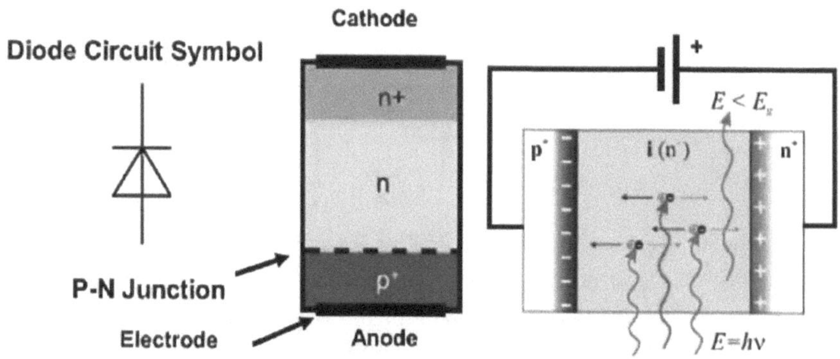

Figure 7.9 PIN diode.

Avalanche photodiodes - APDs amplify the signal during the detection process. The operating principle of a APD is based on the avalanche effect, where a highly accelerated electron excites another electron due to “impact ionization”. However, in the first step a photon must be absorbed and a electron-hole pair has to be generated. The device consists of two regions. In region 1 of the device the electron hole pairs are generated and separated. In region 2 of the device the carriers are accelerated and impact ionized.

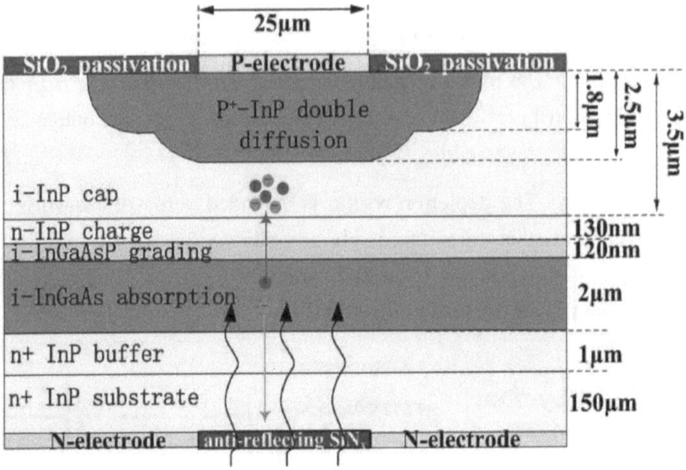

Figure 7.10 Avalanche Diode.

Arriving photons pass through thin n^+p- junction. The carriers are absorbed in a p- region. The absorption leads to the generation of electron-hole pairs in this region. The electric field in the p-region is high enough to separate the carriers. The electric field across the p-region is not high enough for the charge carriers to gain enough energy for multiplication to take place. The electric field, however, in the n^+p-region the electric field is significantly higher, so that the charge carriers (in this case electrons only) are strongly accelerated and pick up energy. The electrons collide with other atoms in the lattice, which leads to the production of new electron-hole pairs ("impact ionization"). The newly released charge carriers again will collide with the lattice to produce more electron-hole pairs.

Schottky diodes - A thin metal layer replaces either the p- or the n-region of the diode. Depending on the semiconductor and the metal being involved, a barrier is formed at the interface of the two materials. This barrier leads to a bending of the bands. Due to the applied voltage the bands can be blended. In the region of the band bending electron hole pairs can be separated.

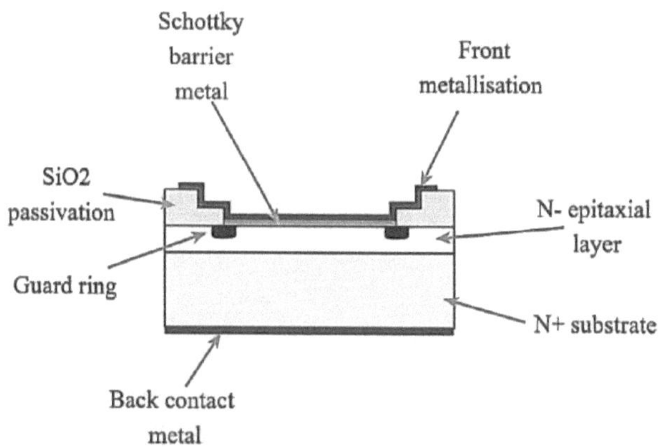

Figure 7.11 Schottky Diode.

7.5.2 Photo conductors

In the case of a photoconductor the resistivity of the device is changed as a function of the intensity and not photocurrent. A voltage is applied to the detector to measure the change in current flow. The photoconductive detector is formed by two adjacent finger contacts which are placed on a semiconducting material. The photoconductive detector is a unipolar device, which means that the current flow is either completely dominated by electrons or by holes.

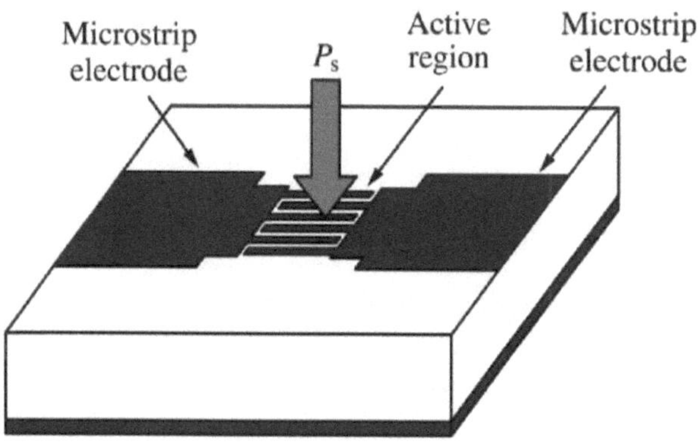

Figure 2.12 Photo conductive detectors.

7.5.3 Time resolved detectors

Pulse excitation source is used. Width of excitation is generally much shorter than the emission process of interest, i.e., much shorter than the lifetime (decay time) of the samples. To measure the lifetime, the time-dependent intensity is measured following the excitation pulse, and the decay time is calculated from the slope of a plot of log I (t) vs. t, or from the time at which the intensity decreases to 1/e of the initial intensity value I (t = 0).

7.5.4 Phase resolved detectors

It is also called frequency domain techniques. Sample is exciting with intensity-modulated light. The intensity of the incident light changes with a very high frequency compared with the reciprocal of the decay time. Following excitation with a modulated signal, the emission is also intensity-modulated at the same modulation frequency. Because the emission from the sample follows a decay profile, there is a certain delay in the emission relative to the excitation. This delay is measured as a phase-shift, which can be used to calculate the decay time. The shape of the frequency response is determined by the number of decay times displayed by the sample. If the decay is a single exponential, the frequency is simple.

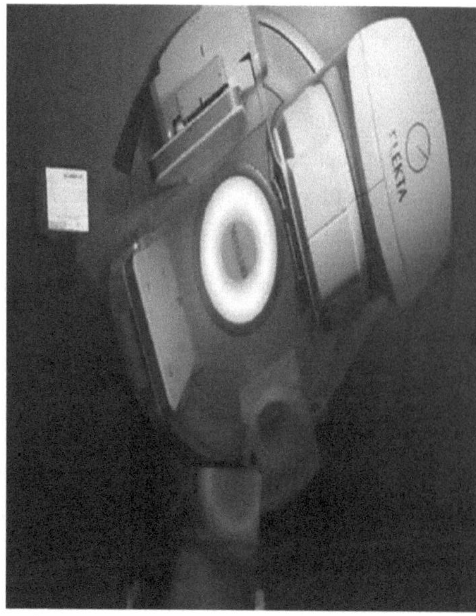

8

CHAPTER

APPLICATION OF RADIATION IN MEDICINE

8.1 RADIATION USED FOR DIAGNOSTIC PURPOSES

In this chapter we shall discuss the use of radiation of different kinds for medical imaging. This includes ordinary x-ray film, the use of contrast media, fluorescent screens, image intensifiers, CT and the use of digital technology to all x-ray systems. In the case of x-rays the source is on the outside of the patient and the detector is on the other side – unless in the case of backscattered x-rays.

We also intend to look in more detail into the use of radioactive isotopes for diagnostic purposes. When isotopes are used, it is always the γ-radiation that gives the information. Furthermore, the isotopes are inside the body – and it is the γ-photons coming out that yield the information. Two types of information are obtained: a). Information about where the isotopes are localized, b). Whether the distribution of activity deviates from normal to an organ or part of the body. We shall give the development of nuclear medicine including the PET-technique.

Both x-rays and isotopes will give a radiation dose to the patient. The doses are rather small, – and should not be of any concern – unless the LNT hypothesis and collective doses are used.

To complete the diagnostic field, we shall mention a couple of other methods such as magnetic resonance (MR or MRI) and ultrasound. In the case of MR electromagnetic radiation is used in combination with a strong magnetic field. Electromagnetic radiation is within the radio frequency field and cannot ionize.

Ultrasound is sound waves with a frequency above 20 kHz.

History of x-ray pictures

The first x-ray picture was taken three days before Christmas 1895 when C. W. Roentgen brought his wife into his laboratory, and they emerged with a photograph of the bones in her hand and of the ring on her finger (the picture is shown below).

Roentgen presented the news on the 28th of December 1895, and the discovery was spread rapidly around the world. About a month later, 23 January 1896, he gave a lecture on the new rays to the Physical Medical Society of Würzburg. During the meeting Roentgen took an X-ray photograph of the hand of the anatomist A. von Kölliker, who was in the audience (see picture below). After this had been done, von Kölliker proposed that the new rays should be called "*Roentgen's rays*", and this suggestion was approved with great enthusiasm by the audience. In Norway and some other countries, we use that name.

The development from this first photo was rapid both about technology and use. We shall give a short history of the development that resulted in sharper and much better pictures.

In an ordinary x-ray photo, the object is placed between the x-ray source and the detector (for example film). The picture is based on the x-rays that penetrate the object and hit the detector – and yields the *electron density in the object.*

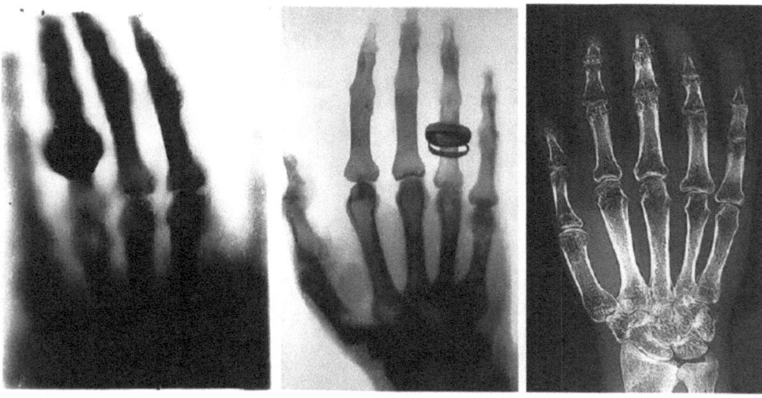

Figure 8.1: Roentgen took an X-ray photograph of the hand of the anatomist A. von Kölliker.

Here we present three pictures of a hand. The two of them are the two first and famous pictures of Mrs. Roentgen (left), von Kölleker (middle). The first one is taken 22. December 1895 and the second one 23 January 1896. You clearly see the improvements. The last one is observed using a digital filter to enhance the details and reduce the noise.

Nikola Tesla and his pictures – shadowgraphs

In the years before 1900 several other physicists worked with equipment like that of Roentgen. We would like to mention the Mult genius Nikola Tesla. He discovered what he called "shadow- graphs" – which in fact was x-ray pictures. The famous one of a foot and shoe is shown here.

Nikola Tesla was born in Kroatia and emigrated to USA in 1884. He is frequently cited as one of the most important contributors to the birth of commercial electricity and is known for his many revolutionaries develop- mints in the field of electromagnetism in the late 19th and early 20th centuries. We can mention that he de- signed the first hydroelectric power plant in Niagara Falls in 1895.

Nikola Tesla invented his own vacuum tube which had only one electrode. Electrons were emitted and accelerated by the electrical field in his "Tesla coil".

When the electrons hit the glass walls, x-rays were produced. Tesla managed to obtain images of the human body with this radiation – the shadowgraphs.

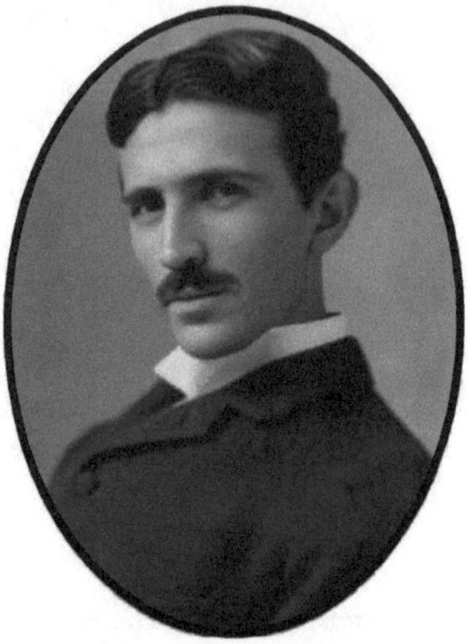

Nikola Tesla (1856 – 1943)

He also sent some of his images to Roentgen shortly after Roentgen published his discovery. Tesla gave Roentgen full credit for the finding and never attempted to proclaim priority. Roentgen, on the other hand, congratulated Tesla for his sophisticated images.

In the magazine "Electrical Review" for 1896 some X-ray observations by Tesla were published. He described some clinical benefits of x-rays – for example, determination of foreign body position and detection of lung diseases. He noted that denser bodies were opaquer to the rays. Tesla even

discovered reflected x-rays which recently have been used (see later).

Nikola Tesla has been honored by calling the SI unit for magnetic field (also known as "magnetic flux density) for "tesla" (abbreviated T). We shall meet this within the field of MR.

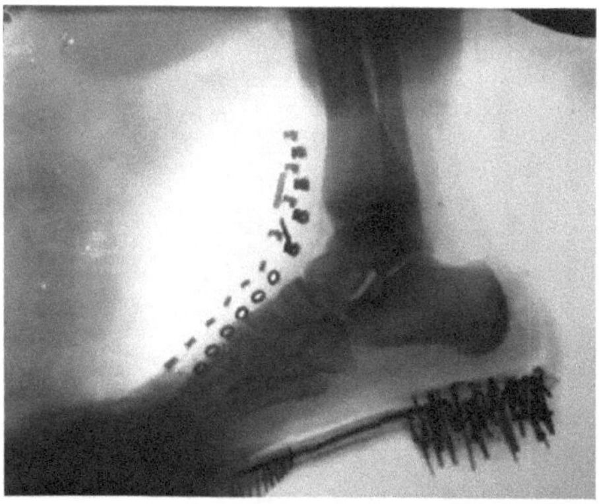

Figure 8.2: Nikola Tesla s famous picture.

8.2 SOME OF THE HIGHLIGHTS FOR X-RAY DIAGNOSTIC

We shall first mention some of the developments in chronological order.

1900 The use of chest x-ray made possible the early detection of tuberculosis. Furthermore, during the next 50 years x-ray pictures and fluoroscopy played an important role in the treatment of tuberculosis. In the period before streptomycin (1947) the only treatment was pneumothorax – an attempt to let the lung rest by accumulation of air in the pleural cavity– and the lung collapsed. The air was absorbed within a couple of weeks, and new air was filled in. To control this treatment fluoroscopy was used. The patient was x-rayed both before and after a filling. The treatment usually lasted for 2 – 3 years and the doses could be quite large. We can note that no dissymmetry was carried out at the time – and the doses now quoted are very much speculations.

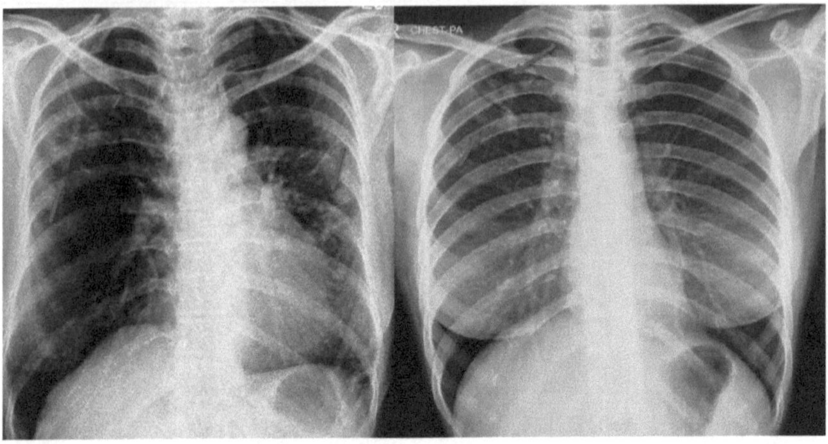

Figure 8.3: x-ray pictures and fluoroscopy played an important role in the treatment of tuberculosis.

The physical basis for an x-ray picture

The x-ray picture is a shadow picture of the part of the body that is between the x-ray tube and the film. Only the x-ray photons that penetrate the object and reach the film can give a signal or blackening of the film. We do not see the photons that are absorbed or scattered.

To see into the body, we must have "something" that can penetrate the body – come out again – and give information. The figure below is an attempt to illustrate the main points for making an x-ray photo.

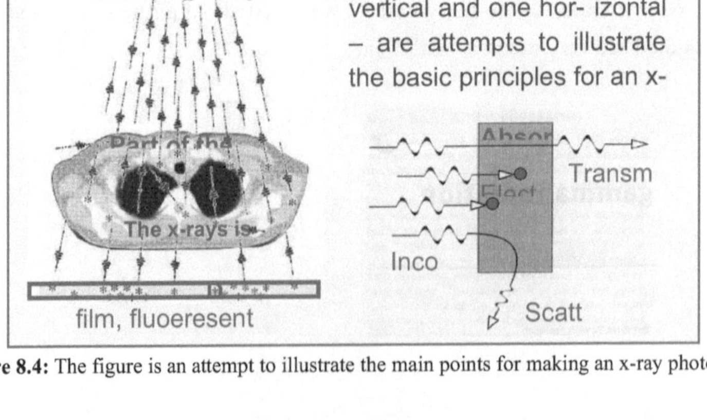

Figure 8.4: The figure is an attempt to illustrate the main points for making an x-ray photo.

1. The x-ray source

We described the basic principles for the formation of x-rays – or rather bremsstrahlung. When electrons with high energy smash into the "anticathode" – a tiny part of the energy is trans- formed into radiation. This implies that the x-ray photons formed, may have several different energies – in fact a whole spectrum is formed (the "Initial spectrum" in the figure below).

X-rays are usually described by their maximum energy, which is determined by the voltage between the electrodes. In x-ray diagnostic the maximum is in the range from 20 kV up to about 120 kV. The x-ray spectrum can be illustrated by the following figure.

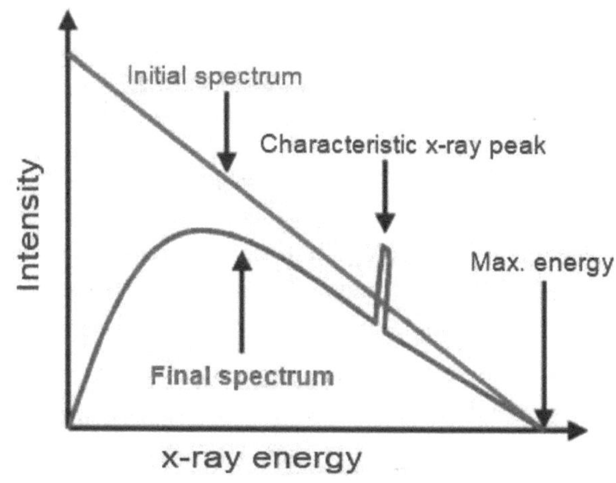

Figure 8.5: The x-ray spectrum can be illustrated.

Here are some details of the radiation from an ordinary x-ray tube. The amount or fraction of the electron energy that is transformed into x-rays from the anode surface is only about a percent of the electron energy. This implies that most of the energy is dissipated as heat, and consequently the anode must be cooled. The probability for transferring electron energy into radiation is proportional to Z. E^2, Here Z is the atomic number of the anode and E is the electron energy. The result is a spec- Trum – in the figure called "initial spectrum"

To use the radiation, it must get out of the X-ray tube. The window absorbs some radiation – mainly in the low energy part. The spectrum changes like that illustrated above – from the "initial spectrum" into the "final spectrum".

The absorption by the window depends on the composition of the window. For example, if low energy x-rays are needed, a beryllium window is used since this window has much lower density than a glass window.

The spectrum also contains characteristic x-rays from dislodging of K- and L-shell electrons from the target. This will not be further discussed when the x-rays are used for diagnostic purposes but is important for x-ray crystallography.

The maximum energy can be changed according to the purpose. It is in the range from 20– 120 keV.

A lot of technological improvements have been made about the x-ray source – probably the most important by William Coolidge – which resulted in stronger (more brilliant) and stable sources.

We are not going to describe all the technological developments about the control of the exposure time – and equipment for the different types of examinations. The maximum energy used depends upon the type of examination. Thus, in the case of mammography the maximum energy is low (below 30 kV) whereas in skeletal and abdominal examinations the energy is larger, between 60 to 85 kV.

Another aspect is that the radiation dose in an examination should be kept as low as possible. Several developments – using intensifying screens have reduced the exposure (see below).

1. Absorption and scattering in the body

The x-ray picture is based on the radiation that penetrates the body and hit the detector (film). The details in the picture are due to those photons that are absorbed or scattered in the body. Since both the absorption and the scattering depend upon the electrons in the object (body) we can say that.

"the x-ray picture is a shadow-picture of the electron density in the body."

On page 30 we discussed the mechanisms for the absorption of x- and γ-rays in matter. Since x-ray diagnostic uses low energy radiation only the" photoelectric *effect*" and the "*Compton scattering*" contribute to the absorption.

The photoelectric effect occurs with bound electrons, whereas the Compton process occurs with free or loosely bound electrons. Both processes vary with the radiation energy and the atomic number of the absorber.

Photoelectric effect – variation with photon energy

For the energy region in question – and for atoms like those found in tissue the photoelectric cross- section varies with E^{-3}. Thus, it is a rapid decrease with the energy in this region.

Photoelectric effect – variation with atomic number

The variation with the atomic number is quite complicated. For an energy above the absorption edge, the cross-section per atom varies as Z^4 (i.e. the cross-section per electron varies as Z^3). It can be noted that the K-shell energy for all atoms in the body (C, N, O, P, and Ca) is below 4 keV. Consequently, for the diagnostic purposes the absorption varies with Z^4 per atom.

Compton effect – variation with photon energy

For the energy range used for diagnostic purposes the Compton effect is rather constant – and de- creases slightly with the energy. Compton scattering is most important for energies above 60 keV. For lower energies the photoelectric effect is by far the most important.

Compton effect – variation with atomic number

The Compton process increases with the electron density of the absorber. This implies that it is almost independent of the atomic number Z.

Conclusion

1. The absorption processes are the photoelectric effect and the Compton scattering.

2. Photoelectric effect depends strongly on the atomic number (Z^4). This implies that the absorption in bones (with an effective atomic number of about 13) is much larger than that for tissue (with effective atomic number of about 7.5). For energies below about 30 keV the absorption is mainly by the photoelectric effect. In this energy region it is possible to see the small variations in electron density in normal and pathological tissue like that found in a breast.

It can be noted that due to the strong dependence of the photoelectric effect with the atomic number we find the key to the use of contrast compounds. Thus, compounds containing iodine (Z = 53) or barium (Z = 56) will absorb the low energy x-rays very efficiently. In angiography the arteries become visible when iodine compounds are used.

3. The Compton process varies slightly with the energy in this range – and is the dominating absorption process for energies above 50 keV.

4. In addition to the absorption processes some photons will be scattered, i.e. elastic scattering. In Rayleigh scattering the photon interacts with a bound electron and is scattered without loss of energy. The probability of this scattering process is proportional to Z2/E. In Thomson scattering the photon interacts with a free electron and the radiation is scattered in all directions. The two elastic scattering processes account for less than 10 % of the interactions in the diagnostic energy range. Tiring is to give some background knowledge of the physics of the x-ray picture.

It is differential attenuation of photons in the body that produces the contrast which is responsible for the information. The attenuation of the radiation in the body depends upon the density, the atomic number and the radiation quality. The absorption of x-rays decreases as energy (kV) increases.

In mammography one is interested in visualizing small differences in soft tissue – and we use low energy x-rays (26 – 28 kV) to enhance the tissue details.

In the case of chest pictures the peak energy must be larger because the absorbing body is very much larger – and some radiation must penetrate the body and reach the detector. It is the transmitted photons that reach the detectors that are responsible for the picture.

3. The detector system

Several different detectors (film, ionization chambers, luminescence and semiconductors) have been used since the beginning of x-ray diagnostic.

For a very long-time film was used. The x-ray picture was created when the radiation was absorbed in the film emulsion consisting of silver halides ($AgBr$ as well as $AgCl$ and AgI).

The emulsion was suspended on gelatin as the supporting medium.

In the usual morning meeting the doctors were often gathered in front of the "light box" to discuss the patients (see illustration).

The absorption in the thin film emulsion is very small. Consequently, to increase sensitivity, intensifying screens were introduced. The screen is usually a phosphor scintillator that converts the x-ray photons to visible light that in turn exposes the film. The introduction of intensifying screens was made already in 1896 by Thomas Alva Edison. He introduced the calcium tungstate screens which were dominating up to the 1970-ties. This material has now largely been replaced by rare-earth metal-based screens. We do not intend to go through the technical details regarding intensifying screens – nor to the many technological details within x-ray diagnostic. However, a few points should be mentioned.

Conventional radiography uses energies between 50 and 80 kV. To ensure that the photoelectric effect is dominant, lower energies are used. Energies lower than 30 kV are used for mammography – which is very effective for seeing details in soft tissue. However, this energy range is only useful for tissue thickness of a few centimeters.

8.3 MAMMOGRAPHY

In mammography the goal is to see the contrast between different density of soft tissue, fat and blood vessels without use of contrast media. The x-ray energy is between 25 and 30 kV to ensure that the photoelectric effect is dominant. This also resulted in absorption of radiation and an increase of the patient dose.

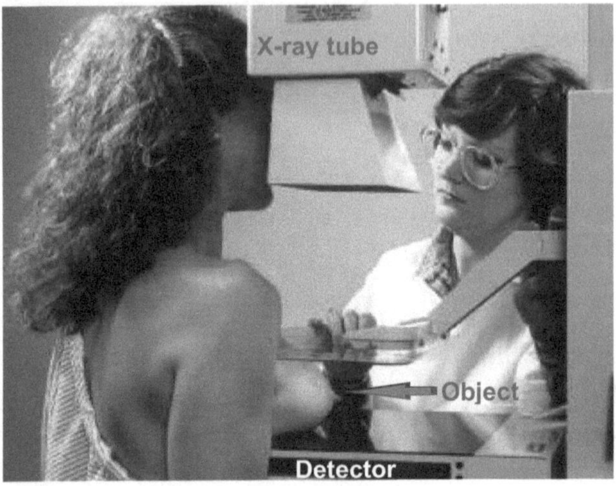

Figure 8.6: The figure shows a mammography machine.

Examples

It is sometimes very convincing to see a mammogram like that shown to the right. It is also amazing that we can see details like this in soft tissue without using contrast media to enhance the difference in electron density.

The next example is shown below. Here you see two mammograms of the same normal breast. The large differences are due to the technique used.

To the left is a modern digital picture whereas the other is a film-based mammography.

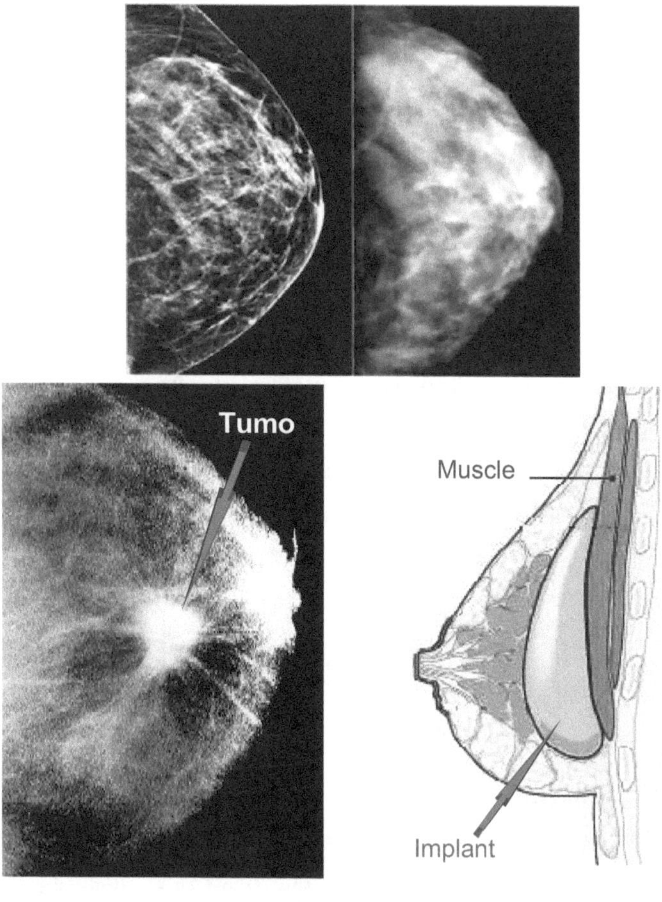

Figure 8.7: A recent digital photo as well as a mammogram.

Implants

It is obvious, even for the layman, that the presence of breast implants does interfere and makes it more difficult to obtain good information with mammography.

The presence of implants affects the way mammograms are done, since additional views are needed during routine screening mammography to visualize all the breast tissue. Implants also makes it more difficult to interpret in some cases.

The lesson to learn from this is that implants could be an impediment to cancer detection. We can conclude that you have to be well trained to give a good description.

8.4 FLUOROSCOPY

With the ordinary x-ray film it was impossible to see any movements. This became possible by using phosphor screens. The transmitted x-rays caused scintillations that was viewed directly. In order to reduce the dose to the doctors the fluorescent screen was backed by lead glass. The whole examination was performed in a dark room and with adapted eyes. The images were faint and low in contrast.

This examination (in Norway known as "gjennomlysning") was widely used in the treatment of lung tuberculosis and pneumothorax treatment.

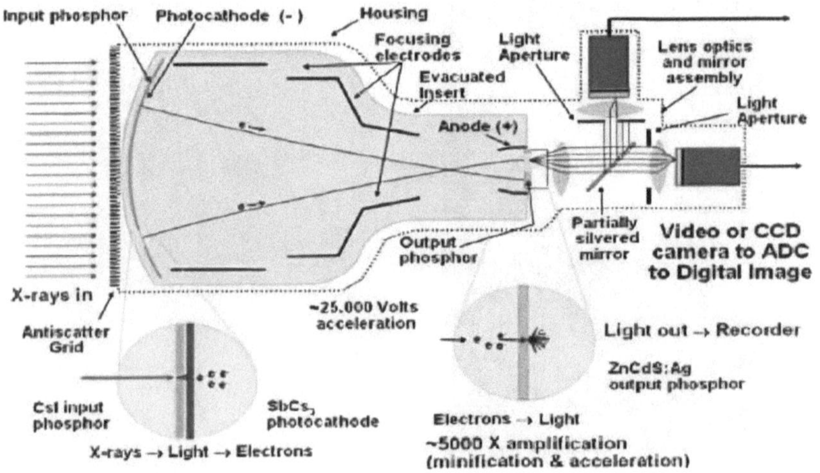

Figure8.8: Fluoroscopy components.

The screens were outdated and "image intensifiers" were introduced (see figure). The x-rays were converted to light by using phosphors (CsI:Na) – and again to photoelectrons. They were accelerated and focused on a smaller fluorescent screen which in turn is coupled to a recorder system; for example a video camera or a film camera.

If the technique is coupled with the use of contrast media it is possible to follow the contrast when it is flowing through the blood vessels. It is thus possible to perform some type of treatment while viewing it.

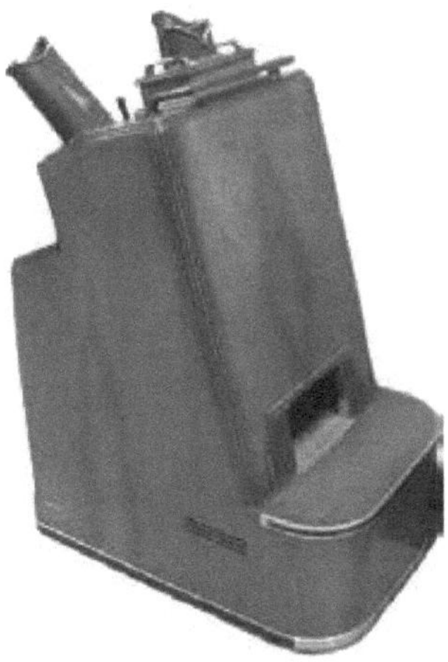

Figure 8.9: The oldest Fluoroscopy device.

Shoe-fitting fluoroscopy

Today it is almost unbelievable that x-rays was used to find the right pair of shoes. However, during the period 1930 – 1950 an x-ray fluoroscope like the one shown was used.

The system consisted of a vertical wooden cabinet with an opening near the bottom into which the feet were placed. When you looked through one of the three viewing ports on the top of the cabinet (e.g., one for the child being fitted, one for the child's parent, and the third for the shoe salesman or saleswoman), you would see a fluorescent image of the bones of the feet and the outline of the shoes.

The machines generally used a 50 kV x-ray tube in the bottom of the cabinet. When you put your feet in the opening, you were standing on top of the x-ray tube. The only shielding was a one mm thick aluminum filter.

Measurements made in recent years indicate that the doses to the feet were in the range 0.07– 0.14 Gy for a 20 second exposure. Doses to the pelvis ranged from 0.03 to 0.17 mGy.

8.5 DIGITAL IMAGING

The technique with digital x-rays was introduced in the 1970's. Analog to digital converters and computers were adapted to conventional fluoroscopic image intensifier systems. Angiographic procedures for looking at the blood vessels in the brain, kidneys, arms and legs, and the blood vessels of the heart all have benefited tremendously from the adaptation of digital technology.

It is reasonable to assume that all the film systems will be replaced by digital x-ray detectors. The benefits of digital technology can be summarized as follows:

1. The x-ray dose can often be reduced to achieve the same high-quality picture.

2. The digital x-ray images can be enhanced and manipulated with computers.

3. The digital images can be sent via network to other computers and hospitals.

4. The digital images can be archived onto compact disks and thus save storage space.

5. The digital images can be retrieved from an archive at any point in the future for reference.

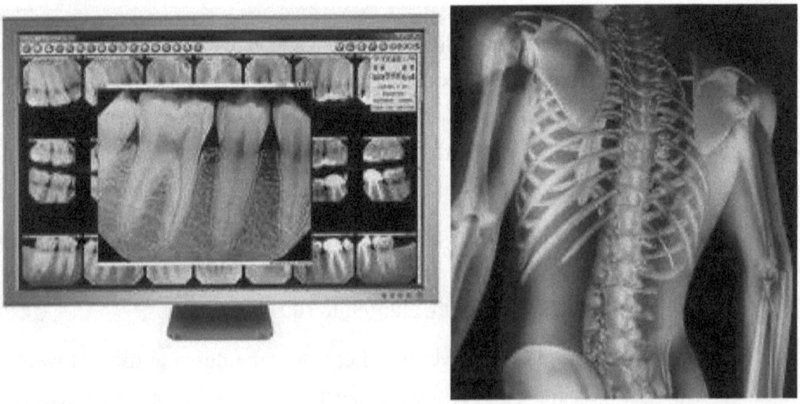

Figure 8.10: The digital x-ray images.

Examples

We have already shown a couple of examples with digital techniques.

On page 173 the picture of a hand is shown together with some old film-based pictures.

On page 182 you can see an example with mammography.

To the right is an example with dental x- rays. The image can be enlarged, which makes it easier to detect the problems.

8.6 CT – COMPUTER TOMOGRAPHY

On page176 we mentioned that the forerunner to CT was called planigraphy – or linear tomography. Let us therefore look into this technique – which played a role in the treatment of tuberculosis in the 1950s and 1960s.

The technique was proposed early in the 1900s by the Italian radiologist Alessandro Vallebona. In Norway professor Marius Kolsrud constructed an equipment in 1948.

The idea is based on the simple principle of moving synchronously and in opposite directions the X-ray tube and the film. Consequently, structures in the focal plane appear sharper, while structures in other planes appear blurred. The lung was shown – slice by slice – and could yield information about the position and extent of the TB infection. To cover a lung about 20 x-ray pictures were required.

The next step was introduced by G. N. Hounsfield and A. M. Cormack

in 1972. The CT or CAT scanner was successful since much smaller contrast differences can be observed. They replaced the x-ray film with a group of small detectors. The signals from the detectors were stored and analyzed mathematically in a computer. The computer rapidly reconstructs an image of the examined cross-section.

Scintillation detectors combined with photomultipliers or photo diodes have been used. We would also like to mention the gas detector. This is like the Geiger detector. To increase sensitivity, the gas detector is filled with pressurized xenon. Xenon is a heavy noble gas with atomic number 54.

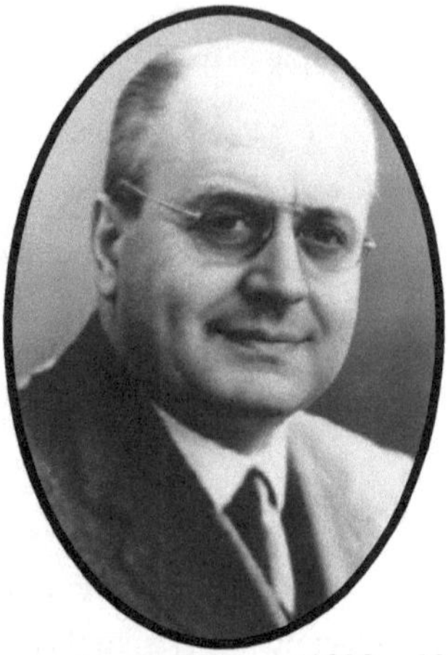

Alessandro Vallebona (1899 – 1987)

Consequently, the photoelectric effect is very efficient. An array of several hundred xenon detectors constitutes the detection system. Since the detector yield analog voltage pulses they have to be digitized by an ADC converter.

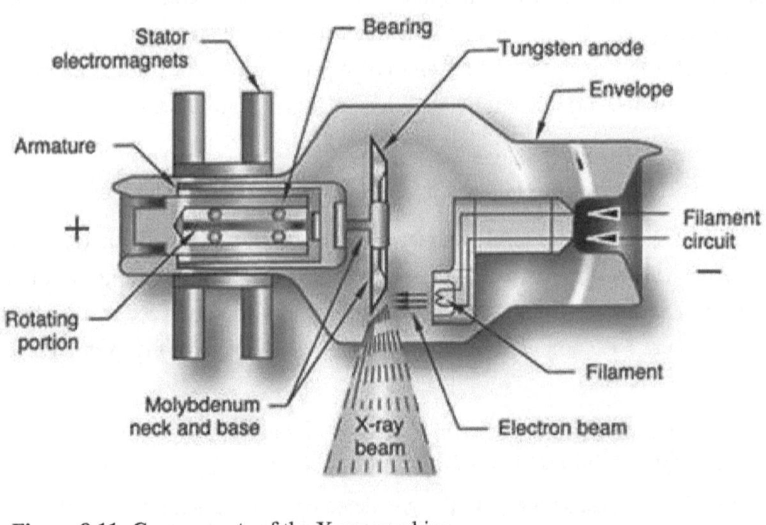

Figure 8.11 :Components of the X-ray machine.

This illustration, taken from Scientific American gives some of the main proper- ties of a CT-scanner.

The technique has been rapidly developed since the first scannerpresented by Hounsfield in 1972.

Both the x-ray tubes, the detector technique as well as the computer presentations with filters etc. have given amazing results.

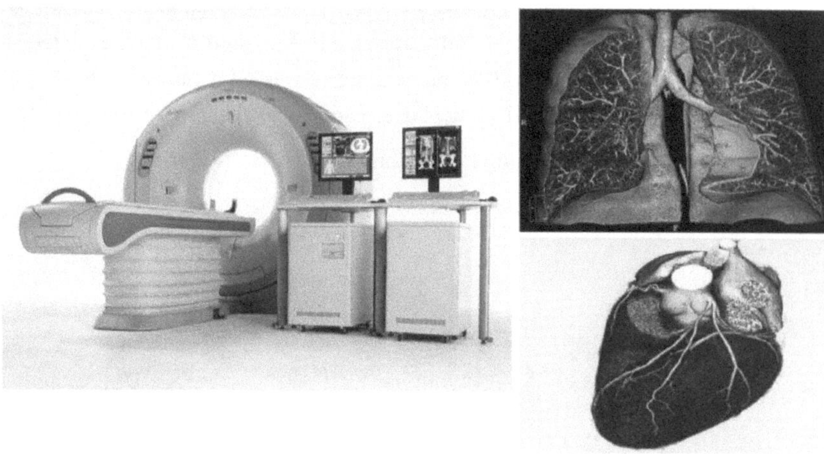

Figure 8.12: A CT-scanner.

The above pictures – and a lot more – can be found on Internet. The examples show the power of this technique.

8.7 BACKSCATTERED X-RAYS – COMPTON SCATTERING

On page 9 we presented a couple of cartoons from more than 100 years ago. These cartoons – given again below – represented a misunderstanding at that time and caused a big smile. The mis under- standing was that some people had the idea that it was possible to take x-ray pictures with reflected x-rays – which means that both the x-ray tube and the film was in the photographer's box (like an ordinary camera). As a result of this some people feared that you could use an x-ray camera to watch people when they changed into swimming suits inside the small cabins on the beach. A London tailor company advertised therefore that they could make *x-ray proof underclothing for ladies*.

Today with the use of Compton backscattering technique all this is a reality – and in fact in use several places for security. Let us therefore give a short glimpse of the technique.

Compton scattering is the key

The Compton process is outlined by the figure. It is a reaction between the x-ray photon and a free or loosely bound electron. The scattered photon has reduced energy. Since both the energy and momentum are conserved it can easily be shown that the energy of the scattered photon, E_S, can be given as a function of the scattering angle θ by the following expression.

$$E_S = \frac{E_\gamma}{1 + \frac{E_\gamma}{m_e c^2}(1 - \cos\theta)}$$

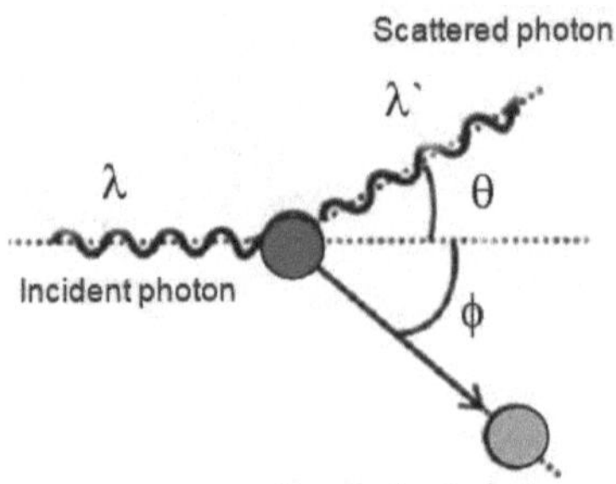

Figure 8.13: The Compton process is outli

For backscattered photons the angle is approximately 180 degrees. Thus the energy of the backscattered photons is reduced by approximately 30 %. The number of backscattered photons are given by the Klein and Nishina formula.

With the knowledge of backscattered Compton radiation, equipment have been developed for observing objects. The x-ray tube and the detector system is now on the same side of the object. The picture is formed by a pencil-shaped beam of x-rays that is sweeping the object. The energy used is approximately 100 keV (100 – 200 kV tubes) which ensures that the Compton process is dominating.

The resolution is (so far) not as good as for ordinary x-rays, but you can easily see objects with an atomic number different from that for tissue. The technique is worked out for security purposes on airports and other places. It is possible to use the technique to see the contents of a closed container through the container walls.

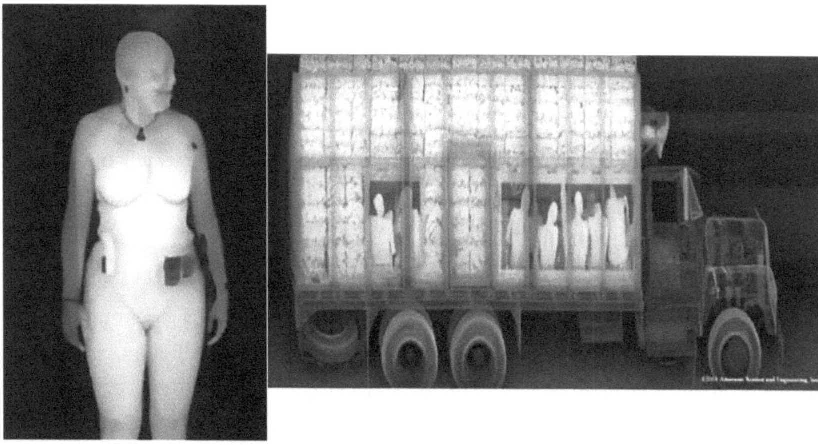

Figure 8.14: The Compton process is technique is worked out for security purposes on airports and other places.

On Internet you can find several backscattered x-ray pictures. The technique is excellent for observing hidden objects on people or the cargo in contain- ers – objects that is not possible to observe with the usual metal detectors.

To the left is a famous picture given in combination with control at airports.

8.8 THE USE OF RADIOACTIVE ISOTOPES NUCLEAR MEDICINE

Radioactive isotopes have been used for more than 100 years in medicine – both for radiation therapy (will be discussed in the next chapter) and for diagnostic purposes. About 90% of the medical use of isotopes are for diagnosis. The most common radioisotope used in diagnosis is technetium-99, but many other isotopes are in use. The thyroid, bones, heart, liver and many other organs can be easily imaged, and disorders in their function are revealed.

MEDICAL OPTICS

Diagnosis

For diagnostic purposes we use radioactive tracers which emit gamma rays from *within* the body. The isotopes are generally short-lived and linked to chemical compounds which permit specific physiological processes to be studied. They can be given by injection, inhalation or orally.

For a number of years, the γ-radiation was observed using a so-called gamma camera. The camera builds up an image from the points from which radiation is emitted. The image can be enhanced by a computer, and abnormal conditions can be observed.

A more recent development is Positron Emission Tomography (PET) which is a more precise and sophisticated technique. It is based on positron-emitting nuclides – usually made in a cyclotron. When this nuclide decays, it emits a positron, which promptly combines with a nearby electron resulting in the simultaneous emission of two γ-photons in opposite directions. The detection gives a very precise indication of their origin. With the isotope F-18 as the tracer, it has proven to be the most accurate non-invasive method of detecting and evaluating most cancers. The reason for this is that F-18 can be added to glucose – and the tumors have an increased rate of glucose metabolism compared to benign cells. PET is also used in cardiac and brain imaging.

Isotopes for diagnosis

Let us point out a couple of important requirements for the use of radioisotopes:

1. Only γ-radiation is used for diagnostic purposes.

For other purposes, i.e. in tracer work, isotopes emitting β-particles can readily be used.

2. The isotopes should have a short half-life for safety reasons and handling. Short in this context is up to a few days.

Due to the requirement of a short half-life mainly or solely artificially made isotopes comes into question. This implies that nuclear medicine started when equipment like cyclotron and neutron sources like the reactor become available in the 1930s and 1940s.

Some of the highlights in the history of nuclear medicine

We shall first mention some of the developments in chronological order.

1924 This year can be considered as the starting point for using radioisotopes as tracers and for biological studies. Georg de Hevesy and coworkers used Pb-210 (one of the isotopes in the Uranium-radium-series) and studied the absorption and elimination of lead, bismuth and thallium salts by animal organisms.

After the start of making radioisotopes in the 1930s O. Chieivitz and Georg de Hevesy administered phosphate labeled with P–32 to rats and demonstrated the renewal of the mineral constituents of bone.

George de Hevesy was awarded the Nobel prize in chemistry for his pioneering work with radioactive tracers.

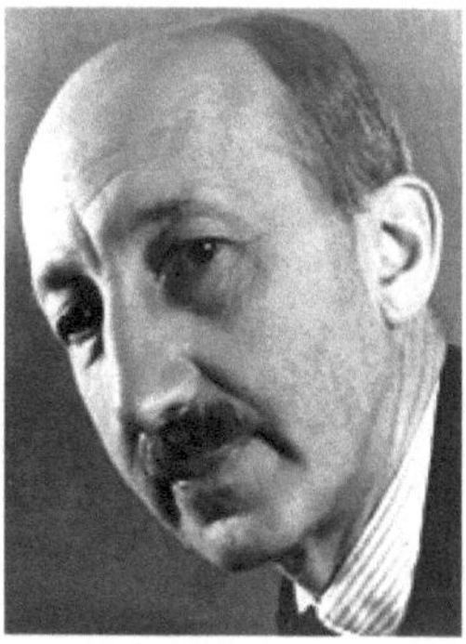

George de Hevesy (1885 – 1966)

8.9 SPECT

SPECT is short for **Single Photon Emission Computed Tomography**. As its name suggests (single photon emission), ordinary γ-ray emission is the source for the information.

The camera or detector rotates around the patient, and the detector will observe the tracer distribution for a variety of angles. After all these angles have been observed, it is possible to reconstruct a three-dimensional view of the isotope distribution within the body. A computer is used to apply a tomographic reconstruction algorithm to multiple projections, yielding a 3-D dataset. This dataset may then be manipulated to show thin slices along any chosen axis of the body, similar to those obtained from other tomographic techniques, such as CT, PET and MR (or MRI).

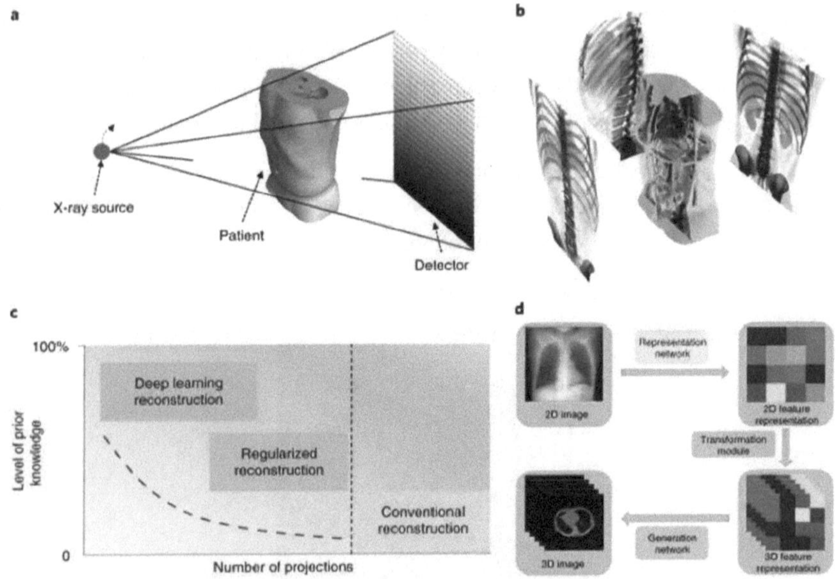

Figure 8.15: Tomographic reconstruction algorithm to the multiple projections.

An example with Tc–99m

In the example shown (to the right), Tc-99m was added to methylene-diphosphonate, which is absorbed by the bone-forming cells (the osteoblasts). The picture makes it possible to study diseases of the skeleton, such as bone cancer.

The doses to both the patient and the medical personnel are small. The strength of the source used for an examination is around a few hundred million Bq (MBq). In the present example 700 MBq was used.

PET – Positron Emission Tomography

The development of positron imaging covered decades and included contributions from different scientists. The technique is based on artificially induced isotopes that emit positrons. To understand this we refer to chapter 2 where we discussed the different ways an unstable nucleus could attain a more stable state. We mentioned that in the ordinary β-decay, a neutron was transformed into a proton and an electron, which was emitted. This is a favorable reaction since the neutron mass is larger than the proton mass. The opposite reaction where a proton is transformed into a neutron is how- ever, a more difficult process. We can, however, attain this goal via two different routes; 1) electron capture and 2) positron emission.

For all natural isotopes, electron capture is the usual process – because the energy between the parent and daughter is less than 2m c2 (m is the electron mass). However, for several artificially induced isotopes positron emission takes place.

The fate of the emitted positron is; after being slowed down, it will meet an electron, and then either annihilate directly, or form a short-lived "positronium atom".

The final process is an annihilation where the mass of the two particles is trans- formed into g-ray photons. Mainly two photons with equal energy, 511 keV, are formed. A very important point is that the photos fly off in opposite directions (see the illustration to the right). This annihilation process represents the basic physical principle for PET. We observe the two photons by detectors 180 degrees apart (coincidence measurements). We know from this observation that the annihilation process has taken place somewhere along the line shown in the illustration.

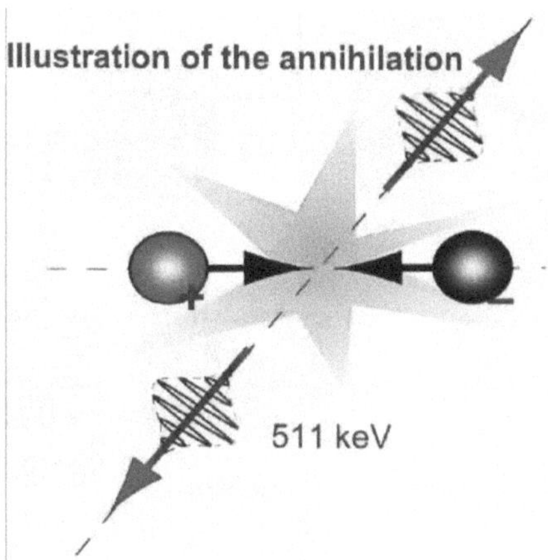

Figure 8.16: Illustration of the annihilation.

PET: We can determine the position of the radioactivity by coincidence measurements of photons with energy 511 keV. One coincidence observation yields a line whereas two or more observations in other directions give a point (or a small area) where the radioactivity has its origin. If we in addition have CT or MR measurements for body reference, we can determine where in the body we find the radioactivity.

PET can give us:

1. Information on how tissue and organs functions on both the molecular and cell level.

2. PET is important to observe cancer – and in particular give information about metastases.

3. With PET it is possible to follow the effect of a treatment.

4. It is also possible to study changes in the brain that follows Alzheimer disease and epilepsy.

In PET we get information on metabolic changes on the cell level. Consequently, PET can to a larger extent observe cancer on an early level – when the changes are on the cellular level. For CT and MR malign changes can only be observed when the structure of the organs and tissue is changed.

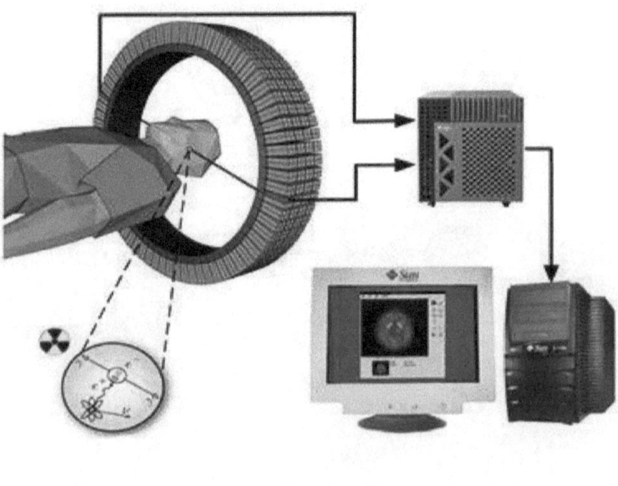

Figure 8.17: PET can to a larger extent observe cancer on an early level.

The illustration from Wikipedia gives a good introduction to PET. The detectors are placed in a ring around the patient. Coincidences for two opposite detectors are measured and a picture is reconstructed. For reference within the body CT or MR is used.

Positron emitters

Only artificial isotopes are positron emitters. Som possible isotopes are given in the table:

8.10 MAGNETIC RESONANCE – MR (MRI)

Today we have other diagnostic methods in addition to, or often in combination with x-rays and radioactive isotopes. The methods in question are magnetic resonance and ultra- sound. For these methods no ionizing radiation is involved, and no absorbed or scattered photons are making the pictures.

What is MR?

The very first MR-picture on a human being was made 3. July 1977 by Raymond Damadian and co- workers in USA (left). The picture obtained was of poor quality and it took hours to obtain. However, despite this it was a sensation and the start of a technique that to- day is very important within med- ical diagnostics.

The field of magnetic resonance started in the 1940s. In 1944 the Russian physicist Yevgeny Zavoisky discovered electron paramagnetic resonance (ESR) and in 1946 Felix Bloch and Edward M. Purcell carried out the first nuclear spin experiments (NMR).

The physics of magnetic resonance

In this book we are interested in the physical background for the different medical techniques rather than to the techniques themselves. Knowledge about x-rays and radioactive nuclides was important for the methods discussed so far. In the case of magnetic resonance (both ESR and NMR) the method is based on units with a magnetic moment. In the case of ESR it implies atoms or molecules with an unpaired electron (we have mentioned ESR in connection to dosimeter on page 80 – 83).

In the case of NMR the technique is based on atomic nuclei with spin – like protons (H-1), deuterons (H-2), C-13, N-14, F-19, Na-23 and P-31. The general MR technique is based on protons in the water molecule.

Let us try to explain the background for magnetic resonance. Units with spin like the electron or pro-ton have magnetic moments. In the case of the electron, it can be written as:

$$\vec{\mu}_e = g\beta\vec{S}$$

Here β is the Bohr-magneton, S is the electron spin and "g" is the spectroscopic splitting factor – which for free electrons is 2,0023. A similar expression is obtained for protons. This implies that we have several small magnets. If these small magnets are placed in a magnetic field B, they will attain energy which depends on the spin state. Thus, for electrons it is given as:

$$E(m_s) = g\beta m_s \cdot B$$

where m_S is the spin quantum number for the electron, which can have two values: +1/2 and –1/2. A figure would help to understand the resonance phenomenon.

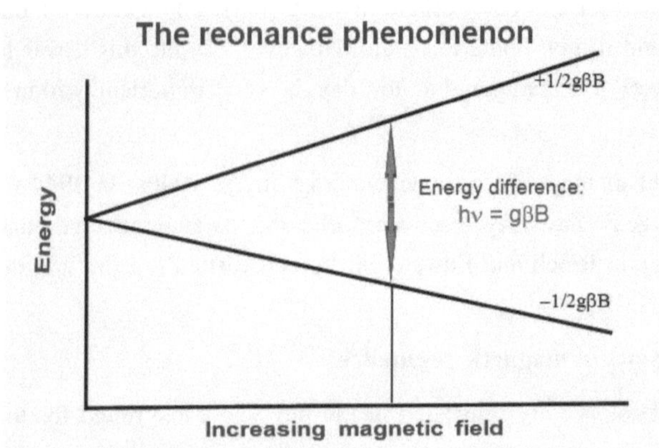

Figure 8.18: The resonance phenomenon.

The figures show that all the small magnets have equal energy as long as the external magnetic field is zero. However, in a magnetic field the magnets will be oriented "with" or "against" the magnetic field. The two states have different energies – and the energy difference increases with the field B as shown. It is possible to induce transitions between the energy states by electromagnetic radiation. The condition for inducing transitions between the energy states is that the energy of the radiation (hν) is equal to the energy difference. A transition from the lower to the higher state yields an absorption. (A transition the other way yields an emission – i.e. the LASER condition).

The conditions for absorption can be written:

$h\nu = g\beta B$ for electrons and $h\nu = g\ \beta_N B_N$ for protons

The figure indicates that we can have resonance at any given frequency as long as the magnetic field follows the resonance condition. We see that the resonance condition is the same for electrons and

protons. However, it is a big difference since $g\beta$ for electrons is much larger than $\beta_N B_N$ for protons.

Thus, a magnetic field of 1 tesla (10 000 gauss) yield resonance for electrons at a frequency of 28 GHz (microwaves with wavelength 1 cm), whereas for protons the frequency is 42.6 MHz (in the radiofrequency region).

Electromagnetic radiation yields transitions in both directions with the same probability. Thus, if the populations of the two levels is equal, the net result would be nil – neither absorption, nor emission. The population of the states follows a Boltzman distribution with the lowest level most populated. The difference increases with increasing magnetic field. This implies that we try to increase the magnetic field and for NMR it is normal to use fields of the order 1.5 tesla (and even up to 7 tesla).

To have a constant absorption, the difference in population must be kept. Two relaxation processes transfer spins to the lower state. Both processes are connected to changes in the proton spin. One process is "spin-lattice" relaxation and the other is "spin-spin" relaxation. The rates of the two processes are measured by relaxation times T_1 and T_2.

We have seen above that the x-ray picture is a shadow of the electron density. In the case of MR the picture depends on the proton density as well as on the two relaxation times T_1 and T_2. It appears that these relaxation times changes when going from normal to pathological tissue – and this can be used in diagnostics.

How is a picture made?

A part of the body is placed in a strong magnetic field. The resonance condition gives the connection between field and frequency. It is therefore easy to understand that it is possible to fulfill the resonance condition for a small volume element. However, it is a long way from a volume element to a picture – and the question is: How is it possible to go from a point (a tiny volume element) to construct a whole picture?

The first solution to this came when Paul Lauturbur tried out his ideas in the early 1970s. He introduced magnetic field gradients and by analysis of the characteristics of the emitted radio waves, he was able to determine their origin. This made it possible to build up images of structures. In 1973 he demonstrated how it was possible to see the difference between tubes filled with water from an environment of heavy water. These very first experiments showed that one could use a set of simple linear gradients, oriented in three dimensions and slowly build up a picture. Peter Mansfield showed how the radio signals could be mathematically analyzed, which made it possible to develop a useful imaging technique.

One of the major practical difficulties encountered with the early MRI, was the time it took to acquire the data. Line-scanning, for example, took typically 10–20 min. The breakthrough came in 1977 when Mansfield introduced the echo-planar imaging. This snap-shot technique meant that in principle complete two-dimensional images could be achieved in extremely short times like 20 – 50 ms.

A modern MR scanner has coils in three directions (see illustration below). They modify the magnetic field at very particular points and work in conjunction with the RF pulses to produce the picture. They are rapidly turned on and off (which causes that banging noise), and the gradient magnets allow the scanner to image the body in slices. The transverse (or axial, or x-y) planes slice you from top to bottom; the coronal (x-z) plane slice you lengthwise from front to back; and the sagittal (y-z) planes slice you lengthwise from side to side. However, the x, y and z gradients can be used in combination to generate image slices that are in any direction, which is one of the great strengths of MR as a diagnostic tool.

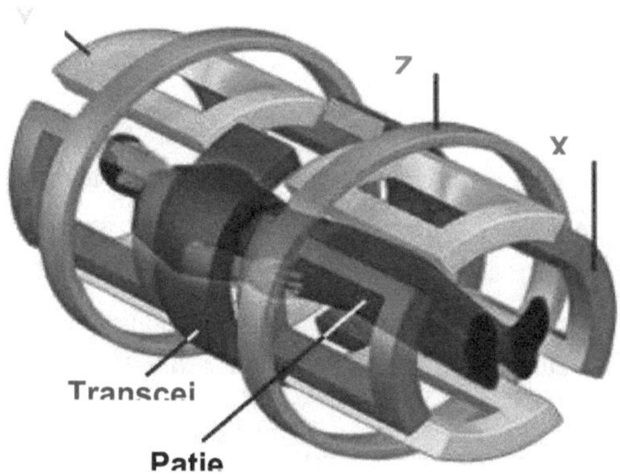

Figure 8.19: A modern MR scanner.

An illustration of the field gradient coils. They usually give off a banging noise. (Illustration taken from Internet)

MR pictures and use in medicine

Most MR scanners in the hospitals use 1.5 tesla magnets. The electromagnets consist of a solenoid cooled down to about 4 K by liquid helium. At such temperatures superconduction is attained and it is possible to send large currents through the solenoid and thus get the large magnetic fields required.

MR can be used to study all different organs in the body. For parts of the body with bones it is difficult to use x-rays to study the tissue around – because the bones absorb the x-rays much more than the tissue. In these cases, MR is very valuable. It has been used to study details in the brain and spine. Brain sicknesses result in changes in the water content which can be visualized in MR. Thus, only a difference in water content of 1 percent can be detected. Multiple Sclerosis (MS) can be studied and followed by MR. The sickness gives infections to brain and spine and with MR it is possible to localize this, and observe the effect of treatment.

Contrast compounds

It is also possible to introduce contrast media in MR. We can mention the element gadolinium (Gd). This is a Lanthanide element (atomic number 64) that is paramagnetic and has the effect that it strongly decreases the T1 relaxation times of the tissues.

Also several vandal compounds are used as contrast agents for MR. These compounds are taken up by, and accumulate in, glycolytic ally active cells, such as rapidly dividing tumor cells. The resulting MR images have excellent resolution and contrast. These compounds also bind to albumin in the blood, allowing for the assessment of blood volume at tumor sites prior to cellular uptake (like imaging with gadolinium), a valuable diagnostic indicator and tool for treatment response in its surroundings.

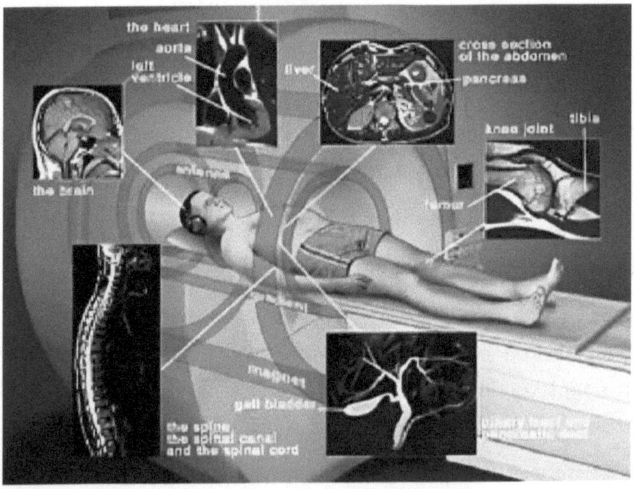

Figure 8.20: Magnetic resonance imaging device components.

8.11 DIAGNOSTIC ULTRASOUND

Ultrasound is sound waves with a frequency above the limit for human hearing – about 20 kHz. For medical use the frequency is in the region from 2 – 40 MHz

Formation of ultrasound

In 1880 Pierre Curie and his brother Jacques discovered that certain crystals (the so-called piezoelectric crystals) can produce a pulse of mechanical energy (sound pulse) by electrically exciting the crystal. Furthermore, the crystals can produce a pulse of electrical energy by mechanically exciting the crystal. This ultrasound physics principle is called the piezoelectric effect (pressure electricity). Crystalline materials with piezoelectric properties are quartz crystals, piezoelectric ceramics such as barium titanate or lead zirconate titanate.

A device that converts one form of energy into another is called a "*transducer*" – and they can be used for production and detection of diagnostic ultrasound.

We are not going into more details about the equipment here, but it is possible to use ultrasound technique to produce pictures of the inside of the body. Since ultrasound images are captured in real-time, they can show the structure and movement of the body's internal organs, as well as blood flowing through the blood vessels. Ultrasound imaging is a noninvasive medical test that helps physicians diagnose and treat medical conditions.

A short history

The origin of technology goes back to the Curies, who first discovered the piezoelectric effect. Attempts to use ultrasound for medical purposes started in the 1940s when they used a continuous ultrasonic emitter to obtain images from a patient`s brain. During the war it was a rapid development within ultrasound. They generated pulse echoes and developed Sonar and Radar. A spin-off from Sonar is ultrasound medical imaging.

The use of Ultrasonic in the field of medicine had nonetheless started initially with its applications in therapy rather than diagnosis, utilizing its heating and disruptive effects on animal tissues.

An excellent review of the history of ultrasound can be found in the following address:

A short description of the technique

In the clinical use of ultrasound, a transmitter produce a short pulse of electrical oscillations (2 – 10 MHz). The transducer converts this to a pulse of mechanical vibrations. The transducer is coupled to the body by a gel and the pulse of ultrasound goes into the soft tissues (speed of about 1500 m per second). The transducer will then sense the reflected, weaker pulses of ultrasound and transform them back into electrical signals. These echoes from different organs are amplified and processed by the receiver and sent to the computer, which keeps track of the return times and amplitudes.

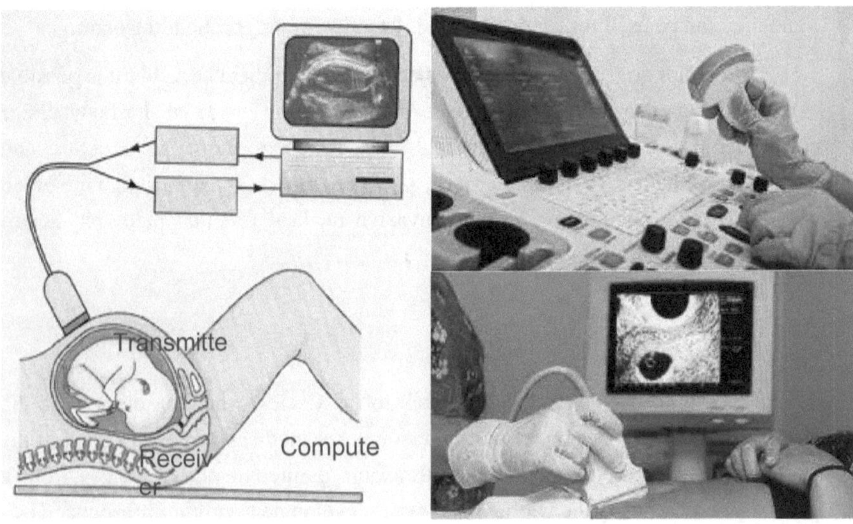

Figure 8.21: ultrasound machine.

The main components of ultrasound

A new pulse is produced and sent off in a slightly different direction (pulse repetition frequency is in the range 2 – 10 kHz). The data from all these pulses are treated by the computer and yield a CT-like image in "real time". You can see how arms and legs of a fetus move or see the heart valve open and close.

A lot of technology is involved in the different parts of the ultrasound technique. However, it is not the purpose of this book to go into detail in this field.

Let us shortly mention that the transducer that transmits and receives the ultrasound energy into and from the body is a key component. It is built up of hundreds of transducers to take a high-resolution real-time scan. Many transducers create a wave front, and the angle of the wave front can be altered by firing the transducers one after another. By changing the angle of the wave front, a three-dimensional image can be built up over a large area.

Doppler ultrasound

The velocity of the blood can be measured by the Doppler effect – i.e. the change in ultrasound frequency. If the ultrasound frequency is 5 MHz and the blood velocity is 20 cms^{-1}, the change in frequency is 1274 Hz if we look along the blood vessel (the frequency shift changes with $\cos\phi$ to the viewing angle) – and can easily be measured.

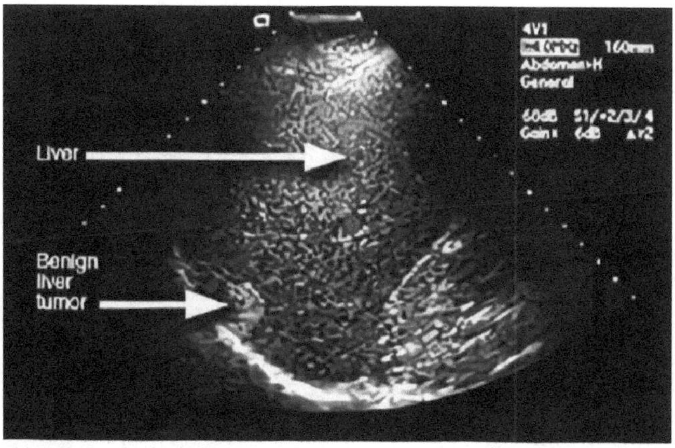

Figure 8.22: Doppler ultrasound.

Side effects

Current evidence indicates that diagnostic ultrasound is safe even when used to visualize the embryo or fetus. In this connection we would like to mention that research in the beginning of 1980s showed that use of clinical ultrasound equipment could result in water radicals (H. and OH.). Furthermore, in work with culture cells exposed to ultrasound resulted in damage (like those known from ionizing radiation).

This implies that if you believe in the LNT-hypothesis where even the smallest radiation dose is deleterious, we have a problem and a possible side effect.

Maybe we should not overdue obstetric ultrasound.

8.12 RADIATION DOSES IN MEDICINE

Each time you are examined by radiation you attain a small radiation dose. The dosesfrom medical use add to the background dose.

In the figure to the right is given the world average use of radiation for medical imaging. It has been a rapid increase since the 1940s. New techniques and methods have been added with the result that the total dose (the collective dose) has increased.

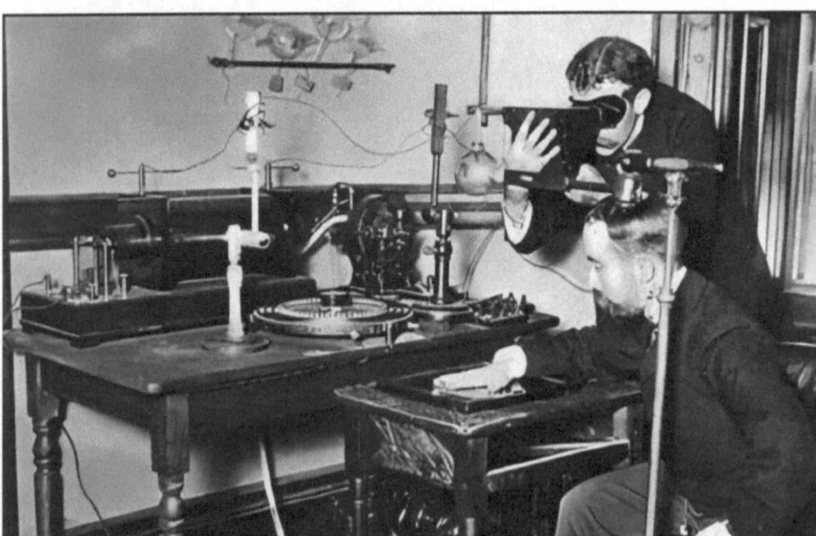

Figure 8.23: The figure shows the use of x-rays for imaging since the start in 1895.

Since the 1950s it has been a goal to keep the doses for each examination as low as possible – to prevent any deleterious effects of radiation.

It may be of interest to attain some information about radiation exposure from diagnostic medical examinations. For this purpose, UNSCEAR have collected a lot of information from all different sources around the world. The Committee concluded that medical applications are the largest man-made source of radiation exposure for the world's population. The doses are in general small and are justified by the benefits of accurate diagnosis of possible disease conditions.

How to observe annual doses?

The dose given in each type of examination has been observed and calculated. Thus, the absorbed dose to each organ or tissue of the body have been obtained. This implies that the effective doses for patients undergoing different types of medical diagnostic have been obtained. Multiplied with the number of examinations yield an effective collective dose in the LNT terminology. From these per capita annual doses can be obtained by averaging the collective doses over the entire population (in-clouding non-exposed individuals).

This procedure yields a world average of 0.4 mSv and for countries like Norway an annual dose per capita of 1.1 mSv.

Will this have deleterious effects?

There is no direct evidence that diagnostic use of radiation ever causing any harm to the public. It is evident that the dose to certain groups of patients may be relatively large, for example for several patients with tuberculosis where chest fluoroscopy was used through 2 – 5 years. Significant doses has also been the result after the use of theorist in the period 1930 – 1950.

However, the collective dose to the public (1.1 mSv to Norwegians) is only a figure that shows the standard of health care and cannot be used to calculate deleterious effects. Some people like the most devoted supporter of the LNT-hypothesis would disagree with this view. According to this hypothesis it is possible to claim that about 250 fatal cancers per year would be the result for Norway with a population of 4.7 million. Do not believe it!

We mentioned two exceptions from the general positive picture. The old use of Thorotrast and the use of fluoroscopy in combination with the pneumothorax treatment for tuberculosis. Let us explore this in some more detail.

Thorotrast

Thorotrast was widely used from 1930 – 1950. It is in the form of thorium dioxide colloid. Thorotrast is retained by the reticuloendothelial system, with a biological half-life of several hundred years, so that such patients suffer lifetime exposure to internal radiation. Some of the decay products, principally the radium isotopes Ra–228 and Ra–224, escape from the colloidal particles and deposit in the skeleton.

The doses involving α-particles may be rather large. The bio- logical endpoints include liver cancer and leukemia and it can be concluded that Thorotrast increased the carcinogenic risk.

Tuberculosis and chest fluoroscopy

In the period 1930 – 1960 many patients with tuberculosis were treated by pneumathorax – air was filled in the cavity of the chest, and the lung was forced to collapse. The aim of the treatment was to give the lungs an opportunity to rest.

To control the air filling the patient was x-rayed both before and after the filling and fluoroscopy was the method. Treatment could last for several years and consequently the number of x-ray examinations could be up to 100 and more. This resulted in a rather large dose to the breasts.

Several TB-patients have been followed up to observe deleterious effects such as breast cancer for women. The results are not easy to understand – see next page.

A Canadian study looked at breast cancer mortality rates for women who had fluoroscopic examinations for tuberculosis, between 1932 and 1952. The results are given in the figure below.

We have several comments regarding this figure. ***First, the dose determination is highly uncertain*** – can probably vary by a factor 2. Second, no information exists about the doses received in the time elapsed since the last examination – i.e. background variation.

Despite these weak points, the data show a surprising decrease in cancer for those who received low doses (34 percent and 16 percent at the dose points of about 15 and 25 centi-Gray).

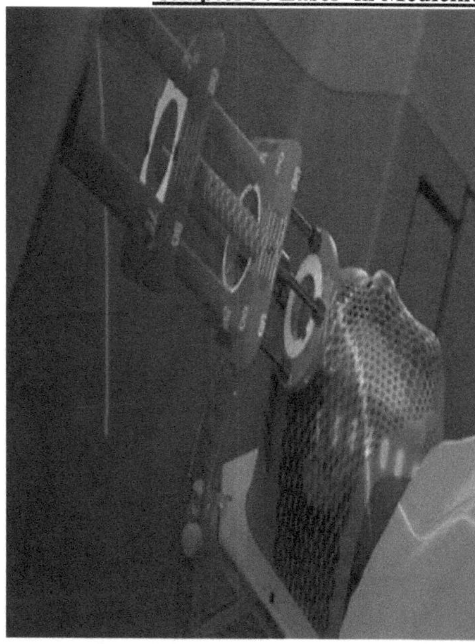

9
CHAPTER

LASER IN MEDICINE

9.1 LASER IN MEDICINE

The use of lasers in medicine began soon the first laser was invented in 1960, when T. H. Maimane produced a laser beam from a ruby crystal.

Laser means light amplification by the stimulation emission of radiation. However, laser light is a unique light source that emits a narrow beam of light of a single wavelength (monochromatic light) in which each wave is in phase with the others near it (coherent light) and collimated beam. These properties make the laser beam a uniquely efficient source of energy. In recent years, the number and variety of applications of laser to biology and medicine have increased rapidly. The laser is based on Einstein's "Theory of Stimulated Emission of Radiation". When an electrical source is directed into the laser optical cavity, which contains the excitation medium, atoms, molecules or ions absorb the thermal, electrical or optical energy.

Electrons are then excited and store an exact Quantum of energy. Atoms in the excited state are unstable and spontaneously emit an equivalent quantity of energy in the form of heat. A small percentage eventually dissipates in the form of heat. A small percentage of spontaneously radiated photons travel along the laser cavity, where they collide with other excited atoms. The collision produces two photons traveling in the same direction and of the same wavelength.

This process is referred to as stimulated emission of radiation (Figure 9.1). The photos resulting from stimulated emission collide with additional excited atoms and more intracavity energy development, as shown in Figure 9.1.

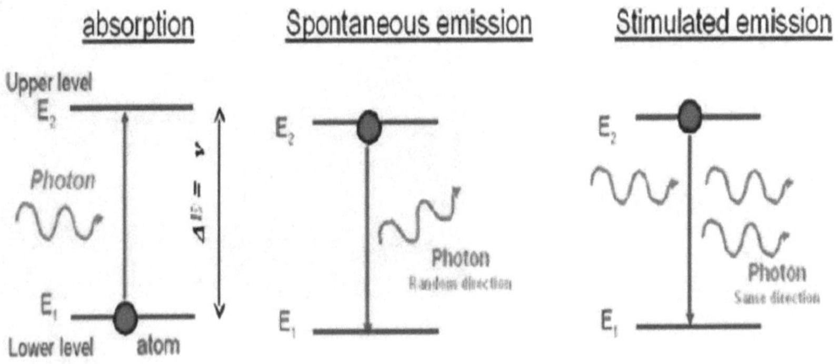

Figure 9.1: Absorption and Emission of photon.

The intensity of the interactivity energy is amplified using parallel mirrors at each end of the cavity, causing even more collisions. A portion of the energy (1 to 20%) is permitted to escape through a partially transparent from mirror (output coupler), as shown in Figure 9.2. The remaining 99 to 80% of light is reflected, and hence the light intensity inside a laser is always higher than the output power.

When an electron makes a transition from higher energy to lower energy state, a photon is emitted. The emission process can be one of two types, spontaneous emission or stimulated emission.

• In spontaneous emission the photon is emitted spontaneously, in a random direction, without external provocation.

• In stimulated emission an incoming photon stimulates the electron to change energy levels. To produce stimulated emission, however, the incoming photon must have energy that exactly matches the difference between the energies of two levels, namely Spontaneously radiated photons travel along the axis of the laser cavity where they collide with other excited atoms. Parallel mirrors at each end of the cavity increase intra-cavity intensity. A portion of light is permitted to escape through the partially transparent front mirror. Laser light is directional or collimated, meaning the beam has low divergence and there is little intensity loss as distance increases.

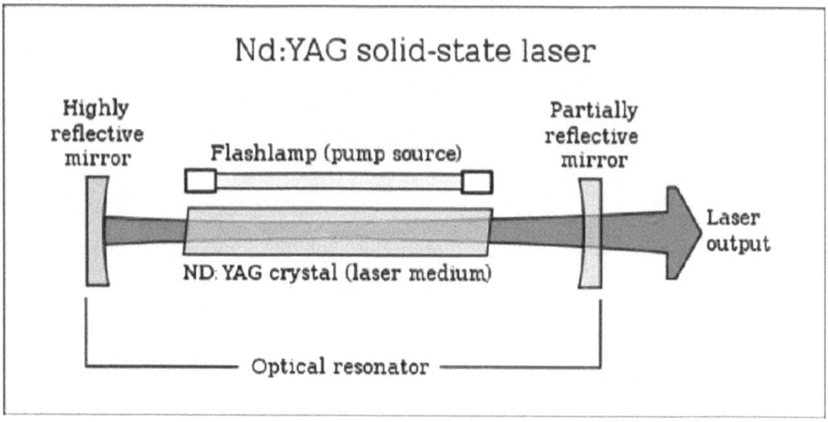

Figure 9.2: Diagrammatic representation of the optical cavity of a laser.

In contrast normal light produces light consisting of photons out of phase with each other (incoherent). It consists of all the colors of the spectrum, with wavelength from 400 nm to 750 nm (Polychromatic) and the light diverges, as shown in Figure 9.3). At 1 m from a filament lamp, the eye receives about 1 millionth of the total light, while the eye can receive 100% of laser light, even at a far distance.

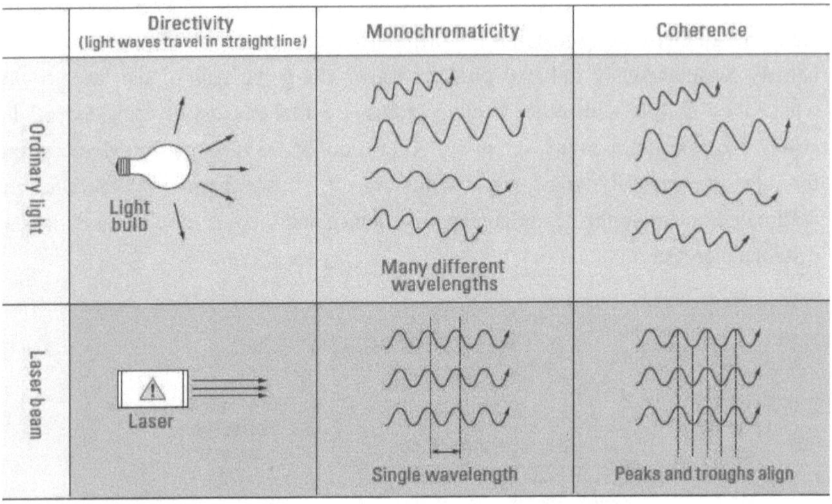

Light produced by lasers is directional, coherent and monochromatic, in contrast normal light is non- directional, incoherent and polychromatic.

Some important points

• **Coherence** is a property of waves that indicates the ability of the waves to interfere with each other. Two waves that are **coherent** can be combined to produce an unmoving distribution of constructive and destructive interference (a visible *interference pattern*) depending on the relative phase of the waves at their meeting point. Waves that are **incoherent**, when combined, produce rapidly moving areas of constructive and destructive interference and therefore do not produce a visible interference pattern.

• **Another way of saying the same thing is that** coherence is a measure of the ability of a light source to produce high contrast interference fringes when the light is interfered with itself in an interferometer. High coherence means high fringe visibility with excellent contrast, (i.e., good black and white fringes, or black and whatever color the light is); low coherence means washed-out fringes, and zero coherence means no fringes.

• **One of the ways of understanding coherence is to predict it.** Suppose one can take a snapshot of the waves and then take another snapshot at a later time. If the two snapshots look almost identical, even with a long-time interval, then we have a high degree of coherence.

• A wave can also be coherent with itself, a property known as **temporal coherence**. If a wave is combined with a delayed copy of itself, the duration of the delay over which it produces visible interference is known as the **coherence time** of the wave, Δt_c. From this, a **corresponding coherence** length l_c, can be estimated as:

$$l_c = \Delta t_c$$

where c is the speed of the light wave.

Coherence time (Δt_c) relates to the finite bandwidth of the source and in general, it is proportional to the bandwidth

$$\Delta t_c \alpha 1/\Delta n$$

where Δ n is the frequency bandwidth. The temporal coherence comes from the monochromaticity of the laser beam. The narrower the line width $\Delta\lambda$ or Δ n of the light source, the better is its temporal coherence.

• If the laser supports the oscillation of multiple longitudinal modes but no higher-order transverse modes, it means that the laser output has finite temporal coherence but perfect spatial coherence. The longitudinal modes in a laser are equally spaced in frequency by c/2L where c is the velocity of light and L is the effective length of the laser resonator. The number of longitudinal modes determines the coherence length of the laser. The relation between the coherence length l_c, the longitudinal mode spacing c/2L and the number of modes N (N>!) is

$$N = [c/2\, l_c\,] / c/2\, L = L/\, l_c$$

• Small coherence lengths are obtained with lasers, which support oscillation over a very wide spectral bandwidth.

• There are certain gas lasers which have very long coherence length of tens of meters, while other lasers, especially Diode lasers have coherence length of the order of millimeters.

• Typically for a commercially available He-Ne laser with 632.8 nm wavelength and 0.01 nm spectral bandwidth, the coherence length is about 4cm or at the most of the order of its resonator because of the presence of many longitudinal modes.

• A frequency stabilized 632.8 nm HeNe laser (a frequency of approximately 473 THz) with a 1 MHz bandwidth would have a coherence length of about 300 meters. In this case, the coherence length is much longer than the length of the cavity because only a single longitudinal is forced to be active at any given time.

• An 800 nm laser diode with a 1 nm spectral width would have a coherence length of about 0.64 mm.

• A 600 nm LED with a spectral width of 60 nm would have a coherence length of around 6 μm.

• He-Ne lasers are also much more spatially coherent than LEDs. LEDs generally have a very short spatial coherence length, typically only a couple of wavelengths.

• In holography, the temporal coherence length determines the maximum depth of the object in a reflection hologram, and the spatial coherence length determines the lateral size. Holography, which is based on interference between light beams, long coherence length enables taking holograms of large bodies, which require greater depth of field. Both the light reflected from the near part of the body, and the light reflected from the far part of the body, will still be coherent with the reference beam.

• Spatial coherence refers to how spherical the wave front is. Does every portion of the wave front appear to have the same center of curvature?

• The requirement for high temporal coherence is in coherent, or heterodyne detection. In these systems, energy reflected off the target is mixed with energy from the original laser to create a fringe pattern. The photos are supposed to maintain the fixed phase relationship for the time needed to hit the target and return in order to have proper contrast in the fringe pattern.

• One of the important applications includes Doppler velocity measurements of the target through the measurements of the frequency shift because of the moving targets. The frequency shift from the target-reflected energy is a function of the target velocity. However, if the frequency of the laser itself is shifting (because of poor coherence) during the time of flight, this creates a broadening or an error in the frequency of the returned beam that limits how accurately one can measure the Doppler velocity.

• Spatial coherence is high for sphere waves and plane waves and is related to the size of the light source. A point source emits spatially coherent light, while the light from a finite source has lower coherence. Spatial coherence can be increased with a **spatial filter**; a very small pinhole preceded by a condenser lens. The spatial coherence of light will increase as it travels away from the source and becomes more like a sphere or plane wave. Light from distant stars, though far from monochromatic, has extremely high spatial coherence.

• Coherence length is defined as the length over which energy in two separate waves remains constant. With respect to the laser, it is the greatest distance between two arms of an interferometric system for which sufficient interferometric effects can be observed.

• Using Michelson Interferometer, one can estimate the coherence length by measuring the maximum path difference between the two beams, which still show the interference pattern.

• Since temporal coherence is a measure of the ability of the radiation to perform interference, because of differences in path lengths between the two beams, it is thus important in interferometry and holography.

• Ordinary light is not coherent because it comes from independent atoms, which emit on time scales of about 10-8 seconds. There is a degree of coherence in sources like the mercury green line and some other useful spectral sources, but their coherence does not approach that of a laser.

Components of atypical LASER

1. The gain medium is a substance that could magnify light through stimulated emission. Light of a particular wavelength is amplified as it travels through the gain medium (increases in power).

2. In order for the medium to amplify light, it must be fed with energy through a process known as pumping. The energy is usually provided in the form of an electric current or a particular wavelength of light.

3. The most common kind of laser receives feedback from an optical cavity, which consists of a pair of mirrors at each end of the gain medium. Light bounces back and forth between the mirrors, passing through the gain medium each time and being amplified.

4. The output coupler, which is usually one of the two mirrors, is partly transparent. This mirror allows some light to escape.

5. The light from the laser may spread out or create a narrow beam, depending on the shape of the cavity (whether the mirrors are flat or curved).

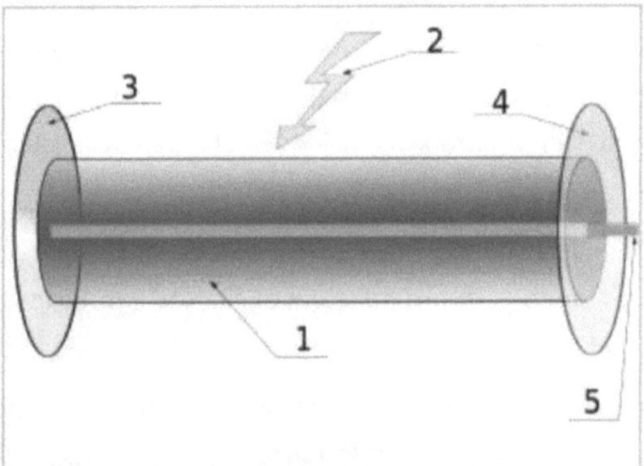

Components of a typical laser:

1. Gain medium
2. Laser pumping energy
3. High reflector
4. Output coupler
5. Laser beam

9.2 IRRADIATION DOSE AND POWER DENSITY OF LASER

Energy contained within light is expressed in joules (J) and its fluency or energy density in joules per square centimeter (J/cm^2). Power is the rate at which work is performed and is measured in watts (W). The power density / irradiance (i.e. light concentration) is the amount of optical energy incident upon a surface, divided by the area of surface being irradiated and is measured in watts per centimeter square (W/cm^2), with the area being defined by the beam spot size (r^2) at the tissue surface. Spreading laser light over a large area leads to a directly proportional reduction in power density as shown in Figure 9.4.

Energy (J) = Power (W) x Time (s) **(9.1)**

Power density (Irradiance) $\left(\frac{W}{cm^2}\right) = \frac{Power\ output\ (W)}{Impact\ spot\ area\ (cm^2)}$ **(9.2)**

The treatment dose is the same as the energy density. Dose refers to the amount of energy per unit area. The dose is the most important treatment parameter. The production of power density and exposure time define the irradiation dose that is measured in J/cm^2. This is an extremely important parameter for laser treatment and biomodulation. Doses that are too low produce no effect, whereas doses that are too high produce no effect or dampen biological activity. Each tissue has an optimal dose that is lases dependent.

Dose (J/cm^2) = Power density (W/cm^2) x Time (s) **(9.3)**

A formula for more formal calculation of energy density (dose) is

Energy density (dose) $(\frac{1}{cm^2}) = \frac{Power\ (W) \times time\ (s)}{Area\ (cm^2)\ of\ spot}$ **(9.4)**

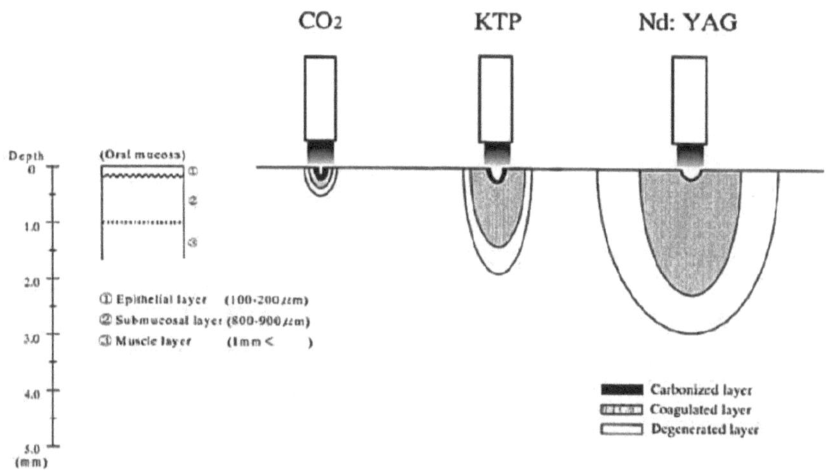

Figure 9. 4: Increasing beam spot size proportionally decreases power density.

Schematic showing a laser beam of 1 W power focused through a lens to a 100 nm spot. As the dimeter of the defocused beam increases, the power density decreases by an inverse square ratio.

9.3 LASER TYPES

Laser consists of three basic components, namely a power source, a lasing or excitation medium and reflecting mirrors (resonating cavity), the generic name of a laser reflects the components/s that make up its active medium, which can be a solid, gas or liquid and determines the wavelength (s) of the radiation produced. Laser light can be described according to whether the beam is continuous (continuous wave, CW), pulsed or quality switched (Q- switched). Lasers that are continuous consist of a constant beam of relatively low steady output power. In pulsed lasers the beam is gated by mechanical shutters or electrically switched, thus the light is emitted in bursts of low energy with peak powers higher than CW. The repetition rate between the pulsed light can be set, typically in the millisecond ranger for surgical lasers and is given in units of pulses per second, or Hertz (Hz).

9.3.1 CO_2 LASERS

A. CO_2 lasers were one of the first gas lasers to be created and is still a powerful laser.

B. CO_2 lasers are the highest-power continuous wave lasers available. They are quite efficient, too.

C. The CO_2 laser produces an infrared beam that has wavelengths centered around 9.6 and 10.6 μm.

Due to water's ability to absorb this light frequency, CO_2 lasers have been helpful in surgical operations. Medical examples include laser surgery and skin resurfacing. It's the best laser for soft tissue with the ability to cut and to control bleeding. photo-thermally CO_2 lasers may replace a scalpel for most operations, and they're even utilized in sensitive regions where mechanical stress might harm the surgical site.

Applications range from gynecology to dentistry, as well as others.

9.3.2 DiodeLASERS

A. Diode lasers are semiconductor deviceslike light-emitting diodes, except that diode lasers are pumped directly with electrical current.

B. Laser diodes can transform electrical energy into light.

C. Diode lasers are finding new applications in dentistry and medicine.

Diode laser is a light emitting diode that uses an optical cavity to amplify the light, which is emitted from an energy band gap that exists in semiconductors. These lasers can be tuned to different wavelengths by varying the applied current , temperature or magnetic field.

They are more appealing to doctors because of their decreased size and price, while also providing increased user friendliness. The wavelengths of diodes vary from 810 to 1,100 nm and are weakly absorbed by soft tissue. Soft tissue is not sliced by the laser's beam but is instead cut by touching a hot charred glass point.

Laser irradiation is very well absorbed at the tip's distal end, heating it to between 500°C and 900°C. The tip is so hot that it may be used to cut delicate tissue and even cauterize or carbonize tissue.

Diode lasers may harm the surrounding tissue if used on soft tissue.

9.3.3 DyeLASERS

A. Dye lasers utilize an organic dye solution as the lasing medium, typically as a liquid.

B. Dye lasing medium typically allows the use of a considerably broader range of wavelengths, which may cover 50 to 100 nanometers or more.

C. The broad bandwidth is excellent for tunable lasers and pulsed lasers. With light adjusted from red to yellow, pulses may be produced as brief as 16 femtoseconds.

D. Another kind of dye may be used to produce more wavelengths from the near-infrared to the near-ultraviolet, although this typically involves changing other optical components, such as dielectric mirrors or pump lasers.

MEDICAL OPTICS

Day laser is the use of_an excitation medium in a liquid suspension in the dye cell. Dye lasers can be tuned to several wavelengths by changing the chemical composition of the dye.

Dye lasers has many applications in medicine, including dermatology, where they are used to level skin tone. The large wavelength range enables an accurate match to specific tissue spectra, such as melanin or hemoglobin, but the narrow bandwidth makes the surrounding tissue less susceptible to harm.

Port-wine stains, scars, and kidney stones are often treated with these kinds of lasers. They are also often used for tattoos removal and in many other purposes.

Laser beams of various wavelengths, powers, and optical properties are used in cosmetology, diagnostics, surgery, and various other medical procedures. The treatment of certain disorders by laser light is controversial. In **ophthalmology** laser are primarily used for **photocoagulation** of retina, that is, heating a blood vessel to the point where the blood coagulates and block the vessel. The minimum amount of laser energy that will do observable damage to the retina is called the Minimal Reactive Dose (MRD), as shown in Figure 9.5.

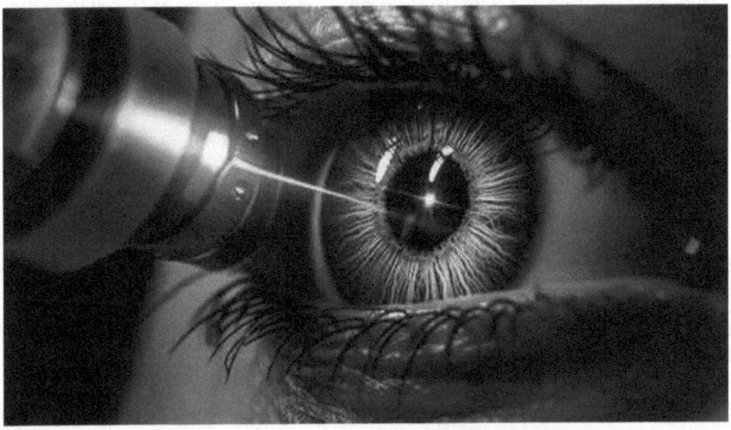

Figure 9.5: Laser beams are almost parallel thus the eye's lens will focus them down to a small spot causing retinal burns.

9.3.4 Ruby laser is a solid- state laser that uses a synthetic ruby crystal as its gain medium. The first working laser was a ruby laser made by Theodore H Maimane at Hughes Research Laboratories on May 16, 1960. Ruby lasers produce pulses of coherent visible light at a wavelength of 694.3 nm, which is a deep red color. A ruby laser most often consists of a ruby rob that must be pumped with very high energy, usually from a flashtube to achieve a population inversion. The rod is often placed between two mirrors, forming an optical cavity, which oscillates the light produced by the ruby florescence, causing stimulated emission.

9.3.5 He- Ne laser is a gas laser which consists of an excitation medium of gas contained in a tube in the optical cavity. When voltage is applied, the atoms in the gas are excited and light is emitted from the output coupler.

Photocoagulation is useful for repairing tears or holes that develop prior to retinal detachment. When the retina is completely detached, the laser is of no help. A complication of diabetes that affects the retina, called **diabetic retinopathy**, can also be treated with photocoagulation.

9.4 LASER INTERACTIONWITH BIOLOGICAL TISSUE

A laser beam is created and directed towards tissue to accomplish a particular job. When energy hits the biological contact, it will interact in one of four ways: reflection, transmission, scattering, or absorption.

• Absorption - Photons are absorbed by certain molecules in the tissue known as chromospheres. To do function, the light energy is transformed into various kinds of energy.

• Reflection occurs when the laser beam bounces off the surface without any penetration or contact. Reflection is often an undesirable result; however, a beneficial example of reflection may be seen when Erbium lasers reflect off titanium, allowing for safe gingiva cutting around implant abutments.

• Transmission is the ability of laser energy to penetrate through superficial tissues and interact with deeper regions. Retinal surgery is an example; the laser treats the retina by passing through the lens. Tissue transmission may also be observed in the deeper penetration achieved with diode lasers.

• Scattering - When laser energy reaches the target tissue, it scatters in a variety of ways. This phenomenon is generally ineffective, but it may be beneficial with specific wavelengths' bio stimulative characteristics.

When laser light strikes a tissue, some of it reflected, while some are absorbed, scattered, or transmitted. A change in the air and tissue (refractive index) produces this phenomenon. Figure 9.6 illustrates this phenomenon. The process obeying the law of Snell:

$$\frac{Sin\ \theta_1}{Sin\ \theta_2} = \frac{n_1}{n_2} \qquad (9.5)$$

Where θ_1 is the angle between surface nor mall in air and the light, θ_2 is the angle between surface normal in the tissue and the ray, n_1 is the refraction index of air, and n_2 is the refraction index of the tissue.

A)

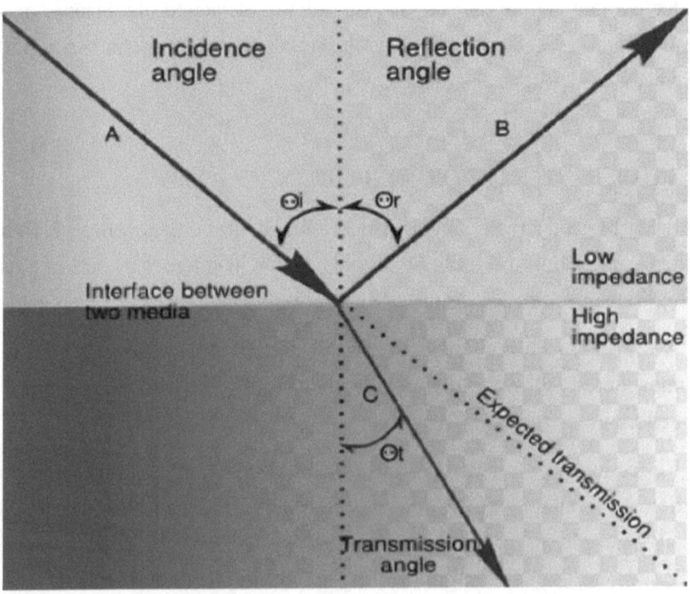

B)

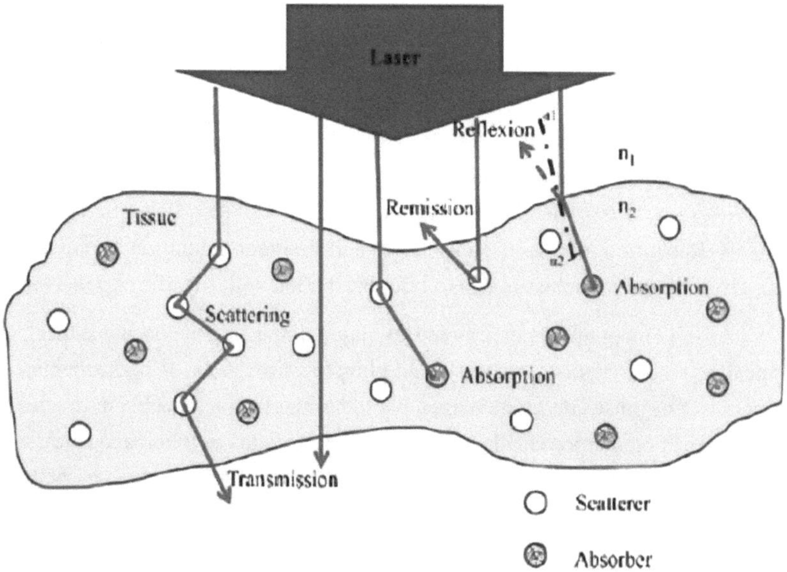

Figure 9.6: Laser light striking a tissue. A) Snell's' law of reflection. B) laser light behavior in a tissue.

The tissue absorbs most of the light, and the energy states of the molecules become quantized. Therefore, photon absorption arises only when its energy becomes equal to the energy difference between such quantized states. This absorption phenomenon creates the desired effect in the tissue. The coefficient (cm^{-1}) characterizes the absorption. The inverse defines the penetration depth (mean free path) into the absorbing medium.

A tissue's scattering behavior is important because it determines the volume of light interaction, which is following by absorption. Scattering of a photon is associated with a propagation expressed by the scattering coefficient (cm^{-1}). The inverse parameter, 1/(cm), is the mean free path length until the next scattering event occurs.

The sum of absorption and scatters, is called extinction, and the relation between absorption (A) and transmission (T), is given by the equation:

$$A = T^{-1} \tag{9.6}$$

9.4.1 Laser – tissue interactions depend on the interplay of irradiation parameters, which are:

i- Wavelength or wavelength band of a laser source.

ii- The physical properties of the irradiated tissue by a particular wavelength or wavelength band irradiance or pulse energy.

iii-Continuous or pulsed laser light wave.

iv-Beam size of the laser on the tissue.

v- Repetition rate, laser pulse length and irradiation duration, or any physical property changes in the tissue due to laser irradiation with specific parameters.

At low energies and/or irradiances, laser tissue interaction are either purely optical or a combination of optical and photobiostimulative or photochemical. As laser power or pulse energy increases, photothermal interactions begin to dominate. Eventually, potomemechaical (sometimes referred to as photoacoustic) effects become apparent when repetitive very short laser pulses are conveyed to the tissue.

Thus, there are five interaction mechanisms associated with the use of lasers in biomedicine, these are:

i- Purely optical, such as fluorescence spectroscopy for cancer screening and high- resolution imaging for optical coherence tomography.

ii- Photochemical (target cells undergo light- induced chemical reactions) such as photodynamic therapy, and photobiostimulative such as laser acupuncture.

iii- Photoablative that causes photodissociation such as molecular bond breaking in tissue.

iv-Photothermal that converts light energy into heat energy, which causes vapourising and heating of a tissue. For example, laser assisted refraction correction by ablation of parts of the cornea as well as for tattoo removal.

v- Photomechanical (photo- acoustic) that induces dielectric breakdown in tissue that is caused by shock wave plasma expanding that results in a localized mechanical rupture, such as laser lithotripsy.

vi-LASER effects on biological tissue

The thermal effect of lasers on biological tissue is a complex process resulting from three distinct phenomena.

1. conversion of light to heat,
2. transfer of heat

3. and the tissue reaction, which is related to the temperature and the heating time.

This interaction leads to denaturation or to the destruction of tissue. The known factors are the parameters of the laser (wavelength, power, time and mode of emission, beam profile and spot size) and the tissue being treated (optical coefficients, thermal parameters and coefficients of the reaction of thermal denaturation).

Laser absorbed by tissue may cause; (Thermal effects).

1. Homeostasis: Any procedure that stop bleeding.
2. Photocoagulation: Heating a blood vessel to point where the blood coagulates and blocks the vessel.
3. Photo Vaporization: To make incisions and vaporize tissue.
4. Sonic: Membrane disruption.

Laser Beam Delivery to Tissue

Laser beams are typically very well collimated. Diffraction causes light waves to spread transversely as they propagate, and it is therefore impossible to have a perfectly collimated beam. The diffraction-limited divergence angle of a Gaussian beam with diameter D and wavelength λ is $\Theta = 4 \cdot \lambda/\Pi \cdot D$. As an example, for an Argon laser emitting a 1 mm wide beam at 515 nm wavelength, the divergence (half-angle Q) is about 0.66 Mrad, ie, the beam spreads by 1.3 mm over a distance of 1 meter.

Using a lens or a concave mirror with focal length f, a laser beam can be focused to a spot with a diameter $d = (4 \cdot f/\Pi \cdot D)\lambda$. The depth of the focal region is: $F = (8 \cdot f^2/\Pi \cdot D^2)\lambda$ (Figure 4). With a f=25 mm lens the same Argon laser beam can be focused to a spot of 16 mm in diameter, having a focal depth of 820mm. It must be emphasized though that exact definition of the spot size depends on the beam profile, which varies in various configurations of laser cavities. For therapeutic laser photocoagulation such tight focusing is usually not required, and laser spots typically vary in diameter between 50 and 500 mm in various applications.

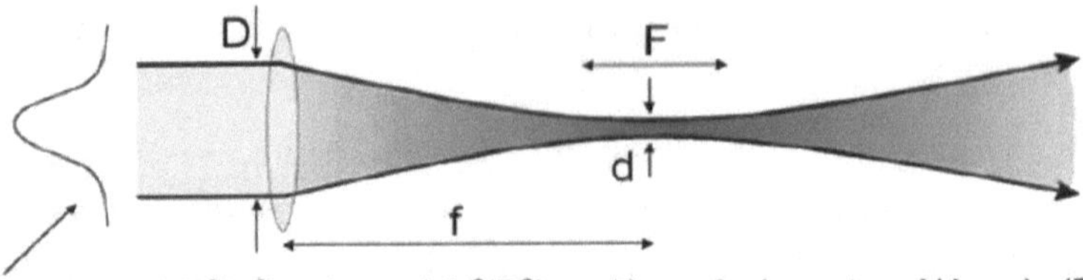

$I(r) = I_0 \exp(-2r^2/w^2) = I_0 \exp(-8r^2/D^2)$ Numerical aperture $NA = \sin (D/2f)$

For a Gaussian laser beam:

Diameter of the focal spot

$$d = \frac{4 \cdot f}{\pi \cdot D} \lambda \cong \frac{2 \cdot \lambda}{\pi \cdot NA}$$

Focal depth

$$F = \frac{8 \cdot f^2}{\pi \cdot D^2} \lambda \cong \frac{2 \cdot \lambda}{\pi \cdot NA^2}$$

Figure 9.7: Laser beam focusing.

As an alternative to a free-propagating beam, laser light can be transported via optical fibers. An optical fiber, schematically shown in Figure 5, typically consists of a core, cladding, and jacket. Light is trapped within the core due to total internal reflection at the interface of core with cladding. To satisfy conditions of total internal reflection, the incidence angle of light at the core/cladding interface should not exceed the critical angle of total internal reflection: $\sin \Theta_{cr} = n_{core}/n_{clad}$, where n_{core} and n_{clad} are refractive indices of the core and cladding, respectively. To satisfy these criteria for total internal reflection, the light should be launched within a so-called acceptance cone, and the sine of its half-angle Θ_{ac} is defined as the numerical aperture (NA) of the fiber: NA = $\sin \Theta_{ac}$ = square root of n^2_{core} - n^2_{clad}.

Typically, the NA is within a range of 0.1-0.2. Optical fibers are often used for delivery of laser light to slit-lamp-based systems and to the intraocular surgical probes.

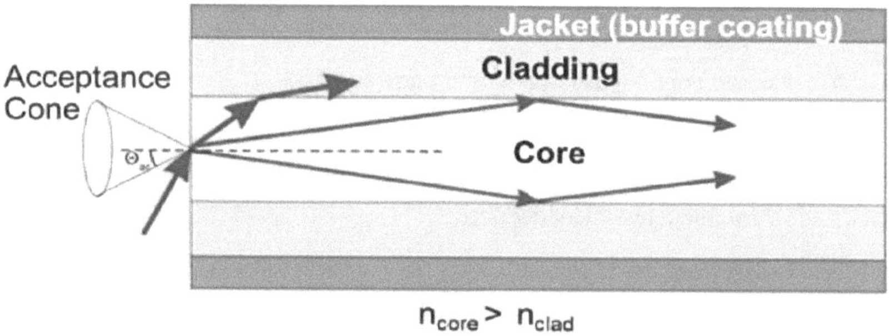

Figure 9.8: Fiber delivery of the laser beam.

Medical applications of LASER

1. Ophthalmology:

a. In ophthalmology lasers is primarily used for photocoagulation of the retina.

b. The amount of laser energy needed for photocoagulation depends on the spot size used.

In general, the minimum amount of laser energy that will do observable damage to the retina is called the Minimal Reactive Dose (MRD).

• Photocoagulation is useful for;

I. Repairing retinal tears or holes.

II. Diabetic retinopathy. (Complication of diabetes that affects the retina)

2. Dermatology:

a. Skin tumor therapy has been attempted by using high energy Focused laser beam.

b. Tattoos removal.

3. Dentistry:

a. Repairing the teeth decay.

b. Bleeding of gums.

c. Ulcers of the gums

4. **Surgery:**

a. Its used continuous lasers of high power.

Example: In Vascular organs such as the liver normal surgery produces a large amount of bleeding. The focused beam of light from laser tends to seal of the vessels and very much less bleeding occurs.

b. Lasers may be combined with fiber optics for some kinds of internal treatment. Example: Lasers are used through gastroscopy in treating stomach ulcers and bleeding

AdvantagesofLASERSurgery

1. No-touch technique.
2. Dry surgical field.
3. Reduced blood loss.
4. Reduced edema.
5. Limited fibrosis and stenosis.
6. Precision.
7. Reduced post-operative pain.
8. It is effective, fast, safe.
9. Painless during its use especially when it is used in eye and dental treatment.
10. Anesthesia is not indicated in eye or dental or some other treatments.

10

CHAPTER

LASERS WITH BIOLOGICAL TISSUES

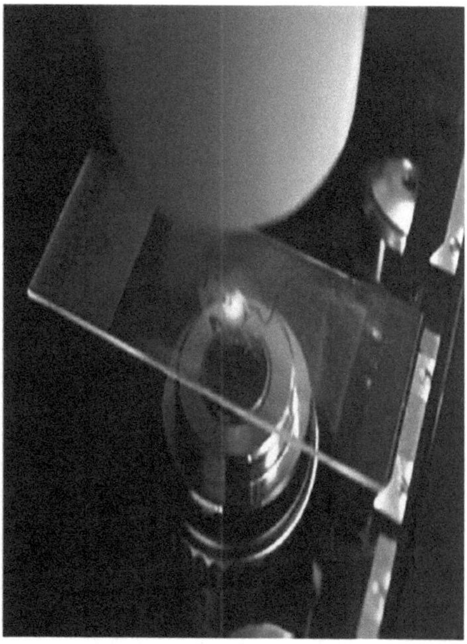

10.1 INTERACTIONS OF LASERS WITH BIOLOGICAL TISSUES

Biological tissues are optically turbid materials: absorption and scattering dominate the interactions of these media, thus enabling an energy transfer process from the laser source to the tissue. The capability of laser light to penetrate a tissue and deposit energy within its volume is the key to numerous therapeutic applications: lasers can be employed to precisely deliver an energy dose to a selected target volume within an organ, e.g. to destroy malignant tissue. In these applications, the spatial distribution of energy induced by the laser is essential for the purpose of predicting successful treatment. Such distribution is described by the volumetric energy density Ev ($J \cdot m^{-3}$) and depends on the incident wavelength as well as on the optical properties of the target.

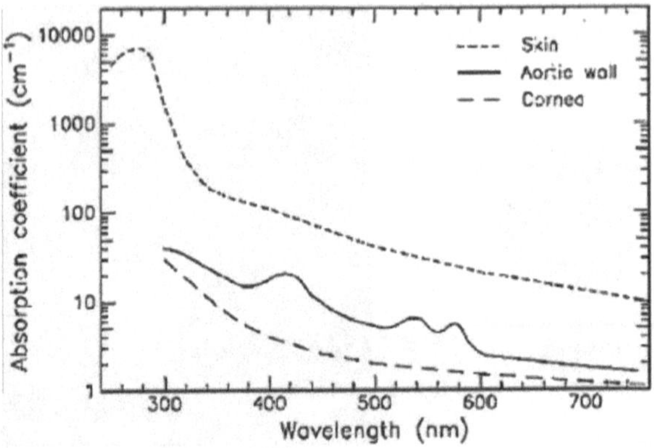

Figure10.1: Wavelength-dependency of the absorption coefficients of skin, aortic wall, and cornea. Reproduced from with kind permission from Springer Science+Business Media.

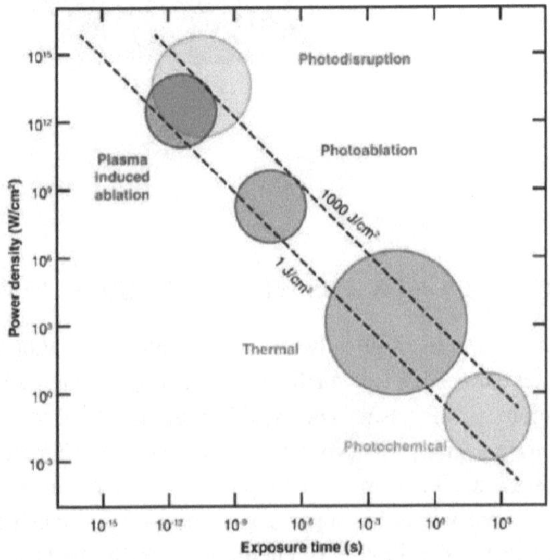

Figure 10.2: Classification of thermal laser-tissue interaction types. Reproduced from with kind permission from Springer Science+Business Media.

Relevant optical properties of tissues include the coefficients of absorption μa (m^{-1}) and scattering μs (m^{-1}). The former determines the fraction of incident energy absorbed by the tissue; the latter is related to how deep laser radiation penetrates the tissue. Both coefficients are determined by the molecular composition of the target. Because different molecules respond selectively to different wavelengths, these coefficients are wavelength-dependent: for instance, Fig. 10.1 presents the absorption spectra of three different types of human tissues, namely skin, aortic wall and cornea. In the considered range of wavelengths, skin presents the largest absorption due to the presence of melanin molecules, which are known to strongly absorb radiation in the visible range (wavelength: 400–780 nm). The absorption of aortic tissue is characterized by hemoglobin, which is also a strong absorber in this range. Conversely, cornea does not have any constituent that presents a significant absorbance, thus resulting almost transparent. In general, different types of tissues present different absorption and scattering coefficients. Numerous works report tabulated values of these coefficients sampled on various tissues and for different wavelengths. Nonetheless, slight variations from the reported values may be observed in practice, due to the inherent inhomogeneity of biological tissues: these may present variations in blood content, water content, fiber development, etc.

Laser energy can act on tissues, inducing alterations at the physical and chemical levels. Diverse effects can be produced, depending on the optical properties of tissues discussed above, as well as on the properties that characterize the laser beam: wavelength, beam intensity and waist. Another important parameter is the total time of laser exposure: this is often used in conjunction with the beam intensity to classify laser-tissue interactions, as shown in Fig. 10.2. Five main interaction classes can be distinguished, namely photo disruption, plasma-induced ablation, photo ablation, thermal interactions and photochemical interactions. It is interesting to observe all these interactions occur for similar values of the applied energy density, i.e. between 1 and 1000 $J \cdot cm^{-2}$. This result shows the practical importance of exposure time, which can be tuned to selectively enable a specific interaction.

To this dissertation, we shall focus on thermal interactions. For further details on the other types of interactions, the reader is referred to.

10.2 THERMAL INTERACTIONS

Thermal interactions constitute a large group of interaction types, characterized by irradiations longer than 1 μs and shorter than 1 min. During these interactions, laser energy is absorbed by the tissue under the form of heat, thereby determining a local increase of temperature. As we shall see later on, several different effects can be produced on tissue, depending on the duration and peak value of temperature achieved. These effects range from hyperthermia (45°C) to vaporization (100 °C) and carbonization (>100 °C).

In the scope of laser surgery, laser-induced thermal effects are especially of importance. Vaporization is the process by means of which laser incisions are conducted: because soft tissues are largely composed by water, their molecules start to evaporate at approximately 100 °C, determining a material removal (ablation) process. Although some laser-induced effects are advantageous, others are considered detrimental. It it the case of carbonization that occurs at temperatures above 100 °C. Carbonization determines the formation of scar tissue, thus diminishing the quality of the surgical procedure. It is important to note that temperature is the parameter that governs the onset of these effects. Therefore, for the purpose of understanding the diverse thermal effects that lasers can produce on tissues, we must establish a model for the spatial and temporal evolution of tissue temperature during laser irradiation. In the following paragraphs we derive the equations that govern the generation of heat within the tissue and see how the generation of heat is related to the variation of temperature. Then, we will review and discuss the diverse thermal effects that lasers can produce on tissues.

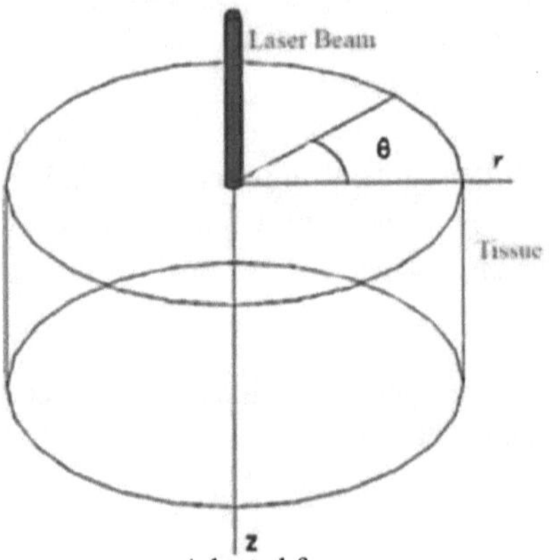

Figure 10.3: Tissue geometry. Adapted from.

Let us consider a sample of homogeneous tissue exposed to a TEM00 laser beam, as depicted in Fig. 10.3. For the sake of simplicity, we assume that the surface of tissue exposed to the beam is plain and normally oriented with respect to it. A cylindrical reference frame (r,ϑ,z) is used to describe the tissue geometry, with z being coincided with the beam axis and r representing the radial distance with respect to such axis. Without any loss of generality, cylindrical symmetry is assumed. The beam intensity inside the tissue is then described by Niemz:

$$I(r,z,t) = I_0 \exp\left(-\frac{2r^2}{\omega^2} - \mu_a z\right) \exp\left(\frac{-8t^2}{\tau^2}\right), \qquad (10.1)$$

where I0 is the beam intensity incident on the surface of tissue, μa is the coefficient of absorption of the tissue, ω is the beam waist, t is the total exposure time and τ is the pulse duration. This model of intensity does not consider the effect of scattering, which can be neglected for most practical applications on soft tissues. One important parameter associated with the spatial distribution of intensity within the tissue is the absorption length, defined as the inverse of the absorption coefficient μa:

$$L = \frac{1}{\mu_a}. \qquad (10.2)$$

The absorption length measures the distance, along the beam axis z, at which the intensity has dropped to 1 / e of its incident value I0.

The rate of heat generation within the tissue $S(r, z, t)$ ($W \cdot m^{-3}$) is proportional to the intensity I, with the coefficient of absorption μa being the proportional factor:

$$S(r,z,t) = \mu_a I(r,z,t). \qquad (10.3)$$

Having identified a model for the rate of heat generation, we now focus on the equations that permit quantify the consequent variation of temperature. If neither phase transitions (e.g. vaporization) nor tissue alterations (e.g. coagulation) occur, a basic law of thermodynamics can be used to model the change of temperature *d*T related to a variation of heat content *d*Q:

$$dT = \frac{dQ}{mc}, \qquad (10.4)$$

where m is the mass of tissue, and c is its specific heat capacity, expressed in $J \cdot kg^{-1} \cdot K^{-1}$. A variation of heat content can occur either because of the energy deposited by the heat source (Eq. 10.3) or due to heat conduction, i.e. the variation of heat content per unit of volume ($\dot{q}$), which is the primary mechanism by which heat is transferred to tissue structures not reached by the laser radiation. Other heat losses such as heat convection and heat radiation can be neglected in first approximation.

It can be shown, by means of the equation of continuity and the general diffusion equation, that the volumetric variation of heat $\dot{q}$depends on the temperature by the following relation:

$$\dot{q} = k\Delta T \tag{10.5}$$

where Δ is the Laplace operator and k is the tissue heat conductivity, expressed in W · m · K. Combining Eq. 10.5 into Eq. 10.4 yields:

$$\dot{T} = \frac{1}{mc}\dot{Q} = \frac{1}{\rho c}\frac{\dot{Q}}{V} = \frac{1}{\rho c}\dot{q} = \frac{1}{\rho c}k\Delta T \tag{10.6}$$

where V is the volume of the tissue (m3), ρ is the tissue density (kg · m−3) and c is its specific heat capacity (J · kg−1 K−1). Equation 10.6 can be extended to account for the heat generated by the laser:

$$\dot{T} = \frac{1}{\rho c}(k\Delta T + S). \tag{10.7}$$

Using the Laplace operator for the cylindrical reference frame, we obtain:

$$\dot{T} = \kappa\left(\frac{\partial^2}{\partial r^2} + \frac{\partial^2}{r\,\partial r} + \frac{\partial^2}{\partial z^2}\right)T + \frac{1}{\rho c}S \tag{10.8}$$

Here, *k* is the temperature conductivity of tissue, which relates both constants, the specific heat capacity (k) and the heat conductivity (c). Azimuth symmetry is evidenced in the expression above. Exact solution of this inhomogeneous differential equation is rather complex. It involves the use of several approximations and assumptions. Numerical methods are commonly used to solve the time-dependent function that describes the temperature *T*(*r*, *z*, *t*).

The diffusion of heat within tissue during laser irradiation is described by the thermal penetration depth dtherm:

$$d_{\text{therm}} = \sqrt{4\kappa t}. \tag{10.9}$$

Analogously to the optical absorption length (Eq. 10.2), this term quantifies the depth at which the temperature has dropped to 1 / e of the superficial value, i.e. with respect to $T(z = 0)$. Equating the optical absorption length with the thermal penetration depth, we obtain the following time-dependent relation:

$$\frac{1}{\mu_a} = \sqrt{4\kappa t} \qquad (10.10)$$

Their solution T_{therm} is called thermal relaxation time. This quantity gives an indication of how quickly a tissue dissipates the heat generated by a laser. For laser exposures shorter than T_{therm}, we have that $L > d_{therm}$, i.e. the diffusion of heat is contained in the volume reached by the laser radiation. By contrast, exposure times longer than T_{therm} determine a significant diffusion of heat also to surrounding tissues, which are not under direct laser irradiation. As we shall see in the following, this result has great practical relevance: it gives a criterion for the selection of the laser exposure time, based on the thermal effects one wants to achieve.

Table 10.1 Thermal effects of laser radiation on tissues. Reproduced from with kind permission from Springer Science + Business Media.

Temperature (°C)	Biological effect
37	None
45	Hyperthermia
50	Reduction in enzyme activity, cell immobility
60	Denaturation of proteins and collagen, coagulation
80	Permeabilization of membranes
100	Vaporization
> 100	Carbonization
> 300	Melting

Having established the equations that govern the thermal response of tissues subject to laser irradiation, we now focus on the different biological effects that a thermal interaction may produce. Depending on the duration and peak value of temperature achieved, different effects like coagulation, vaporization, carbonization, and melting may be distinguished. These effects are listed in Table 10.1, together with the temperature at which they occur. Elevating the temperature of tissue up to 60 °C does not induce any permanent alteration, given that this condition is maintained for a time duration in the range of seconds. Above 60 °C, coagulation occurs. This is a form of irreversible tissue necrosis which causes cells to cease their function. A phase transition is induced at 100 °C: this is temperature at which the free water molecules in the tissue start to vaporize. As the volume of water tends to increase during the transition, a pressure build up occurs. Increasing pressure eventually leads to micro explosions that tear up the fabric of tissue and produce craters. In the literature, this process is commonly referred to as thermal decomposition. Another effect that may occur during thermal interaction is carbonization. This occurs when the tissue temperature rises above 100 °C, i.e. when laser irradiation continues after the water content of tissue has been completely evaporated.

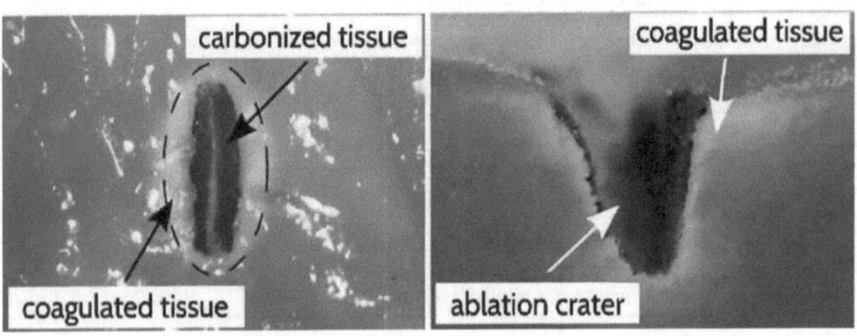

Figure 10.3: Thermal effects of CO_2 laser radiation on soft tissue. Here, the same tissue specimen is shown from a top view (left) and cross-section (right) perspective.

Material ablation can be observed in correspondence with the laser incision line. Dark areas on the edges of the ablation crater indicate that temperatures over 100 °C have been reached, resulting in the carbonization of tissue. Coagulation can also be observed in the surroundings of the laser incision site. The volumetric extent of coagulation has been highlighted in the cross-section image using a fluorescent light source

Medical applications of lasers typically aim to induce one specific thermal effect on tissue. Vaporization is exploited in laser surgery to create ablations and produce incisions on tissue. In practice, several thermal effects might occur simultaneously, depending on the parameters that characterize laser irradiation. The location and extent of each effect follow the spatial distribution of temperature produced during and after the laser exposure. The coincidence of diverse thermal artifacts is represented in Fig. 10.3, which shows a sample laser incision produced with a CO_2 laser on ex-vivo chicken muscle tissue. The incision line was created through repeated scans of the laser beam: the high temperatures induced in correspondence of the laser incidence points determined the ablation of tissue. Carbonized tissue can be recognized in the surroundings of the incision crater, where the temperature of tissue has risen above 100 °C. These areas appear darker in color with respect to normal tissue. Visual inspection of a broader area around the incision line reveals the presence of coagulated tissue. A temperature below 100 °C has been induced in these areas by means of heat conduction.

10.3 APPLICATIONS TO CLINICAL SURGERY

Lasers are employed in several surgical specialties as cutting tools. Their use has gained popularity in those procedures where high accuracy is required, e.g. for the surgical treatment of glottis cancer. With respect to traditional cutting tools, lasers present numerous advantages: they operate in a contact-less fashion, thus ensuring sterile conditions on the surgical site. In surgery of soft tissues, lasers can be tuned to simultaneously cut and coagulate blood, thus preventing excessive blood losses and limiting the need to resort to transfusions; this hemostatic effect further allows to keep the surgical site clean, enhancing the surgeon's assessment of the state of tissues. Furthermore, lasers have enabled the development of new surgical techniques, such as the piece-wise tumor resection introduced by Steiner, which would have been impossible without a tool able to cut and coagulate surrounding tissues at the same time.

The knowledge of the absorbing and scattering properties of tissues is of paramount importance in laser surgery. Clinicians seek to create clean ablations with minimal thermal damage to surrounding tissues. The selection of a laser source with an appropriate wavelength is an essential prerequisite to achieve these goals. The CO_2 laser is often indicated for surgery of soft tissues. These are rich in water, which is a strong absorber of the infrared radiation emitted by this class of lasers (wavelength: 10.6 μm). Alternatively, the solid-state Er:YAG laser (wavelength: 2940 nm) is recommended for the ablation of bony tissue.

For surgical applications of lasers, carbonization of tissues surrounding the ablation site should be minimized as much as possible. It represents a non-intentional damage where healthy tissue that should have been preserved is being compromised, i.e. burned. Carbonization causes a longer recovery time for the patient and may leave scars, diminishing the quality of the procedure. One common strategy to limit the extent of carbonization consists in the selection of laser exposure times shorter than the thermal relaxation time of tissue. In most soft tissues, laser irradiations shorter than 1 μs do not produce significant thermal damage (this simple practical result is referred to as the "1 μs rule"). State-of-the-art CO_2 surgical lasers present minimum pulse durations of a few hundred microseconds, thus potentially enabling thermal damage of surrounding tissues.

Laser surgery requires dexterity to control the laser effects on tissues in order to obtain appropriate global results. These aspects will be discussed in detail in the next chapter. We shall see how the equipment currently in use for laser microsurgeries gives little support to clinicians to detect and understand the effects of laser actions.

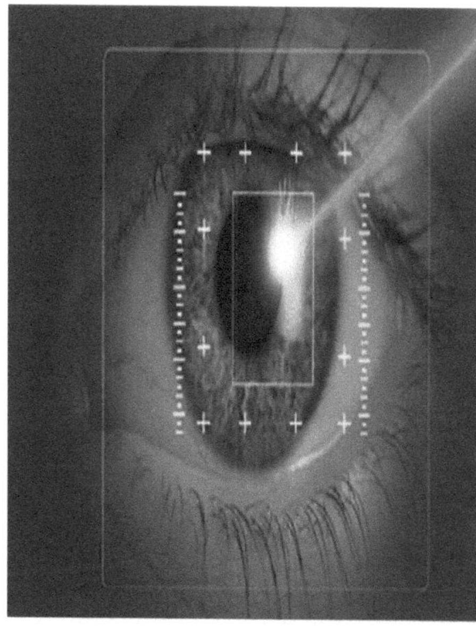

11 CHAPTER

SURGICAL APPLICATIONS OF LASERS

11.1 LASERS IN OPHTHALMOLOGY

Ophthalmology is a branch of medicine and surgery which deals with the diagnosis and treatment of eye disorders. Ophthalmologists are allowed to use medications to treat eye diseases, implement laser therapy, and perform surgery when needed. Lasers have particular use in ophthalmology because the eye can be used as an optical device. The transparency of the front part of the eye, the cornea, allows light such as LASER to reach almost all the tissues of the eye. *Lasers Used.*

Argon blue-green laser (70% blue (488 nm) and 30% green (514nm)).

Frequency-doubled Nd-YAG Laser (532 nm) -treatment of many retinal conditions' proliferative diabetic retinopathy, diabetic macular edema, vein occlusions.

Krypton red (647 nm) - treatment of sub retinal neovascular membrane. Diode laser (805-810 nm) -treatment of Retinopathy of Prematurity (ROP).

MEDICAL OPTICS

Nd:YAG LASER (1064 nm)-produce photo disruption in the eye for the treatment of acute angle closure glaucoma.

Absorption Spectrum

- Melanin absorption in 400-700nm
- Deoxyhemoglobin 555nm
- Oxyhemoglobin 542nm, 577nm
- Xanthophyll < 500nm

Effects of Laser Effects Eye

- Laser coagulation- Thermal effect of the laser radiation is used, therapeutic effect in vascular pathology of the eye: laser coagulation of vessels of iris, cornea, retina, trabeculoplasty, and the effects on the cornea with infrared radiation (1,54-2,9 m), which is absorbed by the stroma of the cornea, to change the refraction. Commonly used is an argon laser.
- Photodestruction (photodiscision) -Dissection of tissues using high peak power of Laser.

Based on an electro "breakdown" of tissue that occurs due to the release of large amounts of energy in a limited volume. In this case, at the point the laser plasma is formed, and this leads to the creation of a shock wave and of microscopic tearing of tissue. Infrared YAG-laser utilized.

Photoevaporation and photoincision - Effect is based on prolonged heat exposure to the evaporation of tissue. Used for this purpose infrared CO_2 laser (10.6 m) to remove surface formations of the conjunctiva and eyelids.

Photoablation (photodecomposition) - Based on the removal of biological tissue. It is an excimer laser operating in the hard UV range (193 nm). Application: refractive surgery, treatment of degenerative changes in corneal opacities, inflammatory disease of the cornea, and glaucoma

Laser stimulation - Low-intensity red light He-Ne-laser. Found that the interaction of radiation with various tissues from complex photochemical processes are shown anti- inflammatory, desensitizing, resolving effects.

11.1.1 Photorefractive Keratomy

It corrects refractive vision errors by changing the shape of the cornea. It alters the contours of the cornea so that it bends light correctly. It is an effective treatment myopia (nearsightedness), hyperopia (farsightedness) and/or astigmatism. PRK completely removes the epithelium to access the cornea, and then the epithelium grows back. It utilizes a type of laser called an excimer laser (Cold UV).

11.1.2 Radial Keratomy

A surgical procedure used to decrease nearsightedness. During the procedure, radial incisions are made in the cornea of the eye with a highly precise diamond blade set to a particular depth. The number of incisions and their location is determined by the degree of nearsightedness. These incisions allow the sides of the cornea to bugle outward and thereby flatten the central portion of the cornea. This brings the focal point of the eye closer to the retina and improves one's distance vision.

11.1.3 Astigmatism Coorrection

Excimer laser can be used to reduce astigmatism when performing LASIK or PRK surgery. The degree of astigmatism currently approved for correction is 0.75 D to 4.0 D. Astigmatism measurements describe to what degree the cornea is non-spherical. The excimer laser reduces the degree of astigmatism by removing corneal tissue in an asymmetric manner. This is accomplished by utilizing an oval-shaped laser beam.

11.1.4 Laser Iridotmy

The technique creates a bypassing hole in the iris to allow fluid trapped behind it to flow to the AC. Fluid blockage occurs due to closure of the ACA or to pupillary block. Argon and Nd:YAG lasers can be used — separately or in combination. Laser parameters for the argon laser are energy = 800 to 1000 mW, diameter = 50 μm, and exposure time = 0.1 sec. A total of 40 to 80 applications is used. For the Nd:YAG laser, energy = 3 to 7 mJ, and four to ten applications are used.

11.1.5 LASIK

LASIK stands for "LAser in SItu Keratomileusis". Excimer laser and the microkeratome are used to alter the degree of near-sightedness in an eye. After anesthetic eyedrops are put on the eye, a suction ring is centered. The suction ring stabilizes the position of the eye and increases the pressure to a level that is needed for proper functioning of the microkeratome. The microkeratome is a mechanical shaver(device) that contains a sharp blade that moves back and forth at high speed. This shaver is placed in the guide tracks of the suction ring and is advanced across the cornea using gears at a controlled speed. This process creates a partial flap in the cornea of uniform thickness. The flap is created with a portion of the cornea left uncut to provide a hinge. After the suction ring and microkeratome have been removed, the corneal flap is folded back on the hinge exposing the middle portion of the cornea. The excimer laser is then used to remove tissue and reshape the center of the cornea. The amount of tissue removed depends upon the degree of near-sightedness that is being corrected. In the final step, the hinged flap is folded back into its original position. The front surface of the eye is now flatter since the flap conforms to the underlying surface. In effect, the change made in the middle of the cornea is translated to the front surface of the cornea.

11.2 LASERS IN DERMATOLOGY

Lasers have been used to treat skin conditions that occurred over 40 years ago . Recent past major advances in laser technology have revolutionized their use in the treatment of many skin conditions and congenital defects.

In pigmented epidermis, melanin absorption is in the optical spectrum (200–1000 nm). In the dermis, there is strong, wavelength-dependent scattering by collagen fibers. In general, between

280 and 1300 nm, the depth of penetration increases with wavelength. Above 1300 nm, penetration decreases due to the absorption of light by water. The most deeply penetrating wavelengths are 650–1200 nm, while the least penetrating wavelengths are within the far-UV and far-IR regions.

Penetration of laser depends upon

1. Absorption and scattering
2. Dept of penetration increases with wavelength
3. Amount of scattering is inversely proportional to wavelength

The ablative laser treatments work mainly on the epidermis (surface skin cells). Non-ablative treatments work solely on dermal collagen (mid-layer of skin) only. Fractional laser treatment works at both the epidermal and dermal layers of the skin.

11.2.1 Applications

- Ablative (Vaporizing) Skin Resurfacing
- Treatment of Vascular Lesions
- Interactions During Treatment of Pigmented Lesions and Tattoos
- Interactions During Hair Removal
- Interactions During Non-Ablative Skin Rejuvenation
- Fractional Photothermolysis
- Laser-Based Diagnostics

11.3 LASERS IN DENTISTRY

The rapid development of laser technology has seen its introduction into various fields of dentistry.

The laser is directed on the rotten area, which contains more water molecules than rest of the tooth. Water molecules in the decay are heated rapidly. The pressure increases and the rotten area "explodes" making a popping sound. The laser kills bacteria in the area leaving the tooth surface sterile.

11.3.1 Classification

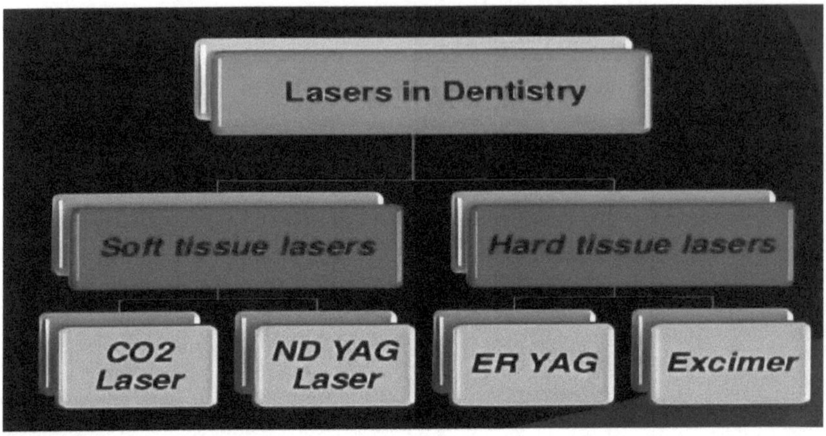

Figure 11.1: Laser classification in dentistry.

11.3.2 Applications

Diagnosis

- Detection of pulp vitality
- Doppler flowmetry
- Laser fluorescence- Detection of caries, bacteria and dysplastic changes in the diagnosis of cancer.

Hard tissue applications

- Caries removal and cavity preparation
- Re-contouring of bone (crown lengthening)
- Endodontic (root canal preparation, sterilization and Apicectomy)
- Laser etching
- Caries resistance

Soft tissue applications

- Laser-assisted soft tissue curettage and peri-apical surgery
- Bacterial decontamination
- Gingivectomy and Genioplasty
- Gingival retraction for impressions
- Implant exposure

11.3.3 Lasers used

CO_2 Laser

1. Mode: vaporization, cutting (>100°C)
2. Specification: 10.6-micron wavelength
3. Used effectively in treating patients with oral lesions with blood dyscrasias.
4. Oral indication: sealing of pits and fissures, welding of ceramic material to enamel, prevention of dental caries
5. Disadvantages: -Cornea at risk -Haemostasias may not be adequate on very vascular area (posterior tongue)

Nd YAG Laser

1. Mode: coagulation (>60°c), central vaporization
2. Specification: 1.06-micron wavelength Can be combined with CO_2 (combo laser) or KTP
3. Oral indications: Coagulation of very vascular lesions or near major blood vessels, Excision in vascular areas such as posterior tongue, Gingivectomy
4. Disadvantages: - Retina at risk - Penetration could cause inadvertent spread - Oedema more than CO_2 laser

Diode Lasers

Compact size and relatively affordable pricing. It is used in both contact and non-contact mode and can function with continuous wave or gated pulse modes. Diode lasers are invisible near infrared wavelengths and current machines range from 805–1064 nm.

Effective for a host of intraoral soft tissue-gingivectomy, biopsy, impression troughing, and frenectomy. Diode lasers also exhibit bactericidal capabilities and can be used for adjunctive periodontal procedures. They also are used for laser assisted tooth whitening. Diode lasers have excellent photobiomodulation.

11.3.4 Advantages

Less pain in some instances (reducing the need for anesthesia)

Reduce anxiety in patients uncomfortable with the use of the dental drill. Minimize bleeding (high-energy beam photocoagulation) and swelling. Reduce bacterial infections (sterilizes the area being worked on) Preserve healthier tooth during cavity treatment.

11.3.5 Disadvantages

Lasers can't be used on teeth with fillings that are already in place.

Lasers can't be used in many commonly performed dental procedures. Eg. lasers can't be used to fill cavities located between teeth, cavities around old fillings, and large cavities. Traditional drills may still be needed to shape the filling, adjust the bite, and polish the filling even when a laser is used.

Do not eliminate the need for anesthesia.

More expensive since the cost of the laser is much higher.

11.4 LASERS IN UROLOGY

Lasers represent one aspect of the continued development and application of light technology in urology. The photo thermal, photochemical, and photomechanical properties of lasers are used for both the diagnosis and treatment of urologic disease.

11.4.1 Applications

- Urologic disorders
- Stones, (holmium laser)
- Benign prostatic enlargement (BPE)
- Bladder cancer
- Kidney cancer
- Urothelial tumors
- Strictures

11.4.2 Urinary Lithiasis

Lithiasis goes by the name Laser lithotripsy also. Pulsed-dye laser (504 nm, 1 μsec) is coupled to a 250-μm quartz fiber for endoscopic stone fragmentation. Concentrically propagating cavitation bubble created at the laser–stone interface, collapsing and producing a photoacoustic shockwave and causing the calculus to fragment. (Nd:YAG) and alexandrite lasers are also effective in fragmenting calculi. Ho:YAG laser has moved to the forefront of laser lithotripsy technology. Laser in combination with miniaturized actively deflectable ureteroscopes to reach the proximal ureter and even intrarenal calculi are also utilized.

11.4.3 Benign Prostatic Hyperplasia

Urinary frequency, incomplete bladder emptying, and nocturia due to enlargement of prostate gland causes hyperplasia.

Laser prostatectomy has 2 main tissue effects - 1. coagulation 2. vaporization.

Coagulation occurs when somewhat diffusely focused laser energy heats tissue to 100°C. Proteins denature, and necrosis ensues. This results in subsequent sloughing of necrotic tissue. This process often initially results in edema. Vaporization occurs when greater laser energy is focused (increased power density) and tissue temperatures reach as high as 300°C. This causes tissue water to vaporize and results in an instantaneous debunking of prostatic tissue.

The transurethral ultrasound-guided laser-induced prostatectomy (TULIP) incorporated a side-firing Nd:YAG laser that used real-time ultrasound monitoring during treatment. It is Expensive and complex. Visual laser ablation of the prostate (VLAP) incorporates endoscopic for the direct application of laser energy (Nd:YAG) to the obstructing prostatic tissue. Technique incorporates a gold alloy tip at the end of the laser-delivery fiber, which allowed right-angle delivery of laser energy directly into the obstructing prostate tissue. Coagulation of treated prostatic tissue created the desired therapeutic effect. Ho:YAG laser has been used to remove obstructing prostate by a combination of the cutting and ablative effects of the laser. The procedure has been associated with little blood loss.

11.4.4 Urological Oncology

Prostate Cancer- Nd-YAG Laser and CO_2 laser

Bladder Cancer- Nd:YAG, argon, and Ho:YAG lasers have all been used in the treatment of bladder tumors.

Nd:YAG laser is the most widely used laser for the treatment of bladder neoplasms. Ho:YAG in the treatment of superficial bladder cancer

Ureteral and Renal Pelvis Carcinoma-Nd-YAG Laser with endoscopy.

11.4.5 Advantages

Immediate relief of symptoms – Rapid evacuation during recovery. Fewer symptoms of irritation and side effects.

The patient usually leaves either the same or the next day. Workable even in outpatients. Rapid recovery.

11.5 LASERS IN OTOLARYNGOLOGY

A medical specialty which is focused on the problems of ears, nose, and throat. It is also called otolaryngology-head and neck surgery because specialists are trained in both medicine and surgery. An otolaryngologist is often called an ear, nose, and throat doctor, or an ENT.

Lasers are tools that are adaptable to certain of the necessary surgical procedures in these regions. The energy in the laser beam exists as focused light and may be used for diagnostic and therapeutic interventions.

11.5.1 Delivery system

Articulated arm - The emerging beam is transferred from the laser aperture in a hollow metal tube, usually known as an articulated arm

Micromanipulator delivery -Device consisting of a system of lenses and a mirror with a joystick attachment. It is attached to the microscope

Hand piece delivery - The beam is focused by the system of lenses and mirrors onto the handpiece at a fixed point some 2 cm from its emergence at the distal end. A guide probe extends from the end of the hand piece.

11.5.2 Lasers used

Ho YAG Lasers

Wavelength: 2,100 nm; Near to mid Infrared wavelength (invisible) Penetration: 3-5 mm; deeper penetration allows for improved tissue coagulation Otolaryngologic Uses:

Lithotripsy (via sialendoscopy), Tonsillectomy, Endonasal and sinus surgery, Laryngeal surgery.

KTP *Lasers*

Wavelength: b532 nm; visible wavelength Penetration: 0.9-1 mm

Absorbtion: skin pigmentation and hemoglobin absortion Otolaryngologic Uses:

Stapedectomy and middle ear surgery, Laryngeal/tracheal surgery, Sinus surgery.

ARGON lasers

Wavelength: 485-515 nm; Infrared wavelength (invisible) Penetration: 0.8-1 mm

Absorption: -absorbed by pigmented tissues and hemoglobin; reflected by tissues white in color Otolaryngologic Uses:

Treatment of skin lesions, stapedectomy

11.5.3 Benefits

Minimally invasive surgery

Minimal bleeding

Minimal postoperative oedema and crusting Revision surgery

Ambulatory surgery Cost benefit

Lasers in Laryngeal Surgery

Lasers are a relatively recent addition to laryngeal surgery. Since their invention, laser use and applications have expanded rapidly. In this article, we discuss the benefits and disadvantages of lasers for different procedures, as well as ways to overcome commonly faced clinical problems. The use of lasers in surgery has offered a time- and cost-efficient alternative to cold surgical techniques, and has been used in the treatment of numerous laryngeal pathologies, including stenosis, recurrent respiratory papillomatosis, leukoplakia, nodules, malignant laryngeal disease, and polyploidy degeneration (Ranke's edema). However, lasers can incur adjacent tissue damage and vocal fold scarring. These problems can be minimized through understanding the mechanisms by which lasers function and correctly manipulating the parameters under a surgeon's control. By varying fluency, power density, and pulsation, tissue damage can be decreased and lasers can be used with greater confidence. The various types of lasers and their applications to the treatment of specific pathologies are reviewed with the intention of helping surgeons select the best tool for a given procedure. Recent applications of lasers to treat benign laryngeal lesions and severe laryngomalacia demonstrate that additional research must be conducted to realize the full potential of this surgical tool.

Cold surgery versus laser surgery

Although good surgical outcomes can be obtained from cold surgery, laser surgery, or a combination of the two, lasers possess some physiological and technical advantages. Besides being convenient and exact,13, 14 lasers offer surgeons an opportunity for unobstructed vision of the operation field14 with minimal tissue manipulation and a longer working distance.15 Decreased risk of postoperative bleeding, increased sterility,14, 16 minimal surrounding tissue damage,14 and better intraoperative.

Comparing types of lasers

Two broad types categorize all lasers: photoangiolytic and cutting/ablating lasers, which differ in their selectivity. Photoangiolytic lasers, such as KTP and PDL, selectively target hemoglobin, while cutting/ablating lasers, such as the CO_2 and Thulium (2 μm, RevoLix Jr, Health Tronics, Austin, TX) are absorbed largely by water.

Lasers are used to treat pathologies such as stenosis, recurrent respiratory papillomatosis (RRP), leukoplakia, nodules, malignant laryngeal.

Laser precautions and safety

Despite the notable benefits, laser surgery is not without disadvantages. Laser heat can increase scarring and cause damage to adjacent tissue.16 With lasers, there is potential for endotracheal explosion, facial burns, mucosal burns, vocal fold webs, stenosis, and glottis incompetence.51 In addition to recognizing when to use certain types and settings of lasers, surgeons should recognize when lasers should not be used. Xu et al17 showed that although lasers are preferred for malignant.

Future

Laser surgery has thus far offered a method of treating early- and medial-stage laryngeal cancer.56 In the future, it may be beneficial to be able to apply lasers to the treatment of advanced cancer. When CO_2 laser supraglottoplasty was found to be an effective treatment for severe laryngomalacia,57 it offered decreased costs, complications, and morbidity when compared to previous procedures, which included tracheotomies and micro dissection. There is much incentive to investigate areas such as.

11.6 LASER TISSUE WELDING

Laser energy is used to induce thermal changes in connective tissue proteins for joining tissues.

It aims to seal wounds and openings in a surgery using laser. Denaturation of tissue proteins occurs because of temperature rise due to absorption of laser light by water molecules and collagen present in the tissue. A new stronger connecting structure is formed by proteins when the temperature is brought down.

Types: Photo thermal TW (no covalent bonding), Photochemical TW (covalent bonding) Coagulation is one of the key processes in tissue welding, and lasers are used to induce this in tissues. Coagulation is the heating of tissues above 50 C and below 100 C to bring about denaturing of biological compounds. Proteins can break away from their quaternary structure and become long tangled fibrous substances.

11.6.1 Lasers used

Infrared: Co_2, THC:YAG, Ho:YAG, Tm:YAG, Nd:YAG, GaAlAs => Water absorption Visible: KTP, Nd:YAG, Argon => Hemoglobin absorption

Depending on the body tissue being soldered, there are various temperature limitations. Optimal temperature for collagen bonding is within 60-80 °C.

Diode lasers used for vascular welding operate at around 80 °C.

Argon lasers used for arterial vein anastomosis heat the tissue to approximately 70 °C. Conventional closure methods • Sutures • Staples • Clips • Fibrin glue.

11.6.2 Soldering

High tensile strength is needed so that the welded tissues do not break apart. Soldering biomaterial is used for this purpose. Albumen is used as a soldering material while performing anastomosis. After the laser heats the tissues in the junction to bring about denaturation along with the soldering biomaterial, the substructure is allowed to cool down. During this step, denaturation through covalent and electrostatic bond formation among the tissues takes place to hold the whole junction.

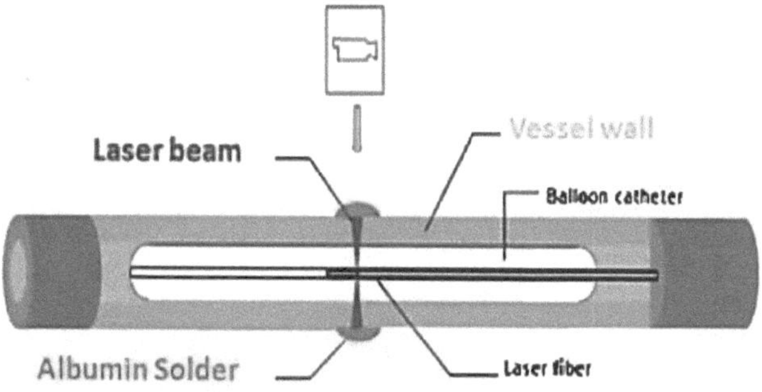

Figure 11.2: Albumen Soldering.

11.6.3 Applications

Cardiovascular surgery: Vascular anastomosis – seals to reduce blood loss during surgeries Thoracic surgery: Seal air leakage after lung surgery, bronchial stump

Dermatology: Skin closure – improved cosmoses, faster healing Gynecology: Repair of fallopian tube

Neurology: Welding of peripheral nerves Ophthalmology: Laser solder closure of cornea & sclera

Urology: Urinary tract closure to prevent water leakage & infection

Advantages Reduced operation time Reduce skill requirement

Reduced suture & needles trauma Reduced foreign body reaction Reduced bleeding Faster healing

Grow back ability and better cosmetic appearance.

11.7 MEDICAL APPLICATIONS

Surgical removal of tissue with a laser is a physical process similar to industrial laser drilling. Carbon-dioxide lasers operating at 10.6 micrometers can burn away tissue as the infrared beams are strongly absorbed by the water that makes up the bulk of living cells. A laser beam cauterizes the cuts, stopping bleeding in blood-rich tissues such as gums. Similarly, laser wavelengths near one micrometer (Neodymium-YAG Laser) can penetrate the eye, welding a detached retina back into place, or cutting internal membranes that often grow cloudy after cataract surgery (Fig. 11.3a). Less-intense laser pulses can destroy abnormal blood vessels that spread across the retina in patients suffering from diabetes, delaying the blindness often associated with the disease. Ophthalmologists surgically correct visual defects by removing tissue from the cornea, reshaping the transparent outer layer of the eye with intense ultraviolet pulses from Excimer Lasers.

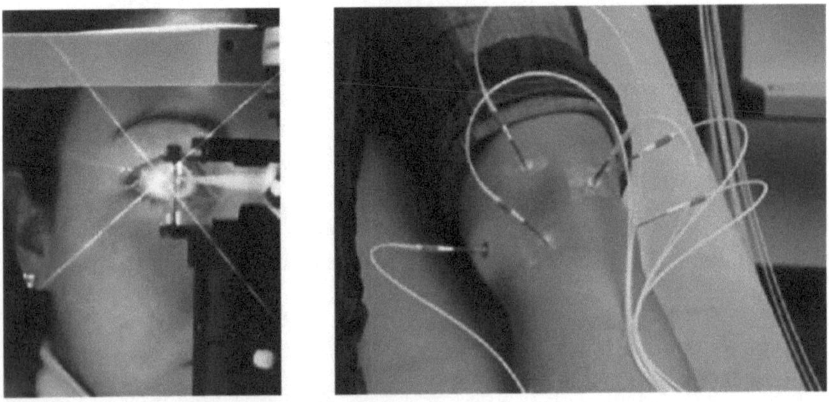

Figure 11.3: (Color online) (a) Schematic of Laser Eye Surgery. (b) Laser energy delivery to precise spots in joints for arthroscopic surgery.

Laser light can be delivered to places within the body that the beams could not otherwise reach through optical fibers like the tiny strands of glass that carry information in telephone systems. One important example involves threading a fiber through the urethra and into the kidney so that the end of the fiber can deliver intense laser pulses to kidney stones. The laser energy splits the stones into fragments small enough to pass through the urethra without requiring surgical incisions. Fibers also can be inserted through small incisions to deliver laser energy to precise spots in the knee joint during arthroscopic surgery (Fig. 11.3b). Another medical application for lasers is in the treatment of skin conditions. Pulsed lasers can bleach certain types of tattoos as well as dark-red birthmarks called port-wine stains. Cosmetic laser treatments include removing unwanted body hair and wrinkles.

11.8 BIOMEDICAL IMAGING AND SUPER RESOLUTION

Confocal microscopy (Fig. 11.4) is a ubiquitous imaging tool for imaging thick specimens in a wide range of investigations in biological, medical and material sciences.

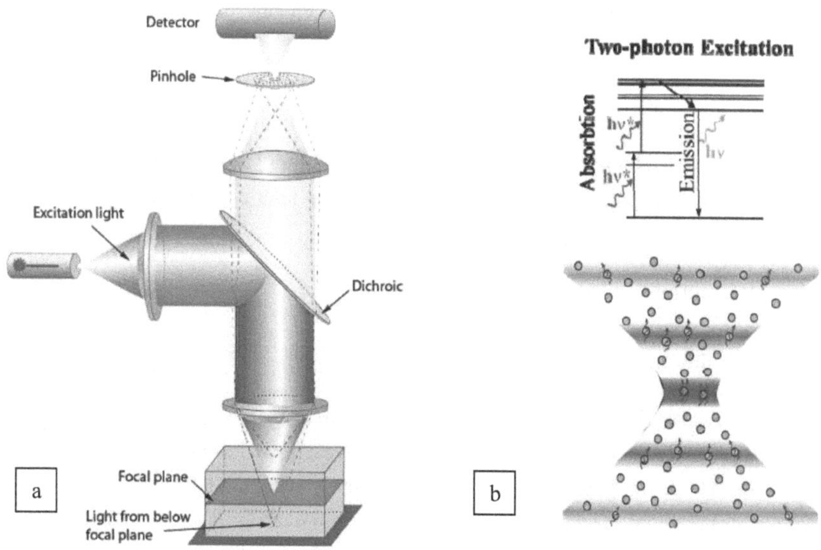

Figure 11.4: (Color online) Schematic of a (a) confocal microscope showing the critical placement of confocal pinhole to ensure all out of plane light is blocked before the detector to result in a sharp image from a thick specimen. (b) For two-photon microscopy, self-aperture occurs.

It uses UV or visible light for the single photon excitation of fluorophore from ground state to excited state followed by deactivation through fluorescence emission which is detected through high quantum efficiency photomultiplier tube (PMT) in the range of near ultraviolet, visible and near infrared spectral region. The basic difference of confocal Light Scanning Microscope with the conventional optical microscope is the confocal aperture arranged in a plane conjugate to the intermediate image plane and thus, to the object plane of the microscope. The PMT can only detect the light that passed the pinhole. As the laser beam is focused to a diffraction limited spot, which illuminates only one point of the object at a time, the point illuminated and the point observed are situated in conjugate planes, i.e. they are focused on each other. The perfection of focused beam, which is connected to the resolution has always been a matter of concern in the far-field fluorescence microscopy. Still, optical microscopy remains the best choice for monitoring live specimens despite the resolution advantage of, say electron microscopes, since the energy deposited in electron microscopy adversely affects the viability of live specimens. This practical compromise implicitly sets resolution enhancement as one of the most important developments in optical microscopy. For a single fluorescent molecule, Ernst Abbe defined a minimum diffraction- limited image having lateral (x, y) and axial (z) dimensions defined by the excitation wavelength (λ) refractive index of the imaging medium (η), and the angular aperture (α) of the microscope objective as:

$$\text{Resolution}_{x,y} = \frac{\lambda}{2[\eta.\sin(\alpha)]} \quad (11.1)$$

$$\text{Resolution}x,y = \frac{2\lambda}{[\eta.\sin(\alpha)]^2} \quad (11.2)$$

where the combined term η • sin (α) is known as the objective numerical aperture (NA). Objectives commonly used in microscopy have a numerical aperture that is less than 1.5 (although new high-performance objectives closely approach this limit), restricting the term α in Equations (11.1) and (11.2) to less than 70 degrees. Therefore, the theoretical resolution limit at the shortest practical excitation wavelength (approximately 400 nanometers when using an objective having a numerical aperture of 1.40) is around 150 nanometers in the lateral dimension and approaching 400 nanometers in the axial dimension. In practical terms for imaging living cells, these values are approximately 200 and 500 nanometers, respectively. Thus, structures that lie closer than 200 to 250 nanometers cannot be resolved in the lateral plane using either a wide field or confocal fluorescence microscope and is known as the Abbe's resolution limit (Fig. 11.5a).

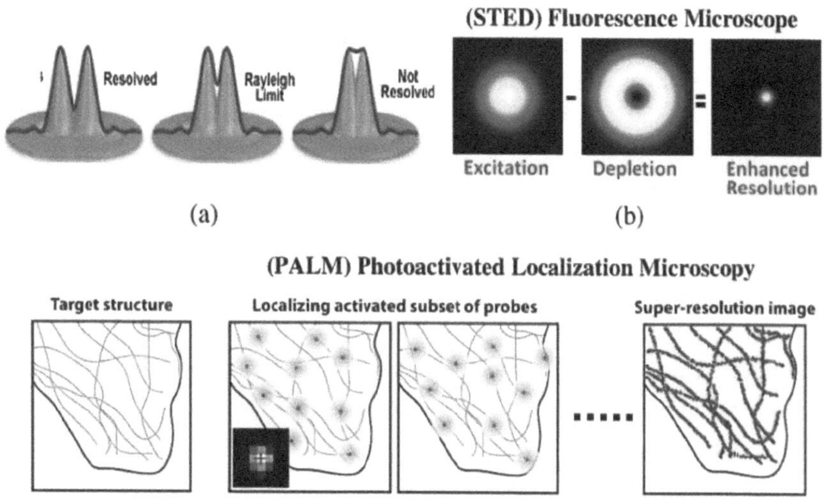

(c)

Figure 11.5: (Color online) (a) Schematic of Abbe's diffraction resolution limit using the Rayleigh criteria where the first diffraction minimum of the image of one source point coincides with the maximum of another. (b) In stimulated emission depletion fluorescence (STED) Microscope, the laser spot size is made smaller by using the depletion effect of fluorophore. (c) In photoactivated localization microscopy (PALM), superresolution is achieved using individual fluorophores that are photoactivated at different times as probe.

The 2014 Nobel Prize celebrated the development of super-resolved fluorescence microscopy that has made visible essential details and movements of the molecules of life. This development conquered the physical limit, described by Ernst Abbe in 1873, implying objects of smaller dimensions than half of the wavelength of light cannot be discerned by opticalmicroscopy. The Prize recognized the very first two ways to surpass Abbe's diffraction limit. The first method to bypass Abbe's limit involved two laser beams shining on the structure of interest in a fluorescence microscope. One beam excites the fluorescent molecules in a volume determined by Abbe's limit (Equations (11.1) and (11.2)). The other beam rapidly brings all the excited molecules, except those in a volume that can be made arbitrarily small, to their ground state before they can emit a photon. When both beams jointly scan the structure, an image with resolution better than Abbe's limit emerges. Stefen W. Hell demonstrated this experiment in 2000 and called it STimulated Emission Depletion (STED) microscopy (Fig. 11.5b). In the second approach, William Moerner and Eric Betzig developed a method where the biological structure is labelled with optically activatable Green Fluorescence Protein (GFP). A weak light pulse activates a small fraction of the GFP molecules, so that all molecules in this fraction are further apart than Abbe's limit and thus can be localized with super-precision. Then, yet another small fraction of the GFP molecules is activated so that also they can be super-localized. This is repeated until many such images were created. Finally, all these images are combined into one super-resolved image with complete structural information. They demonstrated this method first in 2006 and called it Photo Activated Localization Microscopy (PALM) (Fig. 1.5c).

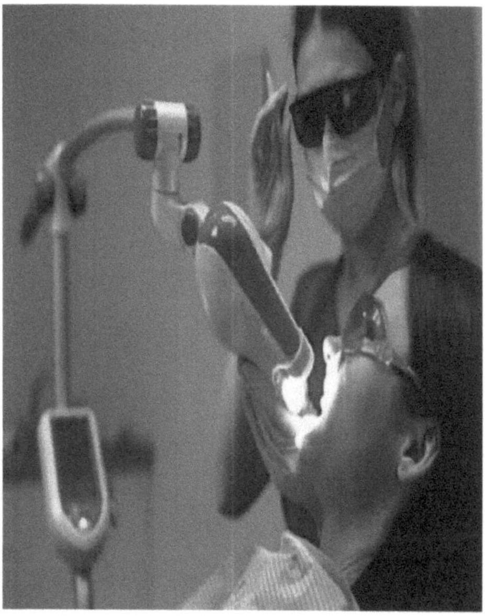

12
CHAPTER

LASER APPLICATION IN ORAL SURGERY

12.1 INTRODUCTION

Laser is a monochromatic, collimated, coherent, and intense beam of light produced by stimulated emission of radiation of a light source. Lasers are classified according to different factors among which is the classification based on laser active medium such as gas, liquid, solid and semi-conductor, which identifies and distinguishes the type of emitted laser beam.

Visible beams (i.e. the Argon laser at 488 or 518 nm) and invisible beams in the inftared range (i.e. CO_2(Carbon Dioxide Laser) , Ho:YAG (Holmium Yttrium Aluminium Garnet), Er:YAG (Erbium substituted: Yttrium Aluminium Garnet), Er-Cr: YSGG (Erbium, Chromium Doped Yttrium Scandium Gallium Garnet), ND:YAG (Neodymium-Doped Yttrium Aluminium Garnet), Diode (Gallium Arsenide) (GaAa)) are used in dentistry. The properties of a specific laser beam, particularly wavelength and the optical characteristics of the target tissue determine the type and the extent of interaction which may occur. Low level laser therapy (LLLT) which has therapeutic effects without inducing a lot of heat is established in clinical dentistry because of its anti-inflammatory, bio stimulant and regenerative effects. Its use has been widely reported with satisfactory results in the literature.

Recently, recently rapid developments in laser technology and better understanding of bio-interactions of different laser systems have broadened the clinical use of laser in dentistry.

Common lasers used in oral surgeries are CO_2, Er. Family, Diode and Nd:YAG. Also, low level lasers are used in assisting with the procedures of disinfection and healing.

CO_2 was the first laser introduced to dental practitioners in the mid-1980s, because of its outstanding cutting abilities and surprisingly, after more than 25 years, it still remains as a desirable choice in facial cosmetic surgeries (10,600 nm).

The Erbium family lasers (Er:YAG 2940 nm and Er,Cr:YSGG 2790 nm) are the lasers mainly used in dentistry for cavity preparation (Paghdiwala 1988, Keller 1989). Their emission wavelengths are perfectly matched to the absorption maximum of water which is a component of oral tissue [5].

Nd:YAG laser, is currently cleared by the U.S. food and drug administration for certain periodontal procedures and some vascular lesions. Its deep extinction length and penetration depth in soft tissue create significant lateral tissue damage, desirable for vascular lesions, but not for other pathology.

Diode laser (810-1064 nm) has become very popular in general dentistry because of their small size, low cost, fiber optic delivery and ease of use for minor surgery of oral soft tissue. The use of low-level Diode laser for noninvasive athermal laser therapy is popular in European countries.

The application of these lasers in surgery in the literature will be surveyed in this review article

12.2 LASER DEVICE COMPONENTS

The laser cavity existing at the center of the laser light consists of three components: an active medium, pumping mechanism and an optical resonator. The active medium is composed of a chemical element, compound or molecules. Lasers are named based on their active medium a) gas (CO_2 laser) (b) solid crystal (Nd: YAG, Er: YAG) (c) solid-state semiconductor (diode laser) d) liquid (not used in dentistry). The pumping mechanism serves to pump energy into the active medium. The (- laser cavity has two mirrors on either side of the optical cavity which acts as an optical resonator (reflects waves back and forth).

Delivery System of Laser

In a target tissue, the laser energy delivery system for shorter wavelength instruments (e.g., diode, Nd: YAG) has small, flexible fiber optic systems with bare glass fiber. The laser wavelength is absorbed by water (e.g., CO_2, Er: YAG) that cannot pass through the conventional glass fibers therefore special fibers are constructed which can transmit the wavelengths, with semi flexible hollow waveguide, or with articulated arms. Water spray is employed in the erbium laser for cooling the hard tissues.

Laser Tissue Interaction

Laser light energy has four different interactions with the target tissue: reflection, transmission, scattering and absorption. Reflection is the first tissue interaction and is simply the beam that is redirected off the surface and influences the target tissue. If redirected to an unintentional target, such as the eye, it could be dangerous. This highlights the importance for every person present in the laser treatment room to wear wavelength-specific safety glasses. Transmission is the second tissue interaction of the laser energy directly through the tissue without any effect on the target tissue. The transmission effect depends upon the laser light wavelength. Scattering is the third tissue interaction in which the laser light weakens the intended energy. It could cause unwanted damage to the tissue by transfer of heat adjacent to the surgical site. Absorption of the laser energy on the tissue depends upon the tissue characteristics such as pigmentation and water content, and the wavelength of the laser.

Tissue Temperature

At the temperature of 100°c, vaporization of water occurs within the tissue, and this process is called ablation. Soft tissue excision/incision commences at this temperature. At temperatures between 60-100°c without any vaporization of tissue, proteins begin to denature. This temperature enables removal of diseased granulomatous without affecting healthy tissue. Edges of the Soft tissue can be welded back at the temperature of 70° to 80°c without applying sutures. At 200°c the tissue gets dehydrated and burned and the final product is carbon, so heat sink occurs as the lasing continues.

12.3 CHARACTERISTICS OF LASER

Wavelength

In dentistry lasers used consist of a diverse wavelength. A beam of a single color (i.e., monochromatic) is generated whenever laser energy is emitted. Each wave in laser light is coherent or identical which means that the amplitude and frequency of all waves of photons are identical. Laser beams emitted by some of the instruments are collimated. But beams that are produced from optical fibers are divergent. Dental laser devices based on emission mode can emit light energy either constantly on or pulsed on and off. The pulsed mode is further divided into gated and free running modes. The three different emission modes (i) continuous-wave mode (ii) gated-pulse mode (iii) free-running pulsed mode or true-pulsed mode.. Lasers are commonly used in dentistry, and their wavelengths are summarized in Table 12.1.

Table 12.1: Common types of lasers used in dentistry.

Laser type	Construction	Wavelength(s)	Delivery system(s)
Argon	Gas Laser	488,515 nm	Optical fiber
KTP	Solid State	532 nm	Optical fiber
Helium-neon	Gas Laser	633 nm	Optical fiber
Diode	Semiconductor	635,670,810,830,980 nm	Optical fiber
Nd:YAG	Solid State	1064 nm	Optical fiber
Er, Cr:YSGG	Solid State	2780 nm	Optical fiber
Er:YAG	Solid State	2940 nm	Optical fiber, Waveguide,Articulated arm
CO_2	Gas Laser	9600,10600 nm	Waveguide,Articulated arm

Penetration Depth of Laser

There are four different interactions in biological tissue, among which degree of absorption determines the performance of a laser and is dependent on its wavelength. Depending on the laser wavelength, it is classified into two types: (i) Deep penetrating: deeper penetration into biological tissue occurs when there is a lower absorption coefficient into the water, such as neodymium-doped yttrium-aluminium- garnet (Nd: YAG) and diode lasers; these laser lights can penetrate and scatter deeply into the tissue. (ii) Superficially absorbed type (shallowly penetrating type): it exhibits a higher absorption coefficient into water such as carbon dioxide (CO_2), Er: YAG and Er, Cr: YAG lasers; these lasers do not penetrate or scatter deeply and laser light is absorbed only in the superficial layer.

12.4 TISSUE ABLATION

1. Soft Tissue

Soft tissue evaporates by the thermal effect, as the photothermal effect is one of the properties of laser on the tissue. A direct photothermal effect has been seen in CO_2 and erbium lasers, which can easily evaporate soft tissue. Nd: YAG and diode lasers create a condition called hot tip by converting its emitting light into heat by refraction or diffuse reflection at the tip end. Thus, secondary thermal effects of the hot tip can incise the soft tissues. The tissue coagulates and gets vaporized with the overheated tip rather than by laser energy itself.

2. Hard Tissue

Based on photothermal interaction, hard tissue ablation with Er: YAG laser has been hypothesized due to the thermo-mechanical effect.[10]Tissue ablation by Er: YAG laser begins with the mechanism of thermal evaporation as this laser is easily absorbed in water within biological tissues. In hard tissue, vaporization occurs when water molecules absorb laser energy, which increases intra-tissue pressure and provokes microexplosions, thus causing the mechanical breakdown of tissue and contributing to the ablation process.

12.5 THERMAL SIDE EFFECTS AND HEMOSTASIS

When a laser deeply penetrates soft tissue, it produces a layer of thick coagulation on the laser surface and exhibits strong hemostasis. Perry et al and White et al. reported that while incising bovine oral soft tissue by Nd: YAG laser at 3-10 W, the width of the coagulation layer was 0.3-0.8 in vitro. Walsh et al reported that in a noncontact mode, when Er:YAG laser incised porcine skin, the width of the thermally changed layer was only 10-50μm. When Er: YAG laser is used with water cooling, it is effectively capable of ablating hard tissues, producing a thermally affected layer approximately 5-30 μm thickness. A major thermal change, such as carbonization, melting, and resolidification has also been seen on the hard tissue, which is generally produced by lasers such as Nd: YAG and CO_2.

Disinfection And Detoxification Effects

The photo thermal effect of lasers enables killing of bacteria. On irradiation by the laser they evaporate, denatured resulting in devitalization or inactivation. During surgery, lasers can create a disinfected field, reducing the risk of infection, and advantageous for postoperative wound healing because of the bactericidal effect of laser therapy. The laser could be effective for debilitating some of the pigmented bacteria (e.g., porphyromonas gingivalis), which is linked with the periodontal disease because Nd: YAG laser shows selective pigmented bacteria absorption.

Biostimulation

Biostimulation (photobiomodulation) is one of the properties of laser therapy for tissues and cells post irradiation. This therapy is related to a photochemical reaction within cells; however, the mechanism is still unclear. Faster wound healing, reduction in inflammation, and relief in pain are the various biological effects of laser irradiation.

Advantages of Laser

- Have bactericidal and detoxification effect
- Less discomfort than conventional approaches
- Minimally invasive

- Usually, no need for sutures
- Tissue easily gets ablated through laser than a conventional scalpel
- Visualization is better at the surgical site due to hemostasis
- Laser provides less post-operative tissue edema and swelling.

Disadvantages of Laser

- High financial cost of laser apparatus
- Improper irradiation can damage teeth and the surfaces of the root
- May also damage the underlying bone and dental pulp

Risk and Precaution of Laser

- Risk and precautions in the clinical use of the laser are summarized in (Table 12.2).

Table 12.2: Risk and precautions in the clinical use of the laser.

Fire safety (continued)

- Do not prepare with flammable skin preparations.
- Use non-reflective instruments.
- Never place hot fibers on dry surgical drapes or towels.
- Use a laser-resistant endotracheal tube during oral cavities, aero digestive tract, or laryngeal procedures. Cover the cuff area with wet cottonoids. Never use a polyvinyl chloride endotracheal tube as it will emit toxic fumes if ignited.
- Good practice shows that when the laser is being used in the perianal area, a saline soaked radiopaque 4 × 4 should be inserted into the rectum to prevent methane gas from escaping which could be ignited by the laser beam and cause a methane gas explosion.

12.6 LASER APPLICATION IN DENTISTRY

The laser has become routine in dental practice. Ablation or vaporization, hemostasis, and the sterilization effect are some of its various characteristics that may serve as either an adjunctive treatment methodology or as stand-alone additions to the dental armamentarium. The current and potential laser application in dentistry are summarized in Table 12.3.

Table 12.3: Active medium of lasers most used in dentistry.

Laser	Abbreviation	Active medium	Hosting medium	Doping atom	Wavelength (nm)
Argon	Ar	Gas	–	–	488 and 514
Carbon dioxide	CO_2	Gas	–	–	9300; 9600 and 10,600
Diode	–	Semiconductor	–	–	445, 635–810 940–980–1064
Potassium titanyl phosphate	KTP	Solid	YAG crystal	Neodymium frequency doubled	532
Neodymium-doped yttrium aluminum garnet	Nd:YAG	Solid	YAG crystal	Neodymium	1064
Neodymium-doped yttrium aluminum perovskite	Nd:YAP	Solid	YAP crystal	Neodymium	1340
Erbium-doped yttrium scandium gallium garnet	Er,Cr:YSGG	Solid	YSGG crystal	Erbium and chromium	2780
Erbium-doped yttrium aluminum garnet	Er:YAG	Solid	YAG crystal	Erbium	2940

1. Scaling and Root Planing

Several studies have been published elaborating the use of laser as an adjunct to scaling and root planing. Numerous studies using lasers (diode, CO_2, Nd: YAG, Er: YAG, and Er,Cr: YSGG) have shown a decrease in inflammation and/or pocket depths. Tucker et al. reported that a CO_2 laser in a pulsed mode at 6 W could eliminate dental plague on the surface of the root. Coffelt et al. observed that in a defocused mode when the CO_2 laser was used at an energy density between 11 and 41 MJ/cm2 destroyed microbial colonies without inflicting undue damage on the surface of the root. Crespi et al reported that pulsed defocus mode CO_2 laser at 2 W, 1 Hz increased fibroblast attachment after root conditioning.

2. Laser Assisted New Attachment Procedure (LANAP) Using Nd: YAG

LANAP was specially developed as an alternative to conventional periodontal surgery and for teeth with severely damaged periodontium. Several evolutions and changes in the name from laser ENAP to LPT to LANAP were done over many years and finally, the definitive LANAP protocol was established.[27] Based on human histologic evidence that LANAP is the only laser procedure which in the absence of a long Junctional epithelium gives the cementum-mediated periodontal ligament attachment and was approved by the United States FDA 510 (K) marketing clearance (K030290). Some studies support new attachment following the use of LANAP **Figure 12.1**.

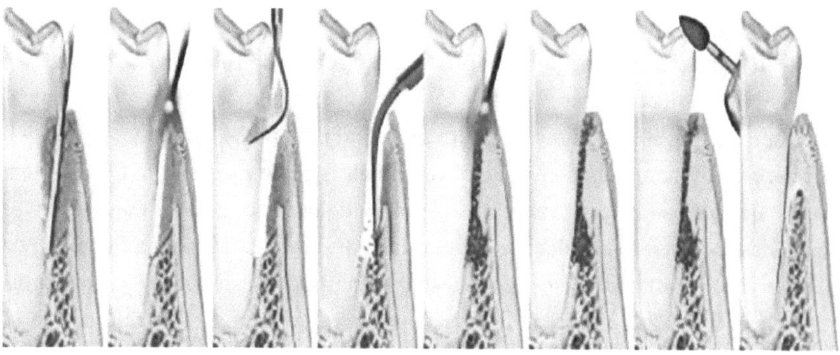

Figure 12.1: Laser assisted with new attachment procedure LANAP protocol.

12.7 DENTINAL HYPERSENSITIVITY

Low output power lasers (helium-neon and gallium/ aluminium/arsenide [diode]) and middle output power lasers (Nd: YAG, Er: YAG, and carbon dioxide) are t used in treatment of dentinal hypersensitivity.[1] Several studies support using lasers in dentinal hypersensitivity. In 1972, Kantola observed craters in dentin which were created while using a CO_2 laser. On analysis with microradiography and electron probe it was revealed that increased levels of calcium and phosphorus existed in the fused or recrystallized dentine walls of the crater compared with normal dentin. One year later, using radiographic diffraction analysis in a follow-up study, Kantola observed that recrystallization had occurred in the laser-irradiated fused dentin and the dentin had changed structurally so that the crystalline structure of normal enamel hydroxyapatite can closely resemble.

Glaucheet *et al.* reported the melting and resolidification of dentin in the presence of craters and cracks using CO_2 laser and Ciaramicoli et al using Nd: YAG laser. Dederich et al were the first to describe melting and recrystallization by the exposure of Nd:YAG laser on root canal wall dentin.

Caries Diagnostics

In the 1980s, the natural green fluorescence of tooth tissue by visual detection method was developed. The method used an argon-ion laser (488nm) excitation wavelength to differentiate bright - green - fluorescing healthy tooth tissue from poorly fluorescing carious lesions. In early 1990, this technique was further refined by replacing argon-ion laser from a xenon-based arc lamp, with the emission light shone through a blue-transmitting filter and known as quantitative light-induced fluorescence (QLF), which quantifies the observed green-fluorescence loss as an indirect measure of loss of mineral by using the digitization of images. 405 nm excitation wavelength which is performed by the QLF system allows quantification and visualization of both intrinsic green fluorescence of dental tissues whereas in calculus, plaque, and advanced caries the red fluorescence is observed. Substantial red fluorescence phenomenon using laser wavelengths between 650 and 800 nm in carious lesions has resulted in a hand-held device to detect dental caries. To limit the possibility of false-positive results, the QLF system is best incorporated as an addition to other diagnostic methods (tactile, visual, and radiographic)

Pulp Diagnosis

Laser Doppler flowmetry (LDF) was developed for the diagnostic measurement of blood flow in the dental pulp40 and to examine blood flow in microvascular systems. This technique uses a low power of 1 or 2 mW from helium-neon and diode laser. There are some limitations to laser Doppler flowmetry. In an anterior teeth region, the enamel and dentine are thin which generally do not create a problem. While in the molar region the enamel and dentin are thick and variability in the pulp position within the tooth may cause variation in pulpal blood flow. There are some problems with laser Doppler flowmetry which was reported by Frentzen et al. that in a posterior region of teeth, it causes inconvenience in acquiring laser reflection. Also in restored teeth, it was difficult to gain laser reflection because of limited transmission. In traumatized teeth excitability of the pulp is reduced, but LDF could present an acceptable alternative to the conventional method of vitality test.

When clinical application improves, and equipment costs decrease, then this technology could be used in a patient who cannot communicate or for young children who may not respond reliably.

Pulp Capping and Pulpotomy

The treatment done with CO_2 laser of the exposed pulp tissues in dogs to achieve hemostasis was first described by Melcer *et al* Shoji *et al.* who applied focused and defocused mode CO_2 laser and a wide range of energy levels (3, 10, 30, and 60 W) to expose the pulps of dogs. There was no damage noticed in the radicular pulp area and coagulation, necrosis, and deterioration of the odontoblastic layer occurred. Jukic *et al.* observed carbonization, necrosis, an inflammatory response, edema, and hemorrhage in pulp tissue by using CO_2 and Nd: YAG lasers with energies densities of 4J/cm^2 and 6.3 J/cm^2. Moritz et al treated a patient in whom direct pulp capping was indicated by using a CO_2 laser of 1W at an exposure time of 0.1-second with a pulse interval of 1 second and was applied until the exposed pulps were not completely sealed and dressed in calcium hydroxide.[47] In the control group, pulps were crapped with calcium hydroxide only. And 1 week later and monthly for 1-year, it was observed that 89% of them had not reported any symptoms and normally responded to the vitality test versus the control group (68%).

Incision/Excision Procedures

A variety of intraoral soft tissue lesions can be treated with laser therapy using continuous and pulsed CO_2 and Nd: YAG systems such as haemangioma, tongue papilloma, tongue lipoma, pyogenic granuloma, lymphangioma, lichen planus, and focal melanosis. White et al proposed that the patient who was treated with the laser excision was well tolerated with no adverse effect.

MEDICAL OPTICS

Removal of oral mucosa lesions

A clinical study described the application of the potassium-titanyl-phosphate (KTP) laser (532 nm), used with low power parameter (1 Watt – CW) to evaluate the intra and postoperative pain. They proposed that KTP laser with low parameters permits us to perform oral surgery with good pain control and good wound healing (Fornaini).

Oral leukoplakia

Oral leukoplakia is a pre-malignant lesion of the oral mucosa [6].

A randomized clinical trial compared the pain and swelling after removal of oral leukoplakia with CO_2 laser and cold knife. They concluded that CO_2 laser caused only minimal pain and swelling, thus suggesting that it may be an alternative method to conventional surgery in treating patients with oral leukoplakia.

A nonrandomized, single-arm, single-site phase 1/2 pilot study determined the safety and efficacy of photodynamic therapy in the treatment of oral leukoplakia with 5-aminolevulinic acid and pulsed dye laser. Photodynamic therapy with 5-aminolevulinic acid and pulsed dye laser could be used to achieve regression of oral leukoplakia. The treatment is safe and well tolerated. An application time of 1.5 hours and laser radiant exposure of 8 J/cm with 1.5-ms pulse time were found to be the optimal settings in this study. The high-power laser used in this study allows completion of laser therapy within 1 to 3 minutes. Further studies are necessary to determine the optimal laser radiant exposure and drug application to maximize the response rate.

The curative effects of photodynamic therapy (PDT) and cryotherapy in the treatment of oral leukoplakia were compared. They found that the advantages of PDT are connected to the minimally invasive and localized characteristics of the treatment with no damage to collagenous tissue structures; therefore normal cells will repopulate these arrangements. PDT is more convenient for patients, less painful, and more esthetic.

A prospective study evaluated clinical healing of a leukoplakia lesion after laser surgery, which was associated with a normal functional status of the new epithelium, also pathological alterations were related to the risk of local recurrence.

They concluded that clinical healing of leukoplakia treated by laser surgery may be accompanied by altered cell turnover in 20% of cases. Ki67, as a marker of proliferative status, may be a prognostic indicator in the mucosa replacing the lesion.

Yang et al. evaluated the associated factors of recurrence in patients who received laser surgery for dysplastic oral leukoplakia. This study suggested that continuous smoking after surgical treatment and widespread multiple-focus lesions are the prognostic indicators for recurrence after laser surgery. Changes in oral habits could be of great importance to the outcome of laser surgery of dysplastic oral leukoplakia.

Lichen planus

Oral lichen planus (OLP) is a common chronic disease of uncertain aetiology. Treatment of patients with symptomatic OLP represents a therapeutic challenge. One study evaluated the efficacy of diode laser (940 nm) in the management of oral lichen planus. Their results demonstrated that diode laser therapy seemed to be an effective alternative treatment for relieving the symptoms of OLP (Misra, 2013 #491).

Low-level laser and CO_2 laser were compared in the treatment of patients with oral lichen planus. They showed that low-level laser displayed better results than CO_2 laser therapy as an alternative or additional therapy.

A clinical report demonstrated the efficiency of Er:YAG laser in reducing symptoms and lymphoplasmocytic infiltrate in case of oral lichen planus (OLP). The parameters used were energy, 80-120 mJ; frequency, 6-15 Hz; non-contact hand piece; spot size diameter, 0.9 mm; pulse duration, 100 μsec (very short pulse) to 300 μsec (short pulse); fluences, 12.6-18.9 J/cm^2; and air/water spray (ratio: 6/5). The use of this wavelength offers several advantages including a good and fast healing process, a very low level of discomfort during and after intervention, and a rapid disappearance of symptoms.

A case report presented a histologically diagnosed oral lichen planus excised by CO_2 laser. CO_2 laser was used to remove the lesion, and the conclusive histopathological diagnosis was oral lichen planus. The patient was followed up over 1 year with no signs of lesion recurrence. The use of the CO_2 laser was found to be useful and effective to treat lichen planus.

Gingival melanin pigmentation

A clinical and histologic study compared surgical stripping; erbium-doped: yttrium, aluminum, and garnet laser; and carbon dioxide laser techniques for gingival depigmentation. They concluded that clinical repigmentation after gingival depigmentation is an outcome of histologic changes in the melanocyte activity and density of the melanin pigments. Surgical stripping for gingival depigmentation remains the gold standard; however, Er:YAG laser and CO_2 lasers can be effectively used but with distinct differences.

Simsek et.al compared the use of diode and Er:YAG lasers in treating gingival melanin pigmentation (GMP) in terms of gingival depigmentation, local anesthesia requirements, postoperative pain/discomfort, depigmentation effectiveness, and total treatment duration. Their results demonstrated the total length of treatment was significantly shorter with the diode laser than with the Er:YAG laser. No melanin recurrence was detected during any follow-up session. They concluded Diode and Er:YAG lasers administered at 1 W both result in satisfactory depigmentation of GMP.

Fordyce granule excision

A surgical lip Fordyce granule excision using a high-power diode laser in a 19-year-old male was reported. The excellent esthetic result demonstrated the effectiveness of both high- and low-intensity laser therapies on the excision of Fordyce granules.

Oral dysplasia

A prospective study evaluated recurrence, residual disease malignant transformation, and overall outcome in patients undergoing such procedure. They demonstrated that recurrence and malignant transformation was mainly identified in erythroplakias and non-homogenous leukoplakias. Laser resection/ablation was recommended for oral dysplasia to prevent not only recurrence and malignant transformation, but also postoperative oral dysfunction encountered by other conventional modalities.

Precancerous lesions

A prospective study evaluated the recurrence rates resulting from different methods of CO_2 laser vaporization. Their results indicated that for CO_2 laser treatment of premalignant lesions of the oral mucosa, the best results could be achieved with the defocused technique. It may be assumed that other methods with lesser penetration of thermal effects did not reach the deeper-lying cells and, consequently, render higher rates of recurrence.

Oral melanoma

A retrospective study surveyed the convenience of laser surgery as optimal treatment for melanoma of the oral mucosa. In their experiment, conservative management with CO_2 laser was adequate for melanomas of the oral mucosa with extraction of the dental organs and curettage of the alveoli to achieve complete surgical resection microscopically without sacrifice of the quality of life. Management of the neck was controversial. They recommend selective therapeutic resection of the neck only if it is found to be clinically positive. Elective dissection had not shown to have an impact on overall survival. (See Table 12.4 for an evidence summary).

Table 12.4: Evidence table summary of different laser used in Removal of oral mucosa lesions.

Study type	Author	year	Sample size	Laser type	Laser parameters	Result
Randomized clinical trial	Lopez-jornet	2013	48	CO_2 laser		The CO_2 laser causes only minimal pain and swelling
Randomized clinical trial	Simsek	2012	20	-gallium aluminum arsenide diode laser	- continuous wavelength of 808 nm, - continuous wavelength	Diode and Er:YAG lasers administered at 1 W both result in satisfactory

				-Er:YAG laser	of 2,940 nm	depigmentation
Randomized clinical trial	Agha-Hosseini	2012	57	low-level laser CO(2) laser		Both methods may be effective in the treatment of OLP
Clinical trial	Kawczyk	2012	85	photodynamic therapy (δ-aminolevulinic acid (ALA)	630-635 nm wavelength	PDT is more convenient for patients, less painful, and more esthetic.
Prospective study	Montebugnoli	2012	13	Nd:YAG laser		clinical healing of leukoplakia treated by laser surgery may be accompanied by altered cell turnover in 20% of the cases
Prospective study	Jerjes	2012	123	CO(2) laser		Laser resection/ablation is recommended for oral dysplasia to prevent recurrence and malignant transformation
Prospective study	Deppe	2012	148	CO(2) laser		CO(2) laser was used in treatment of premalignant lesions of the oral mucosa
Retrospective study	Luna-oritz	2011	4	CO(2) laser		CO2 laser is adequate for melanomas of the oral mucosa with extraction of the dental organs
Clinical study	Hegde	2013	140	CO2 laser Er:YAG laser	(CO2 laser, 2 to 4 W, continuous wave),and "brushstroke" (Er:YAG laser, 180 mJ, 10 Hz, long pulse)	Surgical stripping for gingival depigmentation remains the gold standard; however, Er:YAG laser and CO2 lasers can be effectively used

						but with distinct differences.
Clinical study	Fornaini	2012	52	KTP laser	the KTP laser (532 nm), used with low power parameter (1 Watt - CW)	KTP laser with low parameters permits to perform oral surgery with good pain control and good wound healing
Clinical study	Yang	2011	114	CO(2) laser		Continuous smoking after surgical treatment and widespread multiple-focus lesions are the prognostic indicators for recurrence after laser surgery.
Case report	Misra	2013	1	Diode laser	diode laser (940 nm)	Diode laser therapy seems to be an effective alternative treatment for relieving the symptoms of OLP
Case report	Fornaini	2012	2	Er: YAG laser	energy, 80-120 mJ; frequency, 6-15 Hz; non-contact hand piece; spot size diameter, 0.9 mm; pulse duration, 100 µsec (VSP) to 300 µsec (SP) ; fluences, 12.6-18.9 J/cm(2); and air/water spray (ratio: 6/5)	The use of this wavelength offers several advantages including, a good and fast healing process, a very low level of discomfort during and after intervention, and a rapid disappearance of symptoms.
Case report	de Magalhaes-Junior	2011	1	CO2 laser		The use of the CO_2 laser was found to be

						useful and effective to treat lichen planus.
Non-randomized single arm, single site	Shafirstein	2011	23	Pulsed dye laser		It could be used to achieve regression of oral leukoplakia

12.8 ORAL BENIGN LESIONS

Mucocele

Mucoceles are benign lesions of the minor salivary glands that are common in children. The most frequent localizations of these lesions include the lower lip and the cheek mucosa.

Boj et.al described the case of a 4-mm extravasation mucocele located on the lower lip with an erbium laser. They showed the wound healed excellently and rapidly without sutures. No relapse was observed a year after the surgery. Lasers apply modern technology and are useful for soft tissue surgery in pediatric dentistry, as operations are rapid and wounds heal well without sutures.

Oral mucocele resection with the scalpel versus the CO_2 laser was compared. Their results showed that oral mucocele ablation with the CO_2 laser offered more predictable results and fewer complications and recurrences than conventional resection with the scalpel.

Ranula

Ranulas are mucus extravasation phenomenon formed after trauma to the sublingual gland or mucus retention from the obstruction of the sublingual ducts [24].

Lai et.al presented a case series report on the use of carbon dioxide laser treatment for ranula and a literature review of cases treated using carbon dioxide laser. The authors' experience and reports in the literature indicated that carbon dioxide laser excision of ranula was safe with minimal or no recurrence.

Pyogenic granuloma

Pyogenic granuloma (PG) may develop in the oral cavity of pregnant women. Lindenmüller et al. described CO_2 laser-assisted treatment of a giant pyogenic granuloma of the gingiva. Their results showed the initial wound healing was uneventful. A 12-month follow-up revealed no recurrence of the mass and healthy periodontal tissues.

Gingival hyperplastic lesions removal

Asnaashari et.al applied 810nm Diode laser to remove all gingival hyperplastic lesions. Their results demonstrated that a perfect shaping was obtained after removal of the whole lesion in one session, and no recurrence was observed in 6 months.

Epulis fissuratum

Epulis fissuratum is a pseudo tumor growth located over the soft tissues of the vestibular sulcus caused by chronic irritation from poorly adapted dentures. Treatment indication for these lesions is surgical excision with appropriate prosthetic reconstruction. One study proposed treatment of epulis fissuratum with carbon dioxide laser in a patient with antithrombotic medication. The lesions were excised with CO_2 laser, and no significant complications, such as hemorrhage, pain, swelling or infection, were recorded. They proposed that use of CO_2 lasers is currently the gold standard in the excision of this type of lesion, especially in patients with hemorrhagic diathesis or under antithrombotic therapy.

Treatment of epulis fissuratum with CO_2 laser and prosthetic rehabilitation of three patients with vesiculobullous diseases (VBDs) was presened with Işeri et al. The excision of fibrous tissue was performed with CO_2 laser, and the wounds formed by laser were left open to secondary epithelization. They demonstrated that the CO_2 laser might be a useful instrument in the treatment of soft tissue pathologies in VBDs patients due to minimal damage to surrounding tissue. Use of complete or partial dentures had been considered a practical, economic, and nonsurgical treatment option for patients who have been diagnosed with VBDs.

Lymphangioma

Lymphangiomas are hemorrhagic, rare, benign hamartomatous tumors of lymphatic system which have a marked predilection for the head, neck and oral cavity. Lymphangiomas are congenital lesions and an often present at or around the time of birth (60%).

In A case report, treatment of lymphangioma (a red-purple vesicular appearance, nonulcerated lesion, located on the gingiva of the mandibular alveolar bone) with CO_2 laser was described. CO_2 laser application (focused CO_2 laser beam, 10.600 nm) was performed in a separate operation room at 3 watt (W), continuous wave (CW) with 90-degree angle tip under local anesthesia. They concluded that CO_2 laser therapy can be used as a primary alternative method in the treatment of lymphangiomas. It can be safely used, and recurrence may be less than conventional excision with scalpel. However, long-term clinical follow-up is necessary for the recurrence of the lesion.

Hemangioma

Genovese et al. reviewed the use of surgical lasers in hemangioma treatment. They described the use of GaAs high-potency diode laser in the treatment of hemangioma reduced bleeding during surgery, with a consequent reduction in operating time, and promoted rapid postoperative hemostasis. It was safe for use on large lesions and easy to manage, and postoperative problems, including potential scarring, and discomfort are minimal. (See Table 12.5 for an evidence summary).

Table 12.5: Evidence table summary of different lasers used in oral benign lesions surgery.

Study type	Author	year	Sample size	Laser type	Laser parameters	Result
Clinical study	Yagüe-García	2009	68	carbon dioxide laser	CO_2 laser (5-7 W)	There were no complications or relapses after a minimum follow-up of 12 months
Case report	Monteiro	2012	1	CO_2 laser		The use of CO_2 lasers is currently the gold standard in the excision of epulis fissuratum

Case report	Arslan	2011	1	CO_2 laser	3 watt (W), continuous wave (CW) with 90 degree angle tip	CO_2 laser worked well while making the excision with its hemostatic effect. No recurrence was seen in the two years follow-up period.
Case report	Lindenmüller	2010	1	CO_2 laser		A 12- month follow-up revealed no recurrence of the mass and healthy periodontal tissues.
Case report	Genovese	2010	1	gallium arsenide (GaAs) diode laser	(GaAs) diode laser at 980 nm wavelength, with 4.0 W of power	It is safe for use on large lesions and easy to manage, and postoperative problems.
Case report	Iseri	2009	1	CO_2 laser		There was no recurrent fibrous tissue formation at 1 year follow-up
Case report	Boj	2009	1	Erbium laser		The wound healed excellently and rapidly without sutures.

Case report	Asnaashari	2013	1	Diode laser	810nm	perfect shaping was obtained after removal of the whole lesion in one session.
Case series	Lai	2009	3	carbon dioxide laser		carbon dioxide laser excision of ranula is safe with minimal or no recurrence.

Cancer of Oral cavity

A retrospective study assessed the efficacy of Nd:YAG laser for stage I squamous cell carcinoma of the lip. Their results reported the use of Nd:YAG laser for treatment of Stage I squamous cell carcinoma of lip in accordance with principles of minimal invasive and morbid surgery.

A retrospective study analyzed two hundred thirty-two patients with cancer of the oral cavity were treated by enoral laser microsurgery ± selective neck dissection ± postoperative (chemo) radiotherapy. They concluded that enoral laser microsurgery is an efficient therapeutic option in the treatment of oral cavity cancer. Oncological and functional results are comparable to any other treatment regimen, whereas morbidity and complications tend to be lower.

A retrospective analysis evaluated 296 cases of early glottic squamous cancer with and without the involvement of anterior commissure (AC) treated by trans-oral CO_2 laser microsurgery. Trans-oral laser surgery is an excellent treatment option in patients with early glottic cancer irrespective of whether the AC is involved. Trans-oral laser microsurgery for early glottic cancer involving AC requires adequate exposure, proper assessment, good experience, and advanced surgical skills.

An experimental analysis evaluated tungsten carbide-bur, piezoelectric and laser osteotomies. They concluded that currently, purchase and management elevated costs, minor versatility of use, and long training times for equipment such as Piezosurgery and laser limit their general use but remain advantageous in case of risky interventions near noble structures. Choice of device depends on experience maturated by operator in time, characteristics of operation and patient's clinical conditions.

An experimental study compared thermal changes of the bone surface, procedure time, and volume of the removed bone after drilling with an erbium: yttrium aluminum garnet (Er:YAG) laser (pulse energy, 1,000 mJ; pulse duration, 300 μs; frequency, 20 Hz) versus a low-speed surgical drill. They concluded that the Er:YAG laser produced preparations with regular and sharp edges, without bone fragments and debris, in a shorter time, and with less generated heat. Thermal alterations in the treated surface were minimal.

Luna-Ortiz et al. reported that transoral laser microsurgery was recommended for treatment of soft palate tumors. This treatment could be considered a better option when compared with other modalities such as radio- or chemoradiotherapy which required a longer time of treatment, were more expensive and tend to produce significant toxicity.

Photodynamic therapy (up to three rounds) is a comparable modality to other traditional interventions in the management of low-risk tumors of the oral cavity. Although, sometimes, multiple rounds of the treatment are required, morbidity following PDT is far less when compared to the three conventional modalities: surgery, radiotherapy, and chemotherapy.

A clinical case evaluated the healing of the site after removal of the lesion with use of the laser diode. The laser diodes gave a significant contribution to improving the surgical treatment of tumors of the oral cavity, in fact during the surgery reduce bleeding and surgical time, and while in the process of healing by reduce swelling and post-operative pain and better results appearance without scarring.

Excisional biopsy

A prospective randomized controlled clinical trial evaluated and compared clinical and histopathologic findings of excisional biopsies performed with CO_2 laser (10.6 μm) modes in 60 patients with similar fibrous hyperplasias of the buccal plane. No significant difference was found in the widths of thermal damage zones between the CW and CF groups. The visual analogue scale (VAS) values and analgesic intake were low in the 2 groups. The 2CO_2 laser modes were appropriate for the excision of intraoral mucosal lesions. A safety border of at least 1 mm was recommended regardless of the laser mode used.

A prospective animal study compared operative time and hemostasis of fiber-enabled CO_2 laser (FECL) energy to that of the electrocautery (EC) technique for oral tongue resection. They determined both EC and FECL are effective for resection of the tongue in rats. EC has the advantage of shorter operative time and lower mucosal wound-healing scale scores by postoperative day 3; FECL has the advantages of less intraoperative bleeding, faster return to baseline body weight, and lower mucosal wound-healing scale score by postoperative day 7.

One study compared the conventional surgery with carbon dioxide (CO_2) laser applied on oral soft tissue pathologies and evaluated the effect of collateral thermal damage on histopathological diagnosis. They reported that CO_2 laser is an effective instrument for soft tissue excisional biopsies with minimal intraoperative and postoperative complications and good pain control. CO_2 laser applications are suggested as an alternative method to conventional surgery on oral soft tissues.

12.9 TREATMENT OF ORAL CAVITY VENOUS MALFORMATIONS

Mucosal involvement of venous malformations can cause bleeding, pain, and functional impairment. Treatment options include surgery, sclerotherapy, or laser therapy. A retrospective study surveyed 4 patients (5 subsites) with oral cavity venous malformations treated with the Nd:YAG laser using an underwater technique. Their study demonstrated that the Nd:YAG laser can be a feasible option in the treatment of venous malformations of the oral cavity.

One study reported two treatment strategies using intralesional laser photocoagulation (ILP) for large venous malformations (VMs) in the oral cavity. Treatments included a combination of ILP and transmucosal irradiation, compartmentalization and serial step irradiation. They demonstrated both treatment strategies improved the safety, reliability, and effectiveness of ILP and made the method less traumatic for patients.

Miyazaki et al. described an ultrasound-guided intralesional photocoagulation (ILP) technique using a laser for treatment of deep venous malformations in the oral cavity. ILP is basically a blind operation and has a risk of unintended destruction of surrounding normal tissue; therefore, the authors now routinely use guidance by ultrasonography using a mini probe to improve the safety and reliability of ILP. The authors conclude that ultrasound-guided ILP with a laser is a promising technique for less-invasive treatment of a vascular malformation in the oral cavity.

Álvarez-Camino determined the efficacy of the diode laser in the intralesional treatment of the orofacial venous malformations (OFVM). The advantages associated with the use of non-invasive techniques in the treatment of OFVM, along with the success rate and low number of relapses, showed the use of the diode laser as a therapy to be considered in the treatment of these lesions.

A retrospective study evaluated the safety and efficacy of CO_2 laser resurfacing in the symptomatic treatment of intraoral lymphatic malformations (LM). They proposed CO_2 that laser resurfacing appeared to be both safe and efficacious in treatment of symptoms related to intraoral LM. Intermittent treatments for recurrent symptoms were expected.

Bisphosphonate-associated osteonecrosis of the jaws

Bisphosphonates (BSPs) are used for the treatment of multiple myeloma, metastatic breast and lung cancer, Paget's disease, osteoporosis, hypercalcemia due to malignancy, and many other skeletal diseases. BSPs reduce osteoclastic functions, which result in bone resorption. Bisphosphonates-related osteonecrosis of jaws (BRONJ) is a newly developed term that is used to describe the significant complication in patients receiving bisphosphonates. BSPs are known to exhibit an anti-angiogenetic effect that initiates tissue necrosis of the hard tissue. There is currently no consensus on the correct approach to this issue.

A retrospective study compared the effects of laser surgery with biostimulation to conventional surgery in the treatment of BSP-induced avascular bone necrosis. They reported that there were no statistically significant differences between laser surgery and conventional surgery. Treatment outcomes were significantly better in patients with stage II osteonecrosis than in patients with stage I osteonecrosis. Their findings suggested that dental evaluation of the patients prior to medication was an important factor in the prevention of BRONJ. Laser surgery was a beneficial alternative in the treatment of patients with this situation.

A clinical protocol supported by Nd:YAG low-level laser therapy proposed for extractions in patients under bisphosphonates therapy. Their experience supported the hypothesis that the association of antibiotic treatment and low level laser therapy (LLLT) through Nd:YAG laser (1064 nm--power 1.25 W; frequency 15 Hz; fibre diameter: 320 μm) could be effective in preventing BRONJ after tooth extractions in patients under bisphosphonates therapy.

Surgical treatment with Er,Cr:YSGG-laser was reported in 5 cases of Bisphosphonate-associated osteonecrosis of the jaws. ErCrYSGG laser was successfully applied in surgical treatment of BRONJ. Stable mucosal coverage could be achieved in all of 5 cases. They proposed laser surgery could be considered as a promising technique for the effective treatment of BRONJ [49].

Kan et.al presented the successful management of two dental patients who had high potentials for BRONJ development because of chemo and radiotherapy combined with IV zoledronic acid application. They proposed LLLT application combined with atraumatic surgical interventions under antibiotics prophylaxis is a preferable approach in patients with a risk of BRONJ development. Adjunctive effect of LLLT in addition to careful infection control on preventing BRONJ was reported and concluded.

A prospective study investigated the clinical efficacy of low-level laser therapy (LLLT) for the management of bisphosphonate-induced osteonecrosis of the jaws (ONJ-BP).This study suggested that LLLT would appear to be a promising modality of treatment for patients with ONJ-BP, providing that clinical efficacy is safe and well tolerated, especially by those patients who require conservative treatment. Of course, this needs to be addressed further in larger and randomly controlled studies in different clinical settings.

Vescovi et al. proposed Surgical approach with Er:YAG laser on osteonecrosis of the jaws (ONJ) in patients under bisphosphonate therapy (BPT). They concluded that it was possible to observe that an early conservative surgical approach with Er:YAG laser associated with LLLT, for BP-induced ONJ could be considered as more efficient in comparison with medical therapy or other conventional techniques.

Complications following the removal of mandibular third molars

A prospective, randomized, and double-blind study evaluated the analgesic and anti-inflammatory effects of a low-level laser therapy applied to the wound appeared after the surgical removal of impacted lower third molars. They determined that swelling and trismus at the 2nd and 7th postoperative days were slightly higher in the control side, although not statistically significant differences were detected. The application of a low-level laser with the parameters used in this study did not show beneficial effects in reducing pain, swelling, and trismus after removal of impacted lower third molars.

Amarillas-Escobar evaluated the effectiveness of a therapeutic laser in the control of postoperative pain, swelling, and trismus associated with the surgical removal of impacted third molars. They concluded the use of therapeutic laser in the postoperative management of patients having surgical removal of impacted third molars, using the protocol of the study, decreases postoperative pain, swelling, and trismus, without statistically significant differences.

Aras and Güngörmüş compared the effects of extraoral and intraoral low-level laser therapies (LLLT) on postoperative trismus and oedema following the removal of mandibular third molars. This study demonstrated that extraoral LLLT is more effective than intraoral LLLT for the reduction of postoperative trismus and swelling after extraction of the lower third molar.

12.10 ENDODONTIC SURGERY

An in vitro study evaluated the generated temperature of the Er:YAG laser, with three different pulse durations (pulse duration 50 μs, pulse duration 100 μs, and pulse duration 300 μs) for apicectomy, compared with tungsten bur and surgical saw. Their results showed that laser irradiation with pulse duration 50 μs appears to have the lowest temperature rise and the shortest time required for apicectomy of the three pulse durations. However, Er:YAG laser for apicectomy in all pulse durations could be used safely for resection in endodontics in the presence of sufficient water.

Angiero et al. evaluated the efficacy of erbium lasers for retrograde endodontic treatment, in terms of clinical outcome and therapeutic success. The lasers used in the study were the erbium: yttrium-aluminum-garnet (Er: YAG) laser, wavelength 2940 nm, and the erbium, chromium- doped: yttrium-scandium-gallium-garnet (Er,Cr:YSGG) laser, wavelength 2780 nm. Laser-assisted surgery increases the range of therapeutic approaches in the sphere of retrograde endodontic treatment. The results of this study showed that the erbium laser, used for apicoectomy, results in a high success rate with considerable benefit in terms of clinical outcome and therapeutic success.

Frenectomy

Labial frenula are sagittal fibrous folds of oral mucosa with a periosteal insertion that extend from the lips to the alveolar or gingival mucosa. Occasionally, they assume inadequate size or location and may lead to functional and esthetic limitations. A comparative study evaluated labial frenectomy with Nd:YAG laser and conventional surgery. Their results showed that Nd:YAG laser frenectomies reduced transoperative bleeding, avoiding the need of suturing, and promoted a significant reduction of surgical time in comparison with conventional surgery.

A case series reported the use of ND:YAG laser for labial frenulectomy. Twenty-three patients were treated and afterward controlled. Laser treatment, above all ND:YAG, appeared to be the gold standard technique.

The upper lip frenulum reinsertion, bleeding, surgical time and surgical wound healing in frenectomies performed with the CO_2 laser versus the Er, Cr:YSGG laser were compared. The upper lip laser frenectomy was a simple technique that resulted in minimum or no postoperative swelling or pain, and which involved upper lip frenulum reinsertion at the mucogingival junction. The CO_2 laser offered a bloodless field and shorter surgical times compared with the Er,Cr:YSGG laser. On the other hand, the Er,Cr:YSGG laser achieved faster wound healing.

Fiberotomy

The effects of circumferential supracrestal fiberotomy in vivo (using diode, CO_2, and Er:YAG lasers) on the morphology and chemical composition of the root surface were evaluated. SEM analysis indicated that no thermal changes, including melting or carbonization, were observed following the lasing procedures. They concluded that laser-aided procedures, when used at appropriate laser settings, preserved the original morphology and chemical composition of cementum.

Kim et al. investigated the effectiveness and periodontal side effects of laser circumferential supracrestal fiberotomy (CSF) and low-level laser therapy (LLLT) on orthodontically rotated teeth in beagles. They demonstrated that laser CSF was an effective procedure to decrease relapses after tooth rotation, causing no apparent damage to the supporting periodontal structures, whereas LLLT on orthodontically rotated teeth without retainers appeared to increase the relapse tendency.

Ankyloglossia

One study compared the tolerance of lingual frenectomy regarding a local anesthesia requirement and comparison of postsurgical discomfort experienced by patients operated on with both diode and erbium:yttrium-aluminium-garnet (Er:YAG) lasers. Their results indicated that the Er:YAG laser is more advantageous than the diode laser in minor soft-tissue surgery because it can be performed without local anesthesia and with only topical anesthesia.

MEDICAL OPTICS

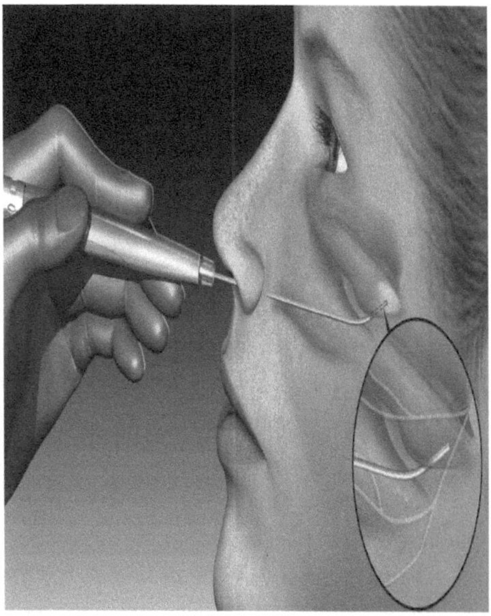

13

CHAPTER

LASER APPLICATIONS IN OTOLARYNGOLOGY

13.1INTRODUCTION

Lasers have been ubiquitous in otolaryngology since Jako and Strong first introduced the CO_2 laser in 1970. Since that time lasers have traditionally been used like a scalpel, able to cut and cauterize precisely. More recently, the role of lasers has been expanded in otolaryngology depending on the specific laser wave-length and dosimeter parameters. Not only can lasers be utilized to extirpate cancer, but also used to recover hearing, improve the air- way, treat epistaxis, and even break up salivary stones for easy removal. The individual characteristics of the laser are important for the specific application. However, the otolaryngologist often works in areas that are either difficult to access using classic methods or require extreme precision, and the mechanism and method for delivering the laser energy is often equally important. In this chapter, we describe the many ways lasers are used in otolaryngology treat both benign conditions to life-threatening diseases. New and innovative applications are also discussed.

13.2 HISTORY OF LASER USE IN OTOLARYNGOLOGY

In otolaryngology, laser has been traditionally used like a scalpel or cautery to precisely incise, cauterize, and coagulate tissue particularly where a collimated beam could provide non-contact and precise tissue ablation for tissue targets that would be difficult to treat using conventional instruments. Over time other applications of lasers have evolved in the head, neck, and upper airway which capitalize not only on the precision realized by the laser, but also on its ability to achieve selective photothermolysis, spatial selective, confined thermal injury, and the generation of photo acoustic waves. By selecting the correct laser wavelength and appropriate dosimeter parameters, surgeons can control both the temporal and spatial evolution of heat within the target site leading to any of the above referenced laser- tissue interactions. Light is variably absorbed and scattered as it propagates through tissue, and the distribution of light in tissue determines the nature of the specific interaction.

As in dermatology, the selection of the appropriate laser in head and neck applications is critically important, and the selection of a specific device and mode of delivery are just as important as wavelength and dosimeter.

The otolaryngologist—head and neck surgeon frequently works in areas that are either difficult to access (e.g. larynx, skull base) or require extreme precision (e.g. middle ear), and in these circumstances laser technology can be extremely valuable. For example, during microsurgery of the vocal fold or stapes, a micromanipulator or microscope-mounted scanner is needed to precisely focus and translate a laser beam as small as 100 mm. In surgery of the subglottic and trachea, flexible optical fibers (fiber optics) or waveguides are used to deliver laser light to these difficult-to- access locations. In minimally invasive laryngeal cancer operations, high power CO_2 lasers (λ = 10.6 μm) are needed to cut tissue while maintaining hemostasis.

13.3 FREQUENTLY USED LASERS IN OTOLARYNGOLOGY

The workhorse in Otolaryngology—Head and Neck Surgery is the carbon dioxide laser. It is used extensively in surgery of the larynx and ear because it can cut tissue precisely, seal small blood vessels and even ablate bone. In cancer surgery, CO_2 lasers may seal lymphatic's potentially reducing the spread of disease. Since infrared light is invisible, the CO_2 laser is always used with a visi- ble aiming beam. The potassium-titanyl phosphate (Neodymium-doped:YttriumAluminum-Garnet), KTP(Nd:YAG) (λ = 532 nm), laser is also becoming used increasingly more commonly in laryngo- tracheal surgery as well as surgery of the oropharynx and nose. The KTP(Nd:YAG) laser is most frequently used for vascular lesions because of its absorption by oxyhemoglobin. In the nose, the KTP(Nd:YAG) laser is most frequently used for treatment of hereditary hemorrhage telangiectasia's (Osler-Weber-Rendu disease). This is a visible wavelength laser and hence easily transmitted using low-cost optical fibers. It can be made to produce a pulsed output beam, also known as giant pulse laser or Q-switching. This allows for the delivery of nanosecond pulses, which leads to less tissue injury to the surrounding structures. Nd:YAG lasers (λ = 1064 nm) are used in otolaryngology as well, however the deep penetration depth of this wavelength has resulted in limited use (primarily for very large venous malformation coagulation in the oral cavity and pharynx); though in contact mode, this laser has applications as a precise cutting device.

The Argon laser (λ = 514 nm) is also used for nasal and middle ear surgery. It is absorbed by hemoglobin and melanin and is generally used in continuous-wave mode. The Holmium: YAG (Ho:YAG) (λ = 2.1 μm) laser is a mid-infrared laser wavelength that is moderately absorbed by water, its principal chromosphere. It is valuable because it has a relatively shallow optical penetration depth like the car- bon dioxide laser but can be transmitted using low-cost silica fibers. Its use in otolaryngology has been very limited thus far due to the lack of availability of these devices in most medical centers. The Erbium:YAG laser (λ = 2.94 μm) is used for middle ear surgery, surgical planning in rhinophyma, and cosmetically for skin resurfacing. It has high absorption in soft tissue and bone and minimal thermally induced peripheral damage. It also has a tolerable photoacous- tic wave effect in the surrounding tissue. Pfalz, Fisch and others have developed Erbium:YAG lasers for middle ear surgery and has more recently been shown to have equal surgical outcomes when compared to the CO_2 laser (Table 13.1).

Table 13.1: Laser applications in otolaryngology

Laser type	Wave length	Penetration depth	Delivery methods	Indications/applications
Argon	514 nm	0.8 mm	Fiber Micromanipulator Focusing handpiece	Ear—Stapes surgery Nose—telangiectasias
CO_2	106,000 nm	30 μm	Articulated arm Micromanipulator Hollow wave-guide scanner Focusing handpiece	Glottis/subglottis/larynx/ oropharynx Benign/malignant Tonsils Lingual Oral cavity/tongue Benign/malignant Nose Turbinate hypertrophy
Erbium:YAG	2940 nm	3 μm	Articulated arm Sapphire fiber	Nose Rhinophyma Cosmetic Laser resurfacing
Holmium:YAG	2120 nm	0.4 mm	Fiber/bare fiber contact Hanpiece	Oral Cavity Lithotripsy Nose Sinus surgery Turbinate hypertrophy
KTP (Nd: YAG)	532 nm	0.9 mm	Fiber/bare fiber contact Side-fire Focusing handpiece Diffuser tip Micromanipulator	Nose Polyps Epistaxis Oropharynx/palatine tonsils Obstructive sleep apnea Vascular malformations Nose Telangiectasias Trachea Stenosis Subglottic hemangioma
Nd: YAG	1064 nm	4 mm	Fiber/bare fiber Contact tips	Vascular malformations Tumor removal (contact mode) Turbinate surgery

13.4 LASERSAFETYINOTOLARYNGOLOGIC APPLICATIONS

As in dermatology, laser safety needs to be considered for the patient, surgeon and surgical staff. The use of a laser near the eyes and in the airway war always rats the diligent practice of laser safety. Blindness burns to the skin, airway injury and death may result if precautions are not taken to prevent these devastating events. The safety pre-cautions and measures to prevent eye injury in head and neck surgery are identical to those used in dermatology, with the exception that the laser dosimeter is often significantly more powerful

than that used to treat the skin. Eye protection measures are reviewed elsewhere. The use of lasers in surgery in the airway presents a major challenge that is unique to otolaryngology—head and neck surgery. Airway fires are a serious risk in laser surgeries involving the airway. Flammable anesthetic gases provide an oxidizing agent that can initiate the fire in the presence of an ignition source such as a laser. The endotracheal tube or other surgical supplies typically used to protect the airway can serve as fuel to propagate the reaction. Specialized laser-safe endotracheal tubes (Fig. 13.2) exhibit prolonged mean times to ignition in comparison to standard endotracheal tubes. Reflective metallic tape wrapped around the endotracheal tube is shown to reduce the risk of ignition of all tubes. Each specific laser interacts differently with these laser-safe endotracheal tubes and many studies have been performed to evaluate the safety of laser surgery in the airway. For example, it has recently been shown that the KTP laser is unable to penetrate even PVC endotracheal tube and suggests that laser safe endotracheal tubes may be unnecessary. However, this laser does interact with the black writing on the endotracheal tube to produce a spark and care must be taken to prevent the KTP laser from encountering these markings.

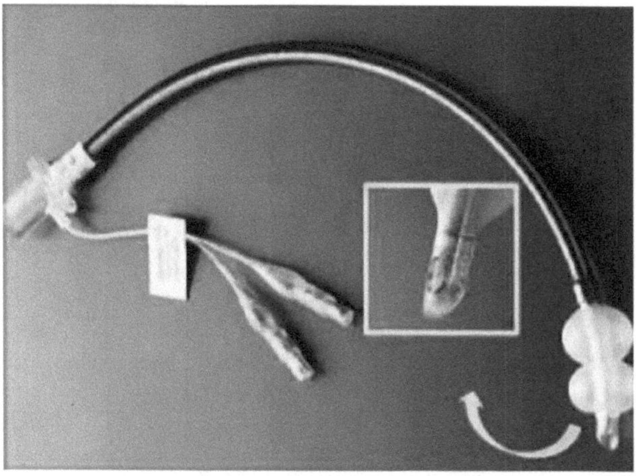

Figure 13.2: Laser-specific endotracheal tube wrapped with reflective metallic tape. Laser-Shield II Endotracheal Tube—Medtronic

13.5 LARYNGOLOGY AND HYPOPHARYNGEAL PATHOLOGY

Jako and Strong pioneered the use of the CO_2 laser in laryngeal surgery in the 1970s. They were among the first to describe the laser excision of early laryngeal cancer. Lasers gained popularity in the 1980s for removal of benign laryngeal lesions such as recurrent respiratory papillomatosis. During this time, Steiner began his seminal work expanding the scope of laryngeal laser surgery to treat more extensive malignant tumors of the larynx and upper-aero digestive tract. His pioneering work is perhaps the greatest contribution to organ sparing laryngeal surgery over the past 20 years and demonstrated the advantages of utilizing microsurgical laser techniques in the treatment of early-stage laryngeal cancer.

The CO_2 laser was the first wavelength used in laryngeal surgery and remains the laser of choice for many laryngeal operations. Recent advances in laser technology, anesthesia, and surgical instrumentation have made minimally invasive laryngeal procedures more common. These new approaches have led to better organ preservation rates, improved post-operative functionality and reduced recovery time.

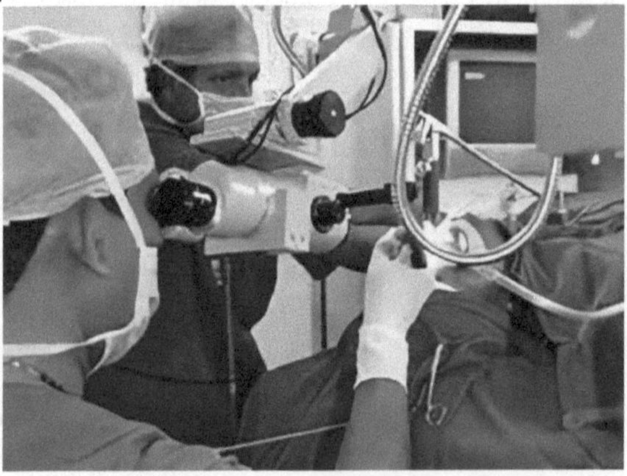

Figure 13.3: Micromanipulator coupled surgical laser with patient placed in suspension (Photograph provided courtesy of Dr. Brian Wong).

Chiefly among these advances, lasers can be precisely focused on providing surgeons with a cut- ting tool capable of incising tissue even at distances of 400 mm. Using a micromanipulator- coupled surgical laser (Fig. 13.3) at 25× to 40× magnification can allow for simultaneous use of both hands as well as focus an extremely accurate laser beam (Fig. 13.4). The line-of-sight lasers that are coupled to the micromanipulator are limited in that they cannot reach around corners, however. Newer hollow waveguides and fiberoptics continue to expand the role of lasers airway surgery. The most used fiberoptic lasers used in otolaryngology at this point in time are the KTP(Nd:YAG) and CO_2 lasers. These lasers can now reach areas that are otherwise difficult to access without performing an open procedure.

13.6 CANCER

Transoral endoscopic laser laryngeal microsurgery depends upon the ability of the surgeon to determine the extent of tumor invasion prior to excision. This can be done by detailed physical examination performed under general anesthesia and imaging studies. The primary objective is to achieve complete resection of the cancer with clear margins, while maintaining as much organ function as possible. Primary goals are to pre- serve swallowing, voice, and airway.

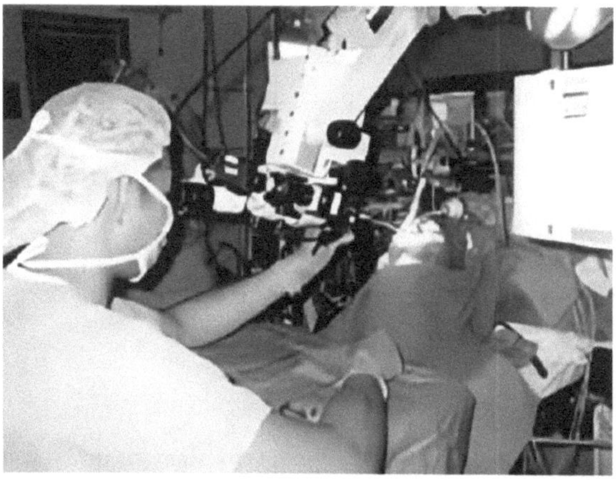

Figure 13.4: Micromanipulator coupled with surgical laser. Note the bimanual instrumentation allowed by placing the patient in suspension (Photograph provided courtesy of Dr. Brian Wong).

While trans oral laser laryngeal microsurgery (TLM) has many advantages such as decreased post-operative morbidity and reduced recovery time. The potential for organ preservation, recurrence or incomplete resection are significant risks. Hence, making the decision to proceed with TLM requires skill and sound clinical judgment. It is generally contraindicated in patients with known extensive invasion into other structures and recurrent cancer in previously irradiated areas. In TLM, tumor is excised piecemeal using a laser, with frozen section guidance, much like Mohs surgery, albeit over complex three-dimensional surfaces with composite tissue structures.

13.6.1 Glottic Carcinoma

The larynx ("voicebox") is composed of the supraglottis, glottis, and subglottis. The glottis includes the vocal cords. Use of the laser to excise glottic cancer is well established for lesions staged at T1 and early T2. For all T2a carcinomas of the glottis, laser excision is recommended regardless of the pattern of the spread of the tumor. Provided the tumor is superficial, it is of limited significance whether the disease involves supraglottis, subglottis or the anterior commissure. The superficial location of the tumor in T1 and early T2 disease allows it to be excised by partial mucosectomy or cordotomy. Laser- assisted endoscopic excision of T3 and T4 laryngeal carcinomas is controversial. Most experts in the field reject the idea of laser microsurgical excision of these advanced tumors unless a classic laryngectomy is not an option due to underlying co-morbid disease. Patients with T3 or T4 laryngeal lesions require the widest possible endoscopic excision followed by post-operative radiotherapy to the primary site and surrounding groups of lymph nodes; however, they more often undergo a classic open total or partial laryngectomy. Steiner groups patients T2b, T3, and T4 together and routinely treat these tumors with laser-assisted endoscopic surgery.

13.6.2 Supraglottic Carcinoma

The supraglottis is the subsite of the larynx superior to the true vocal cords. Supraglottic tumors typically occur either in the suprahyoidepiglottis and false cord area or in the infrahyoid/ epiglottic area. It is relatively rare that small, well-circumscribed tumors are diagnosed in the supraglottic area because the tumors tend to be much more advanced when they start to produce symptoms. Laser resection of early stage supraglottic carcinomas is now more commonly being performed. Tumors in the suprahyoid epiglottis and false cord area are easily removed. Laser excision is indicated because wide margins can be taken without the concern of adversely affecting function. Newer techniques in otolaryngology are now progressing to transoral robotic surgery (TORS) in the resection of early supraglottic carcinomas. Preliminary results show TORS more often had positive margins on pathology, but shorter operative times. This was attributed to improved exposure to TLM.

Infrahyoid epiglottic cancers are difficult to assess preoperatively even with imaging studies and are at risk for infiltrating the preepiglottic space. There are conflicting opinions regarding endoscopic laser resection of carcinoma that involves the preepiglottic space. Iro urges caution and restraint in treatment of T3 staged supraglot- tic cancers with transoral laser surgery. Whereas Rudert believes that even these supraglottic cancers that invade the preepiglottic space are candidates for endoscopic laser resection.

Hypopharyngeal Carcinoma

Pre-resection analysis of the airway during surgi- cal endoscopy under general anesthesia may not be able to identify the true extent of hypopharyngeal tumors. Imaging studies can aid in this endeavor. Tumors involving the piriform sinuses can typically involve the thyroid cartilage, arytenoids, paraglottic and preepiglottic space as well as other soft tissues of the neck with little or no evidence seen on endoscopy. Because of these factors, many laryngologists agree that partial pharyngo-laryngeal resection utilizing only a laser is insufficient for complete eradication of disease and cannot be justified. Classic open surgery (i.e., laryngectomy, laryngopharyn- gectomy) remains the standard of care.

Palliative Therapy

The laser is a useful tool in debulking tumors that obstruct the upper airway and may be an alternative to tracheostomy. Avoiding a tracheostomy greatly improves a patient's quality of life. Palliative airway surgery requires experience and judgment. If too little tumor is respected, the obstruction will persist and ultimately lead to a tracheostomy. However, aggressive resection of tumor may lead to aspiration and the need for a tracheostomy to protect the airway and provide pulmonary toilet. Laccourreye published a 10-year experience describing the use of the CO_2 laser to debulk obstructing endolaryngeal carcinomas in 42 patients for the avoidance of a tracheostomy. Ninety-three percent of patients avoided tracheostomy.

Recanalizing the upper digestive tract by sub- totally ablating hypopharyngeal and esophageal outlet tumors poses a serious risk of hemorrhage and will only provide temporary improvement in swallowing. Placement of a percutaneous gastrostomy tube (PEG) tube is often a safer and better option for these head and neck cancer patients with dysphagia. If palliative laser surgery is considered, one should aim for sustainable symptomatic relief.

13.7 BENIGN DISEASE

The CO_2 laser has a firmly established role in the treatment of benign laryngeal disorders such as papillomas, polyps, vascular malformations and strictures (see Table 13.2). Since Jako and Strong first introduced the CO_2 laser in 1970, several groups, including those led by Shapshay, Zeitels, Ossoff, Steiner, Motta and Rudert, have published extensively their experiences with laser surgery in benign laryngeal disease. The use of other lasers such as the KTP(Nd:YAG) laser and the pulsed dye laser ($\lambda = 585$ nm) has also been reported.

13.7.1 Polyps

Vocal cord polyps are generally unilateral, sessile and appear to be spherical and well circum- scribed. They typically originate at the free edge on the anterior two thirds of the vocal cord (Fig. 13.5). The vocal cords have a delicate subepithelial tissue layer that can be damaged because of repetitive collisions and shearing forces. Voice abuse and chronic inflammation from tobacco smoke irritation are common causes of injury to the vocal cord epithelium and lead to damage within the epithelial basement membrane. A large percentage of patients with polyps are heavy smokers or are exposed to a large amount of secondary tobacco smoke.

When conservative methods (i.e., voice rest, speech therapy, etc.) fail, treatment is surgical removal. It is important to always send the excised polyps for histology to exclude an early malignancy. For this reason, these polyps should never be vaporized with the laser.

Table 13.2: Benign lesions (in laryngology section).

Disorder	Laser treatment
Polyps	CO_2 or KTP (Nd:YAG) laser excision
Papillomas	CO_2 or KTP(Nd:YAG) laser ablation
Vascular malformations	Pulse dye laser photocoagulation
Hemangiomas	CO_2 or KTP(Nd:YAG) laser for coagulation and excision
Vocal cord paralysis	CO_2 laser for enlarging glottic chink
Laryngomalacia	CO_2 laser excision of redundant tissue

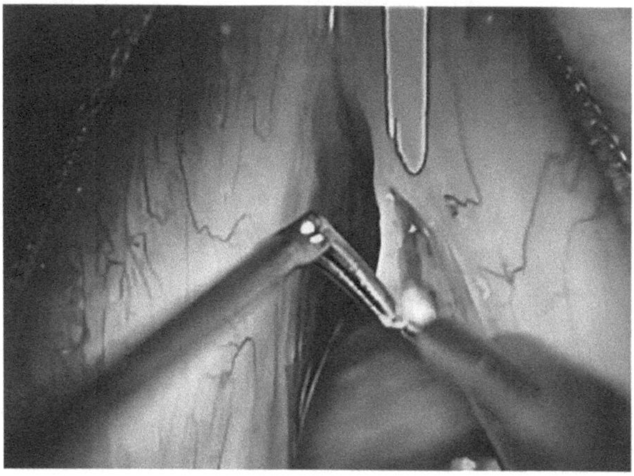

Figure 13.5: Pulsed 532 nm KTP laser assisted subepithelial resection of fibrovascular mass (hemorrhagic polyp) on the middle 2/3 of the left true vocal cord. The green area is refraction from the laser light (Photograph provided courtesy of Dr. Steven Zeitels).

13.8 PAPILLOMAS

Laryngeal Papillomas are typically caused by HPV types 6 and 11 and can affect any age group (Fig. 13.6). The distribution of disease is bimodal, affecting children and middle-aged adults most often. The virus causes formation of benign epithelial papillomas of the larynx. Diagnosis is made with flexible fiberoptic laryngoscopy or microlaryngoscopy. Although papillomas most commonly occur on the vocal cords, the larynx, esophagus and trachea must be comprehensively examined during endoscopy because the papillomas can occur anywhere along the aerodigestive system. While the CO_2 laser is still used to ablate these lesions, the concern over aerosolization of viral particles has made mechanical laryngeal microdebriders an increasingly more common treatment approach. The KTP(Nd:YAG) laser is particularly helpful in surgery for laryngeal papillomas. The advent of fiberoptic cables for the KTP(Nd:YAG) and CO_2 laser has even made it possible to treat papillomas in the clinic with the use of a flexible fiberoptic laryngoscope.

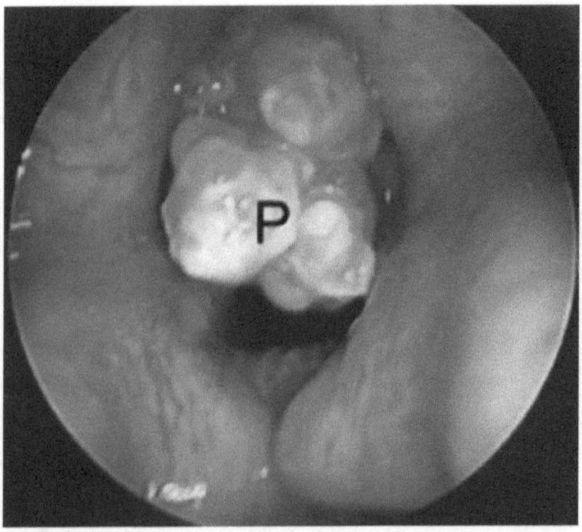

Figure 13.6: Laryngeal papilloma (P) at the level of the glottis (Photograph provided courtesy of Dr. Gupreet S. Ahuja).

13.8.1 Hemangiomas and Vascular Malformations

Subglottic hemangiomas present with persistent cough, hoarseness or stridor, and manifest as red- dish, well-circumscribed masses during surgical endoscopy. Surgery involves primarily vaporization and ablation rather than excision. The CO_2,

KTP or Nd:YAG laser can all be used with low power settings (1–3 W). High power settings can lead to tracheal perforation, pneumothorax or intractable bleeding.

Vascular malformations typically are located in the supraglottic area and are generally asymptomatic. Symptoms of a laryngopharyngeal vascular malformation may include foreign body sensation or mild stridor of unknown origin. Carbon dioxide laser excision or Nd:YAG coagulation is the treatment of choice, though other wavelengths can be used as well with appropriate dosimetry. Use of the Nd:YAG laser has a higher rate of postoperative scarring and stenosis due to the deeper penetration depth of this wavelength but is extremely valuable in treating large vascular malformations where volumetric heating of large regions of tumor is required. These extensive tumors are more commonly found in the oropharynx and oral cavities. Ectatic blood vessels along the vocal cord surface (Fig. 13.7) may alter the pitch and timbre of the voice and can be problematic for singers and other professionals. They are commonly treated using a pulse dye laser and KTP(Nd:YAG).

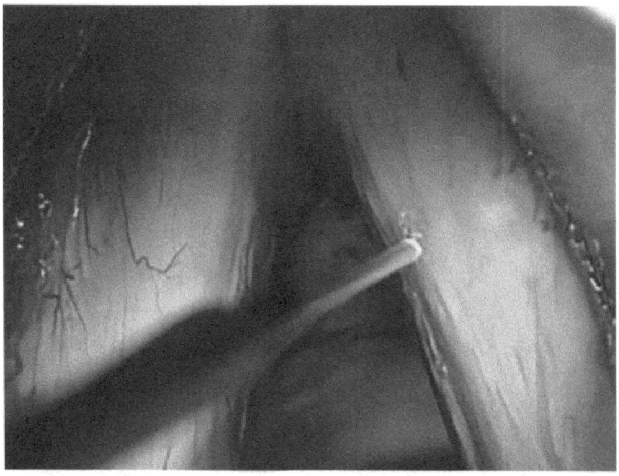

Figure 13.7: Pulsed 532 nm KTP laser assisted photoangiolytic of ecstatic blood vessels in a singer (Photograph pro- vided courtesy of Dr. Steven Zeitels)

13.8.2 Laryngomalacia

Stridor in children is most caused by laryngomalacia, and 60–75% of childhood cases of stridor are associated with laryngomalacia. Approximately 20%

of these cases do not resolve spontaneously or cause symptoms severe enough to require surgical intervention. Dysphagia, apnea and respiratory distress are all indicators for surgical intervention. Laryngomalacia will be discussed in a later section along with subglottic hemangiomas.

13.8.3 Vocal Cord Paralysis

Patients that have bilateral vocal cord paralysis may develop severe respiratory distress and air- way obstruction from the diminished patency of the glottic airway. Vocal cord paralysis commonly presents following surgery where the recurrent laryngeal nerve is inadvertently injured (i.e., during thyroid tumor surgery). In the immediate post-operative period, the patient sometimes develops stridor and respiratory insufficiency. Acutely, treatment may involve intubation and tracheostomy. For long-term treatment, CO_2 lasers can be used to enlarge the glottic chink and increase airway patency. This is challenging surgery because it is important to strike a balance between airway patience and voice quality when enlarging the glottis.

13.9 CONTRAINDICATIONS FOR SURGERY OF BENIGN AIRWAY LESIONS

There are few contraindications to Transoral Laser Microsurgery (TLM) for benign lesions. One important rule is that surgeons should avoid unnecessary disruption or excision of the anterior commissure and the free edge of the vocal cords. Disruption of the anterior commissure may result in change in the patient's voice, extensive scar formation, or an anterior glottic web. If there is epithelial disruption of the free edges of both vocal cords, this can lead to post- operative scarring and webbing. It is imperative that the surgeon only work on the epithelium of one vocal cord at a time to prevent these complications.

13.10 PRE-OPERATIVE MANAGEMENT

In the pre-operative evaluation, patients always undergo an indirect mirror or a flexible fiberoptic laryngoscopy examination to determine the extent of the lesion and vocal cord mobility. Video stroboscopes of the vocal cords may be included in the pre-operative evaluation to determine the dynamics of vocal cord movement. Some patients may undergo diagnostic imaging (CT or MRI of the neck) to determine the extent of disease. Vocal cord polyps warrant a trial of speech therapy for vocal coaching and training in proper voice use prior surgery. Patients with carcinoma of the larynx and recurrent papillomatosis must be strongly encouraged to quit smoking.

The most common parameters for the CO_2 laser beam using a micromanipulator is a 250 mm spot size with a working distance of 350 mm. Laser power is usually below 8 W. In the super- pulse mode, where exposure time is 0.1 s or less, a low power setting of 2–3 W is used. The super- pulse mode is useful in achieving maximum ablation through minimal penetration and maximum energy absorption at the surface of interest. There is almost no charring due to the minimal thermal diffusion in the surrounding areas around the tar- get. In preparation for epithelium incision, microvascular coagulation is required. For this, the laser is typically set for a 0.05 s pulse of 1 W of power using an unfocused beam.

Recently, flash scanner technological originally developed for use in dermatologic applications has been re-purposed and adapted for use in laryngeal microsurgery. This technology spreads the laser energy uniformly over the target area by using two nearly parallel, rapidly rotating mirrors. It creates a uniform area of laser energy approximately 3 mm in diameter in 1 ms. The laser is able to provide surface ablation with little to no chair at a depth of 0.15 mm. The high cost of these systems has limited the broad adoption of this technology.

13.11 DESCRIPTION OF TECHNIQUE

Suspension microlaryngoscopy provides a method in which the surgeon can directly visualize the larynx and its surrounding structures. Gustav Killian was among the first to describe suspension laryngoscopy in 1912 and later developed the Killian-Lynch suspension laryngoscope along with Robert Clyde Lynch. Zeitels showed effective use of suspension laryngoscopy in 120 cases in a prospective assessment. Suspension allows for bimanual direct laryngoscopic surgery. Furthermore, suspension laryngoscopy permits the use of a laryngoscope with a larger bore thereby enhancing exposure. Figure 13.8 demonstrates the positioning of a patient in suspension and Fig. 13.9 shows the normal anatomy of the larynx as visualized under suspension micro laryngoscopy.

With the patient anesthetized and lying supine, the head is fully extended. A rigid laryngeal endoscope is introduced through the oral cavity and past the epiglottis into the larynx until the desired endolaryngeal structures are visualized. The vocal cords should be clearly visualized from the anterior commissure to the vocal process on both sides. The rigid laryngoscope is then stabilized and secured using a suspension arm. Surgery is performed using a microscope with a 400 mm focal length lens or using a Hopkins rod endoscope inserted through the laryngoscope bore. There are several instances that make suspension micro laryngoscopy very difficult or even impossible. Abnormal anatomies such as a short, stiff neck, long or protruding maxillary teeth, dis- placed larynx and lesions or a mass at the base of tongue may limit and prevent suspension laryngoscopy in these patients. Utilizing paralysis is often necessary for successful laryngoscopy.

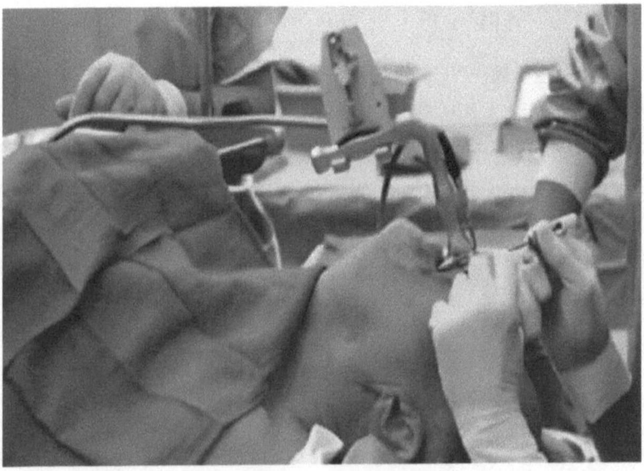

Figure 13.8: Suspension laryngoscopy (Photograph provided courtesy of Dr. Roger Crumley)

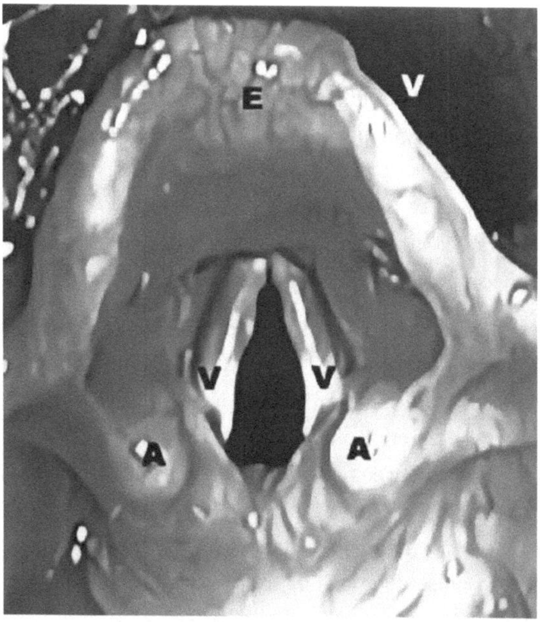

Figure 13.9: View of the glottis through the laryngoscope. An arytenoid, E epiglottis, V (black) vocal cords, V (white) vallecula (Photograph provided courtesy of Dr. Gupreet S. Ahuja)

Suspension laryngoscopy provides a direct airway in which anesthesia may be administered either through an endotracheal tube that is inserted parallel to the laryngoscope or via jet ventilation. This direct airway also provides an unimpeded path for the surgeon to access the vocal cords and other structures in the larynx. When using an endotracheal tube in laser surgery, it is important to use a laser-safe endotracheal tube to minimize the risk of an airway fire. These techniques allow for a minimally invasive approach to laryngeal surgery where traditional approaches have involved large external incisions and significant morbidity.

13.12 LASERS AND LASER DEVICES

Since Jako coupled the carbon dioxide laser to the operating microscope in 1972 for laryngeal surgery, the CO_2 laser has been the wavelength of choice. The

CO_2 laser is used in most operations because of its widespread availability in most medical centers and its efficiency in simultaneously cutting tissue and maintaining hemostasis. Other commonly used lasers in otolaryngology include the KTP(Nd:YAG) laser and the argon laser. In laryngeal surgery, the CO_2 laser is often coupled to a micromanipulator attached to the microscope. This allows the surgeon to use micro- surgical instruments and the laser at the same time. It also provides maximum surgical field visualization with high magnification and an unobstructed view of the lesion. The CO_2 laser has several advantages over conventional surgical instruments that cut or cauterize in that traditional devices may obstruct the field of view or amplify the surgeon's intention tremor via a lever arm of up to 20 cm.

The thermal damage zone when using micro-manipulators introduces limited artifact into the histological assessment, and it coagulates small blood vessels and seals lymphatic channels thus minimizing the incidence of metastases. The diameter of the laser beam, pulse duration and irradiance can be adjusted to produce different tissue effects. Spot sizes between 1 to 4 mm are used for tissue ablation and 0.2–1 mm used for cutting with powers varying anywhere from 2 to 10 W. Some micromanipulators further focus the beam down to an even smaller spot size and combined with short pulse durations or flash scanner technology, can ablate tissue with minimal to no charring just as in skin resurfacing. Morbidity of using the CO_2 laser when appropriate is far less than cold surgery, and the cost effectiveness is much greater.

In certain cases where lesions extend out of the surgeon's visual field, the CO_2 laser can be delivered by a flexible hollow waveguide. However, there are limitations with the use of the hollow waveguide due to its limited angulation, the diameter of the laser spot and the significant and variable loss of power during transmission. Regardless, recent techniques using hollow fiber technology are evolving. Additionally, the KTP (Nd:YAG) laser energy is similarly delivered through a fiber optic cable and various handpieces.

13.13 CANCER

Glottic Carcinoma

T1 and T2a carcinomas of the glottis are typically resected en bloc and clear margins of 1–3 mm is obtained. However, with laser surgery, it is possi- ble to maintain more narrow margins that allow for preservation of vocal function and reduction in post-operative edema.

Transoral Laser Microsurgery (TLM) has yielded good functional results and low rates of recurrence from multiple groups since the 1990s. Studies have shown that it is possible to preserve the larynx in over 92% of cases with a 5 year local control rate that ranges from 80% to 94%. Treatment of early glottic cancer with TLM has a distinct advantage over other procedures in that it maintains the availability of all treatment options for patients with local or secondary tumor recurrence including laser reexcision, radiation therapy or open partial laryngectomy. T2b and T3 carcinoma of the glottis typically involves the vocal cords with supraglottic or subglottic extension. The operative technique using lasers for these tumors involves subdividing the tumor into several pieces for removal. Resection of these tumors may involve the cricoid and thyroid cartilage, the arytenoids, the cricothyroid ligament and any involved laryngeal soft tissue.

The application of laser assisted endoscopic surgery via suspension laryngoscopy draws comparisons to Mohs surgery because resections are driven by frozen section histology. One of the greatest differences between endoscopic laryngeal surgery and cutaneous Mohs surgery lies in the fact that Mohs surgery aims to achieve the best cosmetic result as possible while attempting to remove as little tissue as possible without compromising the tumor resection. In laryngeal surgery, functionality remains essential post-operatively in laryngeal cancer patients. Laser assisted endoscopic laryngeal surgery has potential to allow surgeons to excise cancer piecemeal with frozen section guidance. Frozen section guidance of surgical resections in the larynx is difficult due to the complex geometry of the structures within the larynx, making this radically more complicated than Mohs surgery for cutaneous disease. It is important for the surgeon to carefully label the surfaces of the specimens and work closely with pathologists during surgery. Ambrosch's experience of 167 patients undergoing laser excision of T2b and T3 laryngeal tumors showed a 5-year rate of definitive local control to be 87%. The recurrence free survival rate over 5 years was 62%. None of these patients required a tracheostomy after the primary resection.

Supraglottic Carcinoma

T1 and T2 carcinoma of the supraglottis is defined as tumor that has not infiltrated the pre- epiglottic fat, immobilized a vocal cord, or metastasized to a local lymph node. Vaughan first described carbon dioxide laser resection of supraglottic carcinoma. Since then, Steiner, Davis and Zeitels have used TLM for supraglottic resections. Laser excision of tumors in this area typically involves extensive dissection and removal of involved muscle, cartilage and even portions of the base of tongue and piriform sinuses in advanced cancer. Tracheostomy is unnecessary in most cases due to limited postoperative edema even after extensive laser dissection. However, it should be considered in a procedure with high blood loss or elderly patients with decreased pulmonary function.

There are relatively few reports on laser resection of T1 and T2 cancers in the supraglottis. Ambrosch reports a series of 48 patients with supraglottic T1 and T2 carcinoma in which there was 100% and 89% local control rate for pT1 and pT2 tumors respectively at 5 years. The recurrence free survival rate over 5 years was 83%, and the overall 5-year survival rate was 76%. In patients who experienced a recurrence, none needed a laryngectomy as a secondary treatment. T3 carcinoma of the supraglottis treated with laser excision is not a common practice. Hinni et al. described a series of 117 patients with T2 to T4 lesions treated with TLM. Five- year Kaplan-Meier estimates were local control in 74%, locoregional control in 68%, disease free survival in 58%, and overall survival in 55%. At 2 years 92% had a functional larynx. This study concluded that TLM with or without radiation is a valid treatment strategy for organ preservation.

Hypopharyngeal Carcinoma

Carcinoma located in the hypopharynx carries the worst prognosis of all upper aerodigestive tract tumors. Reasons for poor prognosis lie in the high rate of local recurrence and the increased likelihood of the presence of metastasis in cervical lymph nodes at diagnosis. Though advances have been made in diagnostic imaging, surgery, radiotherapy, and combined approaches, the mortality rate from these tumors does not reflect any improvement in survival. Though there are reports of use of TLM in excision of hypopharyn- geal cancer, there are few that report any treatment results.

Steiner and Ambrosch describe a series of 129 patients with carcinoma of the piriform sinus treated with laser excision. The 5-year Kaplan-Meier survival rate was 71% for stages I and II and 47% for stages III and IV disease and the 5-year recurrence-free survival rates were 95% for stages I and II and 69% for stages III and IV.

13.14 BENIGN LESIONS

Papilloma's

Transoral laser microsurgery of laryngeal papilloma's is done with the laser on a low power set- ting. This has been described by using CO_2, KTP, and pulse dye laser in both an operating room and in-office setting. This allows the surgeon to ablate the disease in a controlled manner that limits disruption of the normal surrounding tissues and ablates only the mucosa affected by the papilloma's (Fig. 13.10). Small islands of healthy mucosa left between the ablated areas promote quicker re-epithelialization. In cases where there is bilateral vocal cord or anterior commissure involvement, a conservative approach is advised. It is better to leave small papilloma's behind than to have postoperative scarring and synechiae of the anterior commissure, also known as an anterior glottic web, which can lead to voice changes. Corticosteroid administration (3 mg/kg Prednisone) preoperatively assists decreasing edema after extubation, even if there has been extensive resection. Figure 5.10a, b show a before and after images of juvenile laryngeal papillomata. Alternatively, microdebriders have been increasingly used to debulk papilloma's and are slowly replacing lasers as the method of choice for treating papillomata.

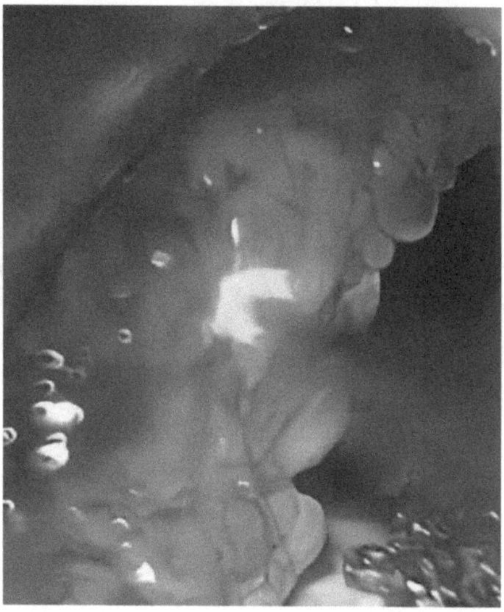

Figure 13.10: Pulsed 532 nm KTP laser photoangiolysis and ablation of glottal papillomatosis (Photograph provided courtesy of Dr. Steven Zeitels).

Laryngomalacia

Anatomically, the cause of the problem in laryngomalacia is an inward collapse of the supraglottic mucosa during inspiration. If conservative measures fail, the surgical treatment for laryngomalacia is supraglottoplasty. Bilateral laser incision of the aryepiglottic folds and the arytenoid cartilage region is the treatment if the cause of the stridor is from shortened aryepiglottic folds. If the stridor is caused by inward col- lapse of the epiglottis during inspiration an epiglottopexy is the surgery of choice. This will be described in more detail in a later section on laser use in the pediatric population.

Vocal Cord Paralysis

The most common laser-based procedure for vocal cord paralysis is unilateral microsurgical laser arytenoidectomy. In Steiner and Werner's experience, excision of the posterior portion of the vocal cords bilaterally with the microsurgical laser offers several benefits. Most of the vibrating parts of the vocal cords and arytenoids cartilage are preserved preventing aspiration while maintaining good voice quality.

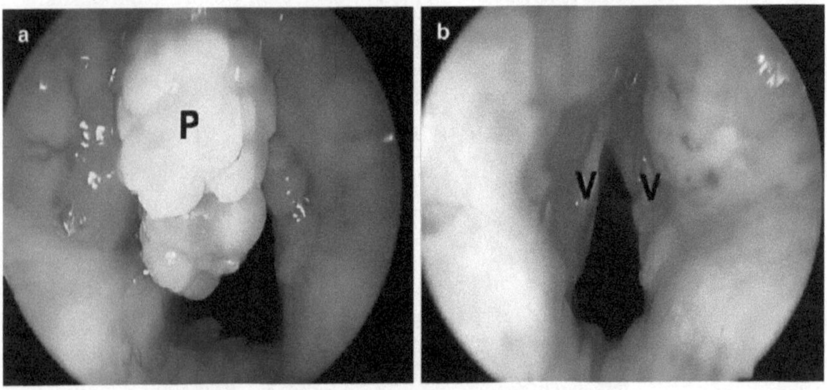

Figure 13.11: Papilloma in the pediatric airway, before (a) and after (b) laser excision.P papilloma, V vocal cords (Photograph provided courtesy of Dr. Gupreet S. Ahuja)

Hypopharyngeal Diverticula

To perform a Zenker's diverticulectomy, the patient is suspended in a similar fashion to that which was described previously. Treatment of Zenker's diverticulum consists of suspending the hypopharynx with a specialized "Weerda" endoscope, then taking down the "party wall" that exists between the herniated pocket and the upper portion of the esophagus. Traditionally, this required a large cervical incision to exercise the diverticulum and perform a myotomy of the cricopharyngeus muscle. The use of the CO_2 laser to take down the party wall endoscopically has been found to be comparable to traditional, open procedures in terms of outcomes. Laser myotomy is improved compared to the traditional approach in that it does not require a neck incision and requires significantly less operative time. Almost 90% of patients report normal swallowing function after undergoing the procedure.

Post-operative Management

Patients who are otherwise healthy and undergo a limited resection are routinely given a single dose of intravenous steroids, observed in the post- operative care unit and discharged on the same day. Patients who have multiple medical problems or have more extensive surgical excisions, and therefore have a higher possibility for airway compromise, are admitted overnight at minimum for airway observation and scheduled steroid dosing. Post-operative antibiotics are not routinely administered. Strict voice rest for the first 48 h is observed followed by modified voice rest (no screaming, no whispering, limited talking) for the next 1–2 weeks. Patients are then monitored in clinics with repeat flexible fiberoptic laryngoscopy exams. Any change in voice, difficulty breathing or weight loss is monitored closely and may necessitate repeated exams and procedures.

In general suspension laryngoscopy is safe for patients as long as the patient has gone through proper pre-operative evaluation by the otolaryngologist and anesthesiologist. There are several situations that preclude the use of suspension laryngoscopy that include anatomy such as a short, stiff neck, long or protruding maxillary teeth, displaced larynx and lesions or mass in the base of tongue. Complications associated with TLM are more pertinent to the use of the laryngoscope instead of the actual laser itself. Difficult intubation or forceful endoscopic suspension can easily chip, loosen, or fracture teeth if the surgeon is not careful with the orientation of the laryngoscope in the oral cavity. In a study of 339 micro laryngoscopy patients, 75% were found to have small mucosal lesions of the oral cavity, oropharynx and lip. Though the injuries were minor, they were a source of major concern for the patients postoperatively.

Other complications associated with laser microsurgery include lingual and hypoglossal nerve palsy. Prolonged displacement of the tongue can cause severe contusion and swelling that often leads to dysphagia and sometimes- permanent dysesthesia (sensory disturbance) in the tongue.

There are many general safety considerations involving the use of surgical lasers in surgery that were discussed earlier in this chapter. In particular to laryngeal surgery where high-powered lasers are used in small, confined areas with flammable gas, the use of caution cannot be emphasized enough. Stray laser light is not a rare event and can cause burns in unwanted areas. It is recommended practice to cover areas beyond the target site to protect them from unwanted burns. Control of oxygen content, inhalation agents, and use of special laser endotracheal tubes in these procedures is important.

Though TLM rarely requires tracheotomy post operatively, it is nevertheless a real possibility in the intermediate and advanced cases. Surgeons must always be aware of certain indicators for tracheotomy. Prolonged compression of the tongue during TLM can cause lingual edema that can lead to airway compromise. Sudden secondary hemorrhage is a major risk in TLM and may necessitate a tracheotomy. Large arteries and vessels should not only be cauterized but clipped as well to avoid sudden secondary hemorrhage.

TLM typically causes the formation of large granulomas if cartilage is exposed by the surgical procedure. These granulomas are perpetuated by small Osseo cartilaginous sequestrate unless they are removed. TLM involving the anterior commissure often results in a round anterior glottis effect, and this often leads to breathiness and hoarseness. Laser surgery for benign lesions in the larynx is relatively safe compared to most other treatment modalities. It is a minimally invasive technique with almost no complications attributed to the laser itself.

Future directions of laser use in laryngology involve new devices for delivery, office-based laser applications, the use of the laser for welding tissue and the creation of lasers that are even more precise than those which are currently available. An important recent technological advance (Omni Guide, Boston, MA) has provided surgeons the use of CO_2 lasers through a flexible fiber referred to as a "photonic band gap fiber." The fiber is placed in a hand piece coupled with a suction that eliminates the need for a micromanipulator and allows the surgeon to have the freedom of a laser cutting tool in his or her hand. The Omni Guide Beam Path has proven useful in the surgery of both benign and malignant lesions in cases where exposure is difficult.

Another new delivery device has recently been described by combining TORS with the CO_2 laser in resecting upper aero digestive tract tumors. Studies to date have been proof-of- concept and no long-term follow-up data has been described. However, these reports have been encouraging. The flexible CO_2 laser provided fine incisions, excellent hemostasis, and minimal peripheral tissue injury. The exposure provided by TORS improved typical exposure and provided more range of motion than typical TLM. Further study must be performed to deter- mine long-term outcomes and cost effectiveness of these powerful tools.

Awake office-based laser surgery is gaining popularity in the treatment of benign laryngeal lesions because of the relative safety of lasers and the quick recovery period post procedure. Though the CO_2 laser has traditionally been the laser of choice for laryngeal surgery, different lasers have been reported to be useful in office-based surgery. In the office, new technologies such as distal chip endoscopy and rare-earth doped fiber lasers have allowed for creative and innovative surgical techniques. Typical diseases treated with these new techniques are dysplasia's and papilloma's. A 585 nm pulsed dye laser was originally the laser of choice for vascular lesions; however the 532 nm pulsed KTP laser has proven to be superior. The use of the Thulium laser (λ = 2013 nm) which mimics the CO_2 laser closely may become useful as an office-based laser as well. Even though otolaryngologists are performing more office procedures that incorporate lasers, the breadth of procedures remains limited for important reasons such as airway compromise, which is poorly handled in the office setting.

13.15 OTOLOGY

Laser applications in otology include the treat- ment of vascular lesions in the external auditory canal (EAC), exostoses in the EAC, debulking of inoperable tumors, Eustachian tube dysfunction, myringotomy/ tympanostomy in otitis media, graft fixation in tympanoplasty, stapedectomy/ stapedotomy in otosclerosis, tympanosclerosis, removal of cholesteatoma, cochleostomy, labyrinthectomy in benign paroxysmal positional vertigo, endolymphatic hydrops and facial nerve decompression. The use of the laser in middle ear surgery is one of the most elegant examples of laser technology use and applications. Perkins pioneered the use of the argon laser in middle ear surgery in the late-1970s performing the first laser stapedotomy for otosclerosis. Otosclerosis is a localized disorder of bone resorption and deposition (remodeling) in the middle and inner ear that causes progressive conductive hearing loss that typically begins in the third to fifth decade of life. This defect in bone remodeling in the vicinity of the footplate stapes and oval window lead to reduced mobility of the stapes and conductive hearing loss. Mechanical causes of hearing loss can be corrected through surgery. Patients with otosclerosis benefited from the laser argon through its precise vaporization of the stapedial tendon, mobilizing the posterior curse of the stapes, and in stapes footplate fenestration. This procedure is called a stapedectomy or stapedotomy and is performed to recreate ossicular chain mobility and decrease conductive hearing loss. Knowledge of middle ear anatomy is critical in obtaining good post-operative results with minimal complications. Avoidance of injury to the facial nerve and the chorda tympani nerve is the standard of care.

DiBartolomeo described other uses of the argon laser in the field of otology. He utilized this laser in the tympanoplasty (repair of the tympanic membrane), stapedectomy, lysis of adhesions and myringotomy (placement of a hole in the tympanic membrane). He describes the "spot welding" technique of the laser that allows for the adherence of a fascial graft placed in substitution of the tympanic membrane onto the soft tissue annulus. Delivery of a laser to the ear and temporal bone can be either via a fiber (KTP and argon) or via a micro-manipulator such as those used with CO_2 lasers.

Eustachian tube dysfunction is a common ear disorder in which patients may experience chronic recurrent ear infections or difficulty in clearing a blocked sensation of their middle ear. A laser myringotomy may be performed to equalize the pressures between the middle and outer ear, and to assist the ear in draining fluid. Some studies have found improvement in postoperative outcomes such as length of temporary perforation and resolution of middle ear effusion. However, it is considerably more expensive.

Laser Eustachian tuboplasty (LETP) is the practice of utilizing a diode or an argonlaser to vaporize select areas of hypertrophic mucosa and submucosa tissue along the length of the Eustachian tube. In a small number of studies with small patient numbers, it has been found that medical management combined with LETP on a select group of patients can be successful in eliminating chronic middle ear effusions.

A cholesteatoma is not a mass made of cholesterol as the name implies. Instead, it is a collection of keratinized epitheliums that is in an abnormal location at the external auditory canal, middle ear, petrous bone or mastoid. It is either congenital in etiology or is acquired due to repeated infection. It is not invasive, but it destroys the bones of the middle ear leading to conductive hearing loss. It can also erode the mastoid bone and tegmen that can possibly lead to a cerebral spinal fluid leak. Therefore, the cholesteatoma needs to be removed in its entirety to prevent progression and recurrence. The use of a laser in this surgery may assist the surgeon in removing the mass in more difficult to reach areas of the middle ear and mastoid. This often requires improved visualization with endoscopy in addition to the use of laser energy directed by curved fiberoptic cables.

Contraindications to laser use for otologic applications include performing a stapedectomy in the presence of active otitis media or in an only hearing ear that responds well to amplification. Additionally, the presence of vertigo and endolymphatic hydrops, certain inner ear malformations or an overhanging facial nerve that completely obstructs access to the oval window niche are contraindications as well. Laser stapedectomy in patients with a perforated tympanic membrane must be postponed until the perforation is fixed. In this case of an overlying facial nerve, preservation of the facial nerve is most important, and conventional instruments are used to perform the operation rather than the laser to minimize the risk of injury.

13.16 PRE-OPERATIVEMANAGEMENT AND LASERSELECTION

Pre-operative management of patients undergoing laser-assisted otologic surgery includes a full history and physical, an audiogram and usually a non- contrast computer tomography (CT) imaging of the temporal bone and internal auditory canal. When choosing a laser to use near a neurosensory organ like the ear, it is important to consider the potential collateral damage. The thermal and photoacoustic effects in laser use are a function of dosimetry and tissue optical and thermal properties. Bones have substantially smaller water content than skin or other soft tissues and visible wavelengths are not well absorbed. In the absence of any distinct chromophore, using an argon or a KTP(Nd:YAG) laser to ablate bone requires an initiator. An initiator absorbs laser light and undergoes pyrolysis. In middle ear surgery, a small droplet of blood or charred tissue placed on the laser target to serve this purpose. Accordingly, there is a risk of thermal injury, as considerable temperature elevations occur within this region, and ablation occurs with at best modest thermal confinement. In contrast, infrared wavelengths are well absorbed by both the hydroxyapatite crystals in bone and the interwoven collagen fibers. Ablation proceeds by the classical mechanisms, though photoacoustic transients may be generated leading to audible pops. These mechanical transients may propagate through the inner ear and may result in injury to the delicate neuroepithelium. In general, shorter laser pulse durations lead to less thermal injury provided the conditions for thermal confinement are met. However, repeated pulses in rapid succession may lead to the buildup of heat in the target site; hence successive pulses should be separated by enough time to allow for complete thermal relaxation. Short pulse laser systems (e.g., Erbium: YAG) generate an acoustic pressure wave that led to a vibration of the ossicular chain that may result in "noise trauma". The heat generated by the laser may also cause "convection currents" that also lead to vibratory stimulations. Both stimulations that can lead to acoustic injury and should be controlled by appropriate dosimeter selection. Regardless, the mechanical transients produced during laser ablation are comparable or even less harmful than the vibratory effects produced using conventional methods to perform surgery.

13.17 DESCRIPTION OF TECHNIQUE

In addition to the argon, CO_2, and KTP laser, more recently the erbium-YAG laser has been used to perform stapedectomy or stapedotomy in patients with otosclerosis. In the stapedectomy and stapedotomy, the stapedial tendon is vaporized with the laser, then the incudostapedial joint is disarticulated using mechanical instrumentation, and the posterior crus is severed with the laser (Fig. 13.12a, b). The anterior crus of the stapes is then fractured manually and the stapes superstructure is removed. The laser is then used to place a single large hole or a set of smaller holes generating a "rosette" type pattern in the stapes footplate to accommodate the prosthesis (Fig. 13.12c). A mobile prosthesis is put into place. Despite multiple recent attempts, no study to date has demonstrated which laser among the three most used in stapes surgery (argon, KTP and CO_2) is best. Recently, erbium: YAG lasers have been developed for use in performing this operation, however the high cost of these lasers has limited broad adoption. The success of laser stapes surgery is based on audiometric analysis (hearing tests) and complication rates.

Smaller cholesteatomas and residual tissue in previously attempted excisions of cholesteatomas have been vaporized with the CO_2, Argon, and KTP lasers with some reports of lower recurrence rates. Laser use is particularly beneficial when removing cholesteatoma from the delicate bones of the middle ear such as the stapes or in removing disease that traverses the obturator foramen of the stapes. When using the laser in this application, its energy is absorbed more by the cholesteatoma than by the bony surroundings. Endoscopic cholesteatoma surgery can be helpful in obliterating cholesteatoma from hard-to-visualize locations such as the sinus tympani. The laser can also be directed towards these locations using a curved, adjustable laser fiber.

Use of the laser in myringotomy and tympanoplasty is currently a boutique interest in otolaryngology, primarily due to cost. Myringotomy is performed by using an Argon, CO_2, or KTP laser directed by a fiber delivery system to create an incision in a patient's eardrum. It is most often performed in patients with chronic otitis media with effusion. Use of the laser instead of a myringotomy knife has shown to be beneficial by preventing the necessity of tympanostomy tube placement; however, laser myringotomy without tube placement only creates a temporary perforation in the tympanic membrane that lasts <6 weeks.

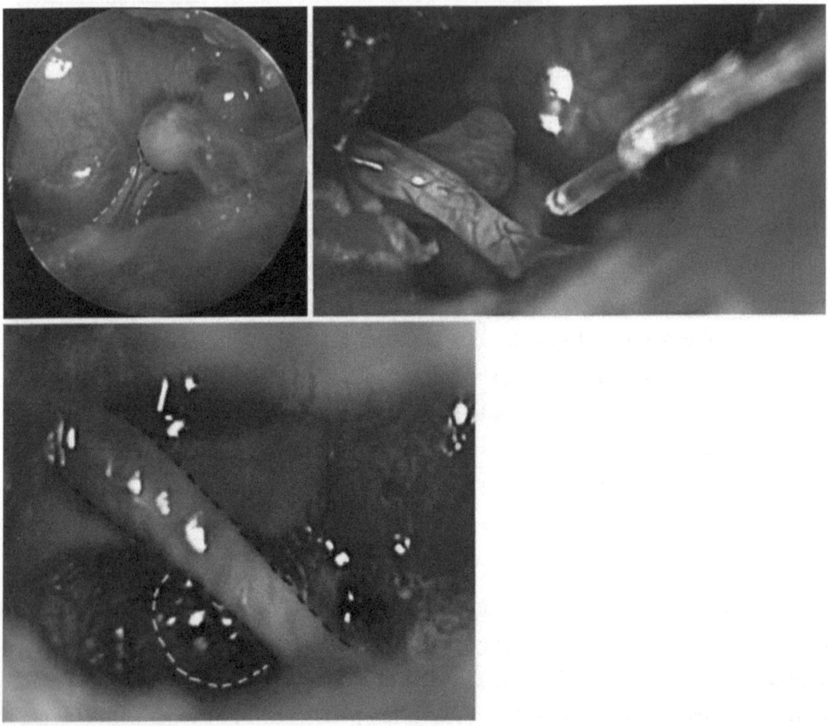

Figure 13.12: (a) In stapedectomy, the stapes tendon (blue dashed line) is vaporized with the laser and the incudosta- pedial joint (black dashed line) is disarticulated. The posterior crus (yellow dashed line) is then severed with the laser. (Photograph provided courtesy of Dr. Hamid Djalilian). (b) Intraoperative image of an argon laser directed at the posterior crus of the stapes after having displaced the chorda tympani nerve from the line of fire. (Photograph provided courtesy of Dr. Hamid Djalilian) (c) Intraoperative image of the oval window after laser stapedectomy. Notice the charred appearance of where the stapes was located (yellow dashed line). Also note the preservation of the chorda tympani nerve (black dashed line). The long process of the incus (blue dashed line) is still intact above and will be used to anchor the stapes prosthesis (Photograph provided courtesy of Dr. Hamid Djalilian)

As with traditional myringotomy, patients with recurrent or persistent episodes of otitis media with effusion may need tube placement at a later date. Office-based laser assisted tympanic membrane fenestration with a hand- held otoscope combined with the CO_2 flashscanner laser, OtoLAM (ESC/Sharplan, Yokneam, Israel) and placement of a pressure equalization tube under local anesthesia has been described as well. Outcomes have shown improvement in hearing and reduced incidence of tube plugging; however, this was performed in a non-randomized population. Again, these systems are very expensive, and the procedure has not been widely adopted.

Tympanoplasty is the repairing of a defect in the eardrum by placing fascia or perichondrium over the defect. In this application, the KTP laser can be used to weld the collagen fibers together along their edges. While promising, neither laser application of myringotomy nor tympanoplasty has been widely adopted due to the extensive cost of the system. CO_2 laser use in acoustic neuroma surgery has shown to be advantageous due to its precision in cutting and coagulating around the facial and vestibular nerves. The use of KTP and Argon lasers for acoustic neuroma excisions has also been noted but are not widely used. Laser use is limited by the size of the tumor, approach to the lesion, and the surgeon's experience. For smaller tumors (2–3 cm), stereotactic radiation is beneficial in preventing further growth of the mass and preserving facial nerve function and hearing.

Laser use in endolymphatic hydrops and labyrinthectomy for benign paroxysmal positional vertigo (BPPV) have been described but have not been adopted due to their potentially high rate of hearing loss compared to traditional surgery. Laser use in the decompression of the facial nerve has also been successfully performed.

Post-operative Management

Most patients are sent home on the same day of surgery. They are told to keep their ear canal and surgical site water free. Packing is frequently left in the external auditory canal for up to 2 weeks for removal by the surgeon at a postoperative visit. A repeat audiogram is per- formed at approximately 6 weeks post-operatively. Patients who undergo cholesteatoma surgery are followed approximately every 4–6 months or more frequently to monitor for recurrence and to adequately maintain the cleanliness of the mastoid bowl. Depending on the surgical approach, a second surgical procedure may be indicated to evaluate for recurrence at 6–12 months postoperatively. Patients with decompression of facial nerve may need post-operative steroids.

13.18 SIDE EFFECTS/COMPLICATIONS

Complications of laser use in otology occur at a rate that is equal to or less than conventional surgical techniques. Noted complications include temporary or permanent hearing loss, intra-operative or post-operative vertigo, cerebrospinal fluid fistula, tinnitus, prosthesis displacement, incus necrosis, fibrosis, postoperative granuloma formation, tympanic membrane fistula facial nerve injury and chorda tympani injury (dysguesia). Accidental fracturing of the stapedial footplate may also occur. As described above, photoacoustic or thermal injury to adjacent structures may occur. The addition of lasers in otologic surgery has been shown to reduce complication rates, but the evidence in comparing various lasers for a specific procedure use is limited.

13.19 PREVENTION AND TREATMENT OF SIDE EFFECTS/COMPLICATIONS

Facial nerve monitoring is the electromyographic monitoring of facial muscles intraoperatively that is proven to be cost effective and reduce the incidence of iatrogenic facial nerve injury during surgery. It is the standard of care in any otologic procedure that is in the vicinity of the facial nerve. Facial nerve monitoring also detects facial nerve injury due to the heat generated by carbon dioxide lasers thereby preventing injury.

Future Directions

Future directions include the adoption of all the above techniques in routine otologic operative procedures. Laser use in acoustic neuroma surgery, tympanoplasty and myringotomy and the use of the laser Doppler vibrometer are all techniques that are emerging as methods that may become standard. Other otologic applications that are being explored include Eustachian tuboplasty for chronic otitis media and Eustachian tube dysfunction and benign paroxysmal positional vertigo.

Oral Cavity and Oropharyngeal Pathology

The carbon dioxide laser is utilized for trans oral resection of T1 and limited T2 squamous cell carcinoma (SCCA) of the oral cavity and tongue. Its advantages in the oral cavity are due to its ability to simultaneously cut tissue and coagulate small blood vessels. Oral cavity cancer has an overall poor prognosis with a high tendency to recur at the primary site and metastasize to the locoregional lymph nodes. However, it has been shown recently to be an effective tool in the treatment of T1 and T2 oral cavity squamous cell carcinoma. The CO_2 laser is also used to remove certain benign lesions such as persistent or suspicious leucoplakia in high-risk individuals and papillomatous lesions.

Uvulopalatopharyngoplasty (UPPP) is a procedure that involves the reduction and removal of soft tissue in the oropharynx, such as the soft pal- ate and the uvula, in the hopes of treating snoring and obstructive sleep apnea (OSA). If necessary, a tonsillectomy is performed as well. In the past two decades, laser assisted uvulopalatopharyngoplasty- plasty (LAUP) with a carbon dioxide laser emerged as an alternative to traditional methods of reshaping the soft palate and uvula and removing this redundant soft tissue to treat snoring. However, it is contraindicated in obstructive sleep apnea, and its efficacy has not been fully proven. Laser midline glossectomy has also been attempted to treat obstructive sleep apnea in patients who failed traditional UPPP.

Zenker's diverticulum is a progressive hernia- tion of mucosa and submucosa through the posterior wall of the esophagus at the junction of pharynx. Patients most commonly complain of dysphagia and the regurgitation of undigested food. Endoscopic laser excision of the wall that exists between the herniated pocket and the upper portion of the esophagus is becoming a more common procedure in otolaryngology instead of the traditional open approach via the lateral neck.

Finally, the recent development of sialendoscopy has led to the treatment of recurrent sialoadenitis caused by sialolithiasis with the Ho:YAG laser. Preliminary studies have shown improvement in symptoms following sialendoscopy with removal of sialoliths. Results thus far do not show a difference in outcomes depending on the salivary gland affected. In the case of large sialolithiases, laser lithotripsy is necessary to remove the sialolith. Laser lithotripsy with the Thalmium: YAG laser has also been described.

Pre-operative Management

Pre-operative management of squamous cell carcinoma of the oral cavity includes imaging studies of the head and neck and flexible fiberoptic laryngoscopy in the office to determine the extent of the lesion and assist in planning the surgical approach. Prior to starting the excision, the patient undergoes a direct laryngoscopy, esophagoscopy and bronchoscopy to rule out synchronous primaries and to stage the neoplasm.

To determine whether a patient has sleep apnea or simply bothersome snoring prior to an LAUP, he or she may undergo a polysomnogram. This may determine if it is more appropriate to perform an LAUP, radiofrequency ablation of the posterior tongue, a traditional UPPP, or one of many other sleep procedures.

A swallowing study is frequently performed prior to a Zenker's diverticulectomy to diagnose the condition. Before the procedure, the oral cavity, hypopharynx and supraglottis are examined thoroughly to rule out any other causes of dysphagia.

Preoperative noncontrast CT scan in patients with recurrent sialoadenitis can evaluate for sialolithiasis. Typically, stones >4 mm would indicate the potential need to use the Ho:YAG laser intraoperatively.

Description of Technique

For safety and access when using a laser in the oral cavity, patients commonly undergo nasotracheal intubation for enhanced surgical access and exposure. The mouth is retracted open by placing a bite block between the teeth or a Dingmans mouth gag. The laser can be controlled by a micromanipulator while the operating field is visualized through an operating microscope or alternatively a handheld fiber optic hand piece can be utilized like a scalpel.

T1 and limited T2 oral cavity carcinoma is excised utilizing a carbon dioxide laser with margins acquired and sent for intra-operative frozen section to confirm the complete excision of neoplasm. Depending on the presence of neck disease as well as the size, location, and depth of invasion of the mass, patients may undergo a unilateral or bilateral neck dissection. Two to five-year follow- up for local control of stage I and II oral cavity carcinoma has been reported to range from 60% to 100%. Local control rates for stage III and IV oropharyngeal carcinoma treated with laser excision and post-operative radiotherapy are reported to be around 50%. This is reduced to 34% for stage III and IV carcinomas located on the floor of the mouth. Disease- free survival for 5 years for previously untreated T1 and T2 oral tumors is reported to range from 80% to 88%. Patients who have undergone selective neck dissections or post-operative radiation therapy and who have stage III or IV disease tend to have lower survival rates.

Patients who have disease located in the tonsil or tongue base have a worse prognosis than those who have more anteriorly based carcinoma of the oral cavity regardless of the technology utilized in its resection. This is attributed to the fact that posteriorlybased oral cavity SCCA is more difficult to detect and is therefore discovered later in the course of the disease at more advanced stages. Resection of tongue carcinomas by CO_2 laser oftentimes allows for the wound to be closed by primarily or it is left to heal by secondary intention without flaps or reconstruction. This can result in less postoperative scarring and tethering of the tongue than traditional surgical methods thereby allowing for more tongue mobility.

Laser assisted uvulopalatopharyngoplasty has been demonstrated to treat patients with snoring. As described above, LAUP) reshapes the soft pal- ate and uvula, removing redundant soft tissue that may lead to snoring. When comparing thermal damage to the soft palate by the CO_2 and Nd:YAG lasers, Laranne did not find any appreciable differences. The use of both the CO_2 and Nd: YAG lasers to treat snoring have been supplanted by office-based radiofrequency (RF) ablation of the palate and base of tongue. While RF ablation may not significantly benefit OSA and repeat treatment may be necessary, patients have experienced success in the reduction of snoring with RF ablation of the soft palate, tongue, uvula and infe- rior turbinates with less associated morbidity from the procedure.

Oral exposure in sialendoscopy is ideally per- formed with both a cheek retractor as well as a bite block. Technique is slightly different depending on if submandibular or parotid sialendoscopy is performed, but the overall concepts are the same. First dilation of the papilla is achieved using lacrimal probes. Once the duct is catheterized with a guide wire, further dilations using the Seldinger technique are performed until the introducer can be catheterized. This introducer stays in place throughout the procedure. The endoscope is then guided through the introducer to diagnose the obstruction, which is typically stenosis versus sialolith. There is a working port that can feed baskets and wires into the duct to capture and remove sialoliths. Alternatively, medicines such as kennalog can be introduced through the working port to decrease postoperative inflammation. When sialoliths are too big to be removed with a wire basket, lasers are utilized to first break up the stone into smaller components that can be removed. It is important not to force a stone that is impacted, as it may result in the avulsion of the duct or breakage of the basket. This procedure is still in its infancy and limited in patient numbers. Long-term follow up with large patient populations has not yet been described.

13.20 POST-OPERATIVE MANAGEMENT

Patients with extensive resections of SCCA in the oral cavity or those who have SCCA involving the base of tongue are typically kept in an intensive care unit setting overnight for airway monitoring. Occasionally, if swelling is severe, the patient remains intubated and is administered steroids until the edema subsides. Rarely, a tracheotomy is necessary if the patient cannot be intubated or if the airway obstruction is anticipated to be long-term. Any patient with surgery performed in the oral cavity is placed on a liquid diet post-operatively and slowly advanced to a soft diet on which he or she remains for at least 2 weeks. The oral mucosa heals quickly, and patients are encouraged to drink as much fluids as they can handle to decrease xerostomia, infection and post-operative pain.

Patients who have undergone a Zenker's diverticulectomy are sometimes placed on a full liquid diet for at least 2 weeks or the decision is made to feed the patient by tube feeding exclusively until a negative gastrograffin swallow study is obtained. These patients are watched closely for symptoms that may indicate a dehiscence of the operative site and mediastinitis including chest pain, shortness of breath or the return of dysphagia.

Postoperative care following sialendoscopy is minimal. The decision to put the patient on post- operative antibiotics is made on an individual basis. The patient is encouraged to maintain strict oral hygiene.

Side Effects/Complications

Complication rates are significantly higher (90%) in patients with oral SCCA who have been previously irradiated than those who have not had radiation treatments (10%). Complications reported in patients who have received radiation therapy include uncontrolled pain, bleeding, infection, delayed healing and edema. As discussed above, patients may have post- operative edema of the tongue and oral cavity soft tissue leading to airway obstruction. When obstruction is severe enough, intubation or a temporary tracheostomy may be warranted.

Post-operative bleeding in any oral cavity laser procedure is rare but may be insidious in onset and potentially life threatening. If suspected, the patient must be carefully examined, and if found, the patient must be brought back to the operating room to control the bleeding.

Complications of both open and endoscopic Zenker's diverticulectomy include post-operative fever with or without mediastinitis, esophageal injury and need for re-operation. Generally, the use of the laser is less morbid than the open procedure. Temporary edema of the affected gland is an expected postoperative outcome. Infection of the affected gland is the most common potential side effect of sialendoscopy. Ductal perforations are possible and are typically treated with a salivary stent for 2 weeks. In addition, a rare but significant complication is the fixation of the wire basket within the duct and inability to remove it from the gland. If this is to happen, the case must be converted to an open procedure with open exploration and possible excision of the gland to free the foreign body from the gland.

Prevention and Treatment of Side Effects/Complications

Complications of oral cancer excisions can be minimized by obtaining good visualization of the surgical field and by obtaining adequate hemostasis intraoperatively. Encouraging fluid intake by mouth is important in preventing post-operative pain and dehydration. Airway obstruction may be minimized with post-operative steroids; however, the primary concern is in preventing an emergent situation. This is averted by thorough preparation and close monitoring of the patient in the immediate postoperative period.

Currently, the use of the laser in head and neck SCCA is limited by the size, location and stage of the disease. Future therapeutics that may lead to the improved treatment of advanced head and neck cancer include interstitial laser therapy (ILT) with the Nd:YAG laser. Laser use in the tissues involved leads to an increase in thermal energy at the site. This is currently only used pal- illatively. Chemotherapeutic agents, such as cisplatin are activated by this thermal energy and create a more precise and minimally invasive technique to ablate higher-staged or unresectable neoplasms. This has been shown to be effective in mouse models and in one case report. Further study is necessary to determine the role in cancer treatment.

Photodynamic therapy (PDT) has been proposed as a potential adjuvant treatment of head and neck cancers and pre-cancerous lesions. PDT takes advantage of energy that has been created by the absorption of laser light in that it can induce specifically directed photo- chemical changes in tissue. Photosensitizers are administered to a patient, accumulate in targeted tissues and undergo light-induced chemical reactions that may lead to selective tissue necrosis and cell death. To date, in the field of otolaryngology, photodynamic therapy has been attempted in patients with soft palate squamous cell carcinoma, recurrent nasopharyngeal carcinoma, early laryngeal malignancies, and laryngeal papillomatosis. Dosing and distribution of the photosensitizer has been difficult to track and quantify. Additionally, patients may experience symptoms of overstimulation such as anaphylaxis if exposed to daylight or neon light during treatment. However, the pilot studies show potentially promising results.

Rhinology

The area in which lasers are most commonly and successfully used in nasal surgery are in patients who have persistent recurrent epistaxis due to intranasal hereditary hemorrhagic telangiectasias (HHT). HHT is an autosomal dominant condition of the vascular tissue that presents in a person at the ages of 20–40. Friable angiodysplastic lesions that bleed easily and are millimeters in size can present anywhere but often are located on the mucosa of the nasal cavity, tongue, lips and cheeks. Patients frequently present epistaxis as the first sign of the disease.

Other areas of rhinology that are utilizing lasers, albeit in a limited fashion, include functional endoscopic sinus surgery (FESS), rhinophyma reduction, inferior nasal turbinate reduction, choanal atresia and laser cartilage reshaping. Choanal atresia can be either bilateral or unilateral. Bilateral conditions are typically addressed within the first few days of life because the neonate, who is an obligatory nasal breather, is unable to breathe unless actively crying, which forces the neonate to breathe through the mouth. This obstruction can potentially be remedied with laser ablation.

Hypertrophic inferior nasal turbinates can cause uncomfortable nasal congestion, a closed nasal airway and obligate oral breathing that can lead to obstructive sleep apnea and snoring. Along with LAUP described above, some patients may also undergo laser reduction of the inferior turbinates with a KTP, Nd:YAG or Ho:YAG laser.

Contraindications of laser use in nasal surgery include refractory nasal epistaxis and large sinonasal tumors. Concurrent treatment of bilateral lesions is contraindicated as it may lead to necrosis of the septum and the creation of a septal perforation.

13.21 PRE-OPERATIVE MANAGEMENT

Patients with chronic recurrent epistaxis undergo a thorough work-up for coagulopathic disease prior to surgery. A full history and physical are performed which includes looking for cutaneous and intra-oral telangiectasias that may need to be addressed. Nasal endoscopy is performed to evaluate for the presence of tumor. Prior to undergoing FESS, patients obtain a computerized tomography (CT) scan of the paranasal sinuses to determine the extent of the disease and for anatomic surgical planning.

Description of Technique

In HHT, the argon, KTP(Nd:YAG), and more recently diode lasers can be used to photocoagu- late these telangiectasias. Low power settings are used for each laser wavelength so that irradiation creates blanching and coagulation of the lesion. While patients often report improvement after one treatment, recurrent treatments are often necessary and more often the rule rather than the exception. Figure 13.13 illustrates the use of a KTP (Nd:YAG) laser and side-firing fiber aimed at a telangectasia on the anterior nasal septum.

Lasers can also be used in recurrent epistaxis due to other causes. The most frequent site of epistaxis in patients without HHT is Kiesselbach's plexus, located on the anterior septum. This area can be cauterized using laser energy, however, is much more expensive than traditional cautery techniques.

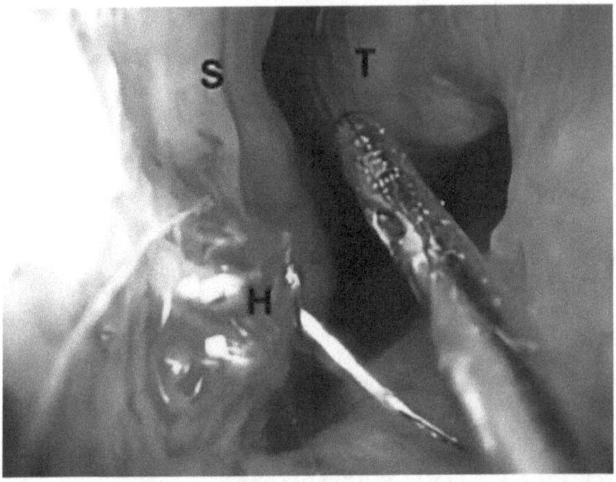

Figure 13.13: Laser vaporization and hemostasis of a Hereditary Hemorrhagic Telangiectasia (H) along the septum (S). The inferior turbinate (T) can be seen along the lateral wall of the nasal cavity (Photograph provided courtesy of Dr. Brian Wong).

Functional endoscopic sinus surgery is a procedure that is performed most in patients with chronic sinusitis or nasal polyposis. Caution must be observed when working within paranasal sinuses because of the proximity to the globe, optic nerve, carotid arteries and skull base. Newer fiber optic-based laser delivery systems have expanded the ability to use lasers in the sinonasal cavities.

When compared to cold or hot steel techniques in rhinophyma reduction, laser use leads to less intraoperative and postoperative bleeding, easier procedures and less discomfort.

Unilateral choanal atresia is often treated any- where from several weeks after birth up to age 12. After the atretic area is opened, a nasal stent is placed and left in for weeks to months. The KTP(Nd:YAG) and the Ho:YAG lasers have been used to treat this condition. While the CO_2 laser was the first to be described, it has fallen out of favor for this application due to the challenge of inserting a relatively large handpiece into the posterior nasal cavity. Reports have found lasers to be beneficial in the treatment of choanal atresia due to the decreased rates of re-obstruction and diminished risk of complications associated with the procedure.

Side Effects/Complications

A possible complication of laser treatment of hereditary hemorrhagic telangiectasias is the creation of a nasal septal perforation. To avoid this, laser irradiation is not targeted on adjacent septal surfaces in the left and right nasal cavity simultaneously, and treatment may be broken up into multiple separate operations. In any intranasal procedure in which a laser is used, stenosis due to scarring or synechiae may occur, this can be pre- vented by conservative use of the laser when treating adjacent septal and lateral nasal wall lesions. Laser use in surgery involving the septum has thus far been limited due to the potential risk of septal perforation. Ablative procedures have been performed and work well for septal spurs and other obstructive deformities.

Future Directions

Recently, laser cartilage reshaping (LCR) has been developed as a non-ablative way to reshape nasal septal deformities. The benefits of laser use in reshaping the cartilage of the ear in otoplasty has also been explored. LCR involves the use of photo-thermal heating both the septal mucosal and cartilage without the need for incisions. In laser cartilage reshaping, specimens are held in mechanical deformation and then heated using laser radiation. Heat generation accelerates the process of mechanical stress relaxation, which allows tissue to remain in stable new shapes and geometries. Although the mechanisms underlying laser cartilage reshaping have not been completely identified, numerous animal studies have investigated the various biophysical mechanisms underlying shape change, and this method is showing great promise in the field of otolaryngology.

13.18 PEDIATRIC OTOLARYNGOLOGY

As discussed previously, choanal atresia is a condition present in neonates that can be treated by using a laser directed toward the imperforate area.

The treatment of juvenile onset recurrent respiratory papillomatosis with a CO_2 laser has also been described in a previous section. Other conditions that are present in the neonate and pediatric populations that may be treated with a laser include laryngomalacia, vallecular cysts, subglottic stenosis and subglottic hemangioma.

Laryngomalacia most often presents in the neonate as "noisy breathing". The classification falls under three types. Type I is the most common and least serious. It is characterized by the intermittent prolapse of redundant supraglottic mucosa. Type II laryngomalacia is defined by shortened aryepiglottic folds, and type III is identified by a posteriorly displaced epiglottis. Types I and II can be treated with a CO_2 laser as previously discussed.

Congenital subglottic stenosis is the membranous or cartilaginous narrowing of the larynx at the cricoid area without previous intubation or trauma and may present with biphasic stridor, dyspnea, recurrent croup or other airway difficulties during the first few months of life. In Fig. 5.13a, the airway obstruction produced by the stenotic airway segment (subglottis) is readily apparent. The CO_2 laser was used to excise portions of this obstructive lesion to improve air- way patency (Fig. 13.14b). The use of the carbon dioxide laser to treat congenital subglottic stenosis is mostly historical due to the possibility of restenosis at the initial site or at a more distal site. More recently, KTP(Nd:YAG) laser has been shown to be helpful in conjunction with open laryngotracheal reconstruction in these patients to ablate portions of thickened cricoid cartilage. Vallecular cysts may also present with noisy breathing and airway obstruction. Their etiology is unknown. Laser excision of vallecular cysts (Fig. 13.15a) is routinely practiced with a high success rate. Typically, a CO_2 laser is used to cut the margins of the cyst, facilitating either removal or marsupialization (Fig. 13.15b).

Subglottic hemangioma presents in a similar fashion to subglottic stenosis with stridor, hoarse- ness, cough, failure to thrive secondary to dysphagia and cyanosis. Cutaneous hemangiomas are present in 50% of patients with subglottic disease, and therefore suspicion should be high in any patient with these symptoms and a history of a cutaneous lesion. Subglottic hemangiomas enlarge rapidly as they undergo proliferation, and appear smooth, spherical, and often blue hued masses on the subglottic wall (Fig. 13.16a). They present twice as often in girls compared to boys and are typically diagnosed in the first few months of life. While they do spontaneously involute, subglottic hemangiomas have potential for airway obstruction. To prevent airway compromise, aggressive treatment is warranted, and the laser plays an integral role in this. Tracheostomy may still be required in the short term.

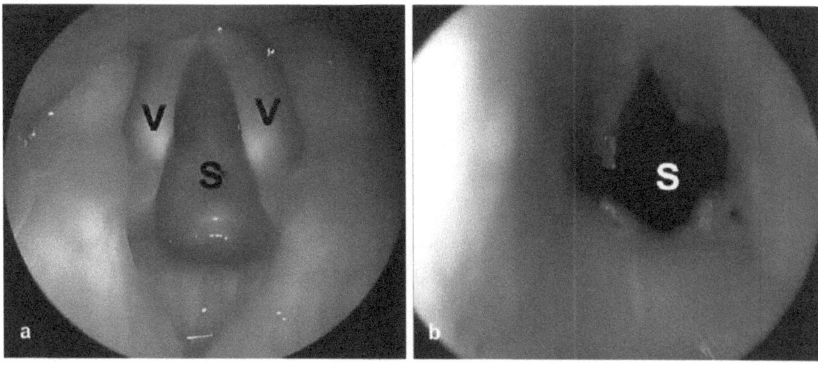

Figure 13.14: Subglottic stenosis (S) in a pediatric patient before (a) and after laser extension from a subglottic view (b). V vocal cords (Photograph provided courtesy of Dr. Gupreet S. Ahuja.

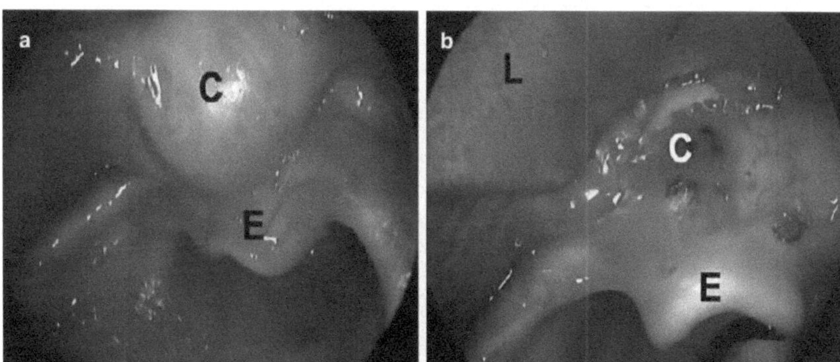

Figure 13.15: Vallecular cyst (C) in a pediatric patient before (a) and after (b) laser excision. E epiglottis, L Blade of laryngoscope (Photograph provided courtesy of Dr. Gupreet S. Ahuja).

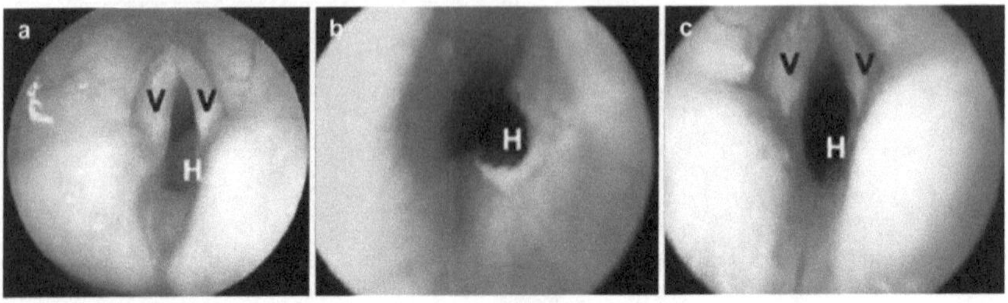

Figure 13.16: Subglottic Hemangioma (H) in a pediatric patient before (a), after laser excision from a subglottic view (b) and after laser excision from a supraglottic view (c). Note how the airway has increased patency and that the lesion was not circumferential. V vocal cords (Photograph provided courtesy of Dr. Gupreet S. Ahuja)

Both laser myringotomy and cholesteatoma excision have been described in previous sections. Laser myringotomy with or without placement of pressure equalization tubes under local anesthesia will reduce the risk of general anesthesia that is typically employed in this procedure. Laser use in creating a myringotomy may also decrease the incidence of tube plugging, persistent bleeding and other complications associated with this procedure. However, these observations have yet to be demonstrated in a large randomized prospective study. Cholesteatoma excision may be assisted routinely by using lasers and endoscopy in the areas that are anatomically difficult to access.

Pre-operative Management

Laryngomalacia in a neonate is most often diagnosed using flexible fiberoptic laryngoscopy. Some neonatess might require nasogastric tube feedings due to the risk of aspiration that is associated with this condition. Severe laryngomalacia may necessitate intubatation while awaiting surgery due to frequent oxygen destruction. Patients may also be placed on peri-operative H_2 blockers or proton pump inhibitors for treatment of gastroesophageal reflux disease, a frequent co-morbid condition that can exacerbate symptomatology. Techniques In type I laryngomalacia, the CO_2 laser is used to per- form a supraglottoplasty and exercise or reduce the aryepiglottic folds. Type II laryngomalacia may be treated by using the CO_2 laser to divide the aryepi-glottic folds. The CO_2, Nd:YAG and KTP(Nd:YAG) lasers have been suggested as possible methods to remove hemangiomas in the sub- glottis (Fig. 13.16a) due to their ability to exercise and coagulate these vascular lesions. The KTP(Nd:YAG) laser is favored in this application because it is more easily delivered to the area via flexible fiberoptics and is readily absorbed by hemoglobin. Figure 13.16b is an image of the subglottic region after laser treatment of a hemangioma. Figure 13.16c is a panoramic image of the larynx showing both the supra and subglottic airway after the hemangioma was removed. Most treatment methods produce some degree of subglottic stenosis. However, the stenosis grade typically does not require tracheostomy.

Post-operative Management

All pediatric patients who undergo laser surgery of the airway are sent to the pediatric or neonatal intensive care unit post-operatively for airway observation. Whereas patients who undergo subglottic hemangioma excision via an open approach will receive tracheostomy, those in whom a laser is used for ablation often do not. Steroids are given to reduce the formation of edema in the airway mucosa. Frequent serial examinations with flexible fiberoptic laryngoscopy is performed to monitor supraglottic edema, stenosis and hemangioma recurrence.

Side Effects/Complications

Possible adverse events that may occur when treating both laryngomalacia and subglottic hemangiomas include tracheal stenosis, granuloma formation and airway compromise. All these events may lead to intubation of the patient post-operatively and in extreme circumstances, tracheostomy is necessary. Other complications include aspiration, pneumonia, subcutaneous emphysema, bleeding that may require re- exploration and mediastinitis. Additionally, sub- glottic hemangiomas or stenosis may recur post-operatively. In the immediate post-operative period, patients may experience dysphagia leading to malnutrition and require a feeding tube for supplementary alimentation.

Prevention of Side Effects/ Complications

Tracheal stenosis may be prevented by performing excision of subglottic lesions in a quadrant approach thereby minimizing the chance of circumferential scar formation. An airway emergency is prevented by preparation and monitoring in an ICU setting post-operatively. To prevent aspiration and malnutrition, a prophylactic nasogastric feeding tube is placed intra-operatively and left in until the patient demonstrates safe and adequate consumption of food and drink.

Conclusion

Laser applications in otolaryngology—head and neck surgery are extensive and diverse. While most used in laryngology and otology, laser applications are being developed for use in all areas of the head and neck including the oral cavity, oropharynx, external nose, paranasal sinuses, cranial base, and the pediatric population. As new devices and delivery systems are developed, new applications will evolve. One element that is critical in all areas of application is laser safety, and this should take the utmost importance when planning and undertaking any procedure.

Lasers are used to treat both malignant and benign laryngeal diseases ranging from cancer to vocal cord paralysis. Middle ear applications have focused on primarily treating conductive hearing loss (stapes surgery), though in recent times new applications include the treatment of Eustachian tube dysfunction and cholesteatoma. Lasers are used to exercise tumors in the oropharynx and oral cavity because they precisely cut and coagulate tissue. In rhinology, treatment of hereditary hemorrhagic telangiectasias is a commonplace and elegant example of laser therapy for non-cutaneous vascular lesions. In children, the laser may be used to ablate subglottic hemangiomas, correct laryngomalacia and excise atretic choanae. Laser applications in otolaryngology continually develop and evolve with a plethora of new devices, procedures and applications are emerging each year.

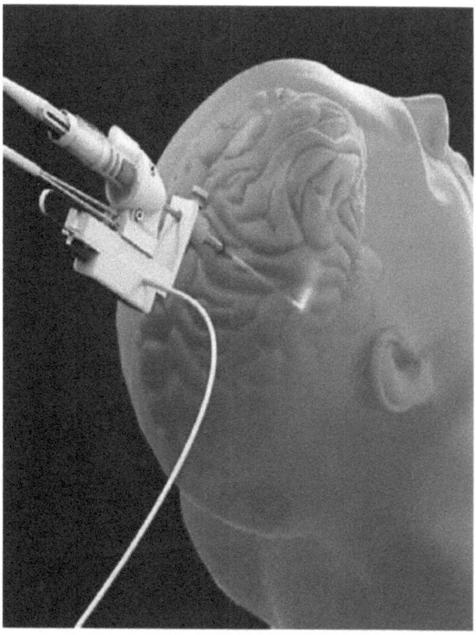

14 CHAPTER

NON THERMAL DIAGNOSTIC APPLICATIONS

14.1 OPTICAL COHERENCE TOMOGRAPHY

Optical coherence tomography (OCT) is a non- invasive imaging test. OCT uses light waves to take cross-section pictures of your retina. Each of the retina's distinctive layers is visible. It can map and measure their thickness. These measurements help with diagnosis. Provide treatment guidance for glaucoma and diseases of the retina. These retinal diseases include age-related macular degeneration (AMD) and diabetic eye disease. It obtains high resolution cross-sectional images of the retina. The layers within the retina can be differentiated and retinal thickness can be measured to aid in the early detection and diagnosis of retinal diseases and conditions. OCT uses rays of light to measure retinal thickness. No radiation or X-rays are used in this test, an OCT scan does not hurt and it is not uncomfortable. Optical Coherence Tomography uses technology that is best compared to ultrasound, except that it employs light rather than sound and thereby achieves clearer, sharper resolution. Employs near-infrared light (1.3 μM) to probe micrometer- scale structures inside biological tissues. It shows real time image for intravascular structure. It gives high resolution and good tissue characterization.

Principle

OCT images are obtained by measuring -echo time and intensity of reflected light. It is also called optical ultrasound. It gives Optical properties of ocular tissues, not histological section. Laser output from OCT is low, using a near- infra-red broadband light source. It measures backscattered or back-reflected light. The source of light: 830nm diode laser.

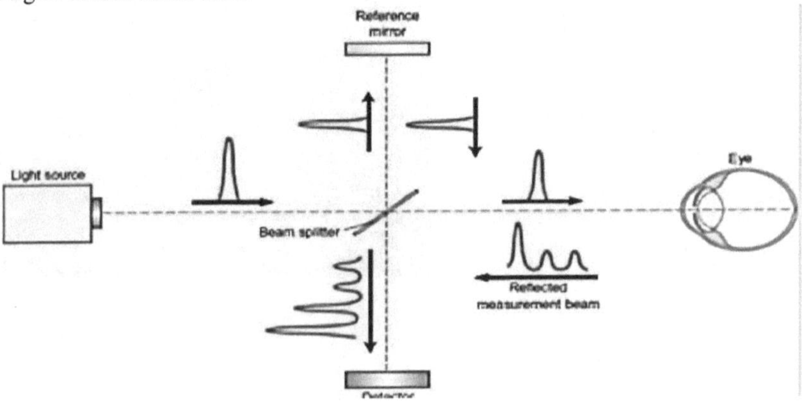

Figure 14.1: Measuring set up.

Technique is called Low coherence interferometry or Michelson Interferometer

A beam of light passes through semitransparent mirror that splits the beam into two. These two beams are then thrown on two equidistant mirrors; reflected light from these mirrors is then picked up and summed up by a detector. The equidistant mirrors reflect the light wave in same phase; however, if one of the mirrors is moved by a distance less than the wavelength of the incident light, the reflected lights from the two mirrors will then possess a phase difference. This phase difference then produces an interference pattern at the level of the detector. The resulting interference patterns are used to reconstruct an axial A-scan, which represents the scattering properties of the tissue along the beam path. A moving beam of light along the tissue in a line result in a compilation of A-scans with each A-scan having a different incidence point. From all these A-scans, a two-dimensional cross-sectional image of the target tissue can be reconstructed, and this is known as a B-scan.

Technique

Quality images can be taken even with a 3 mm pupil; otherwise dilatation is recommended. The patient is seated comfortably in front of the OCT machine with chin positioned on the chin rest. He is asked to fixate on the fixation target. The internal fixation (green color light) target is the commonly used fixation target. After fixation the operator selects the desired scan and aligns the instrument so that fundus image and scan beam is displayed on the screen.

Scan Protocols

Line -scan simply scans in a single, straight line. The length of the line can be changed as well as the scan angle.

Raster – Scans in parallel straight lines Circle- scans in a circle instead of a line.

Radial - scans 6 consecutive line scans in a star pattern

Types

Time Domain OCT - Image resolution and acquisition speed are inversely related

Spectral Domain OCT - Simultaneous increase in imaging speed and resolution can be brought about by spectral domain OCT

Advantages

Broad dynamic range High resolution

Rapid data acquisition rate Compact portable structure Acquisition of 4-8 frames /second.

14.2 ELASTOGRAPHY

Elastography is a non-invasive medical imaging technique that helps determine the stiffness of organs and other structures in your body. It maps the elastic properties and stiffness of soft tissue. Also gives information about if the tissue is hard or soft will give diagnostic information about the presence or status of disease. It measures movement or transformation of tissue in response to a small applied pressure. Elastography techniques have been developed for both ultrasound and MR imaging.

Basic method of elastography involves applying a mechanical force to the tissue, internally or externally, and imaging the stiffness by analyzing the spatial deformation caused by the stimulation over a period of time. Palpation is the most common and primitive method for understanding the changes in the stiffness of the tissue.

Principle

Elastography is a tissue elasticity imaging, important to understand the general principles which govern the behavior of an elastic material when acted upon by an external force. When external forces are applied to objects made up of elastic materials, they undergo a change in shape and size.

STRAIN is a relative change in shape or size of an object due to externally applied forces. STRESS is the internal force (per unit area) associated with strain

HOOK'S LAW states that strain is directly proportional to stress for a linearly isotropic elastic material

Ultrasonic Elastography

It is based on high frequency compressional waves or ultrasound waves; morphological images of organs can be re-constructed.

The technique computes the difference between pre-compressed and postcompressed ultrasound signals to calculate the axial displacement occurring in the tissue. It is classified into quasi-static method and dynamic method on the basis of application of the external force.

a) Quasi-static method involves application of constant stress on the required region. The two- dimensional cross-correlation of the ultrasound images yield the displacement and the strain generated by the applied load. Drawback associated with this method is that it is difficult to find the Young's Modulus since the stress distribution is unknown. Technique is hence considered qualitative.

(b)Dynamic method involves application of time varying force which can either be a short transient mechanical force or an oscillatory force of fixed frequency. The shear waves which are basically low frequency (10Hz to 2000Hz) mechanical waves are directly proportional to the shear modulus of the medium. The dynamic method can yield quantitative and higher resolution Young's Modulus mapping when compared to the quasi- static method.

Magnetic Resonance Elastography

A special Magnetic Resonance Imaging (MRI) technique to assess the propagation of mechanical waves through a medium thus, deducing the stiffness of the medium. Magnetic Resonance Elastography (MRE) uses mechanical shear waves of a single frequency which are synchronized with the magnetic resonance pulse sequence. A magnetic resonance imaging technique called phase contrast MRI is used to image the tissue motion due to the propagation of the shear waves. This technique is based on conventional MRI.

Optical Coherence Tomography

OCE is a non-invasive imaging method that can gives more details than ultrasound or MRI. Using light source to image biological tissue, OCE is considered generally safe compared to CT scan and other radiographic imaging modalities which involve with ionizing radiation. More affordable and time efficient compared to MRI. Tissue exhibits varying degrees of viscoelasticity (time-dependent response to a load), poroelasticity (presence of fluid-filled pores or channels), and anisotropy, as well as a nonlinear relationship between elasticity and the applied load.

Laser speckle technique used for the mechanical characterization of tissue has many advantages of being non-contact, non-invasive as well as in providing high resolution. This method is aimed at computing relative strain in tissue by tracking the laser speckle pattern obtained by illumination of coherent light on the deformed tissue. Optical elastography has a disadvantage of lesser penetration depth compared to other modalities.

Optical elastography is done by tracking the speckle pattern obtained by illuminating the region of interest during the application of deformation. A reference image of the speckle pattern before deformation is acquired and then the movement in the speckle pattern due to deformation is tracked by acquiring subsequent images for each stage of deformation. The tracking of the speckle pattern is done by image processing algorithm which gives the corresponding relative strain that occurred in the region of interest due to deformation. High speed sampling of the speckle pattern is required to track the movement during deformation and hence, the system requires to acquire speckle images at a high frame rate.

Applications

Dermatology, Oncology, Opthalmology Cardiology

14.3 LASER INDUCED FLUORESCENCE IMAGING

Laser Induced Fluorescence (LIF) is an optical spectroscopic technique where a sample is excited with a laser, and the fluorescence emitted by the sample is subsequently captured by a photo detector. Usually lamp excitation is replaced by a laser source. LIF spectroscopy was first developed by Richard Zare in 1968 for the detection of atoms and molecules in the gas phase.

Principle

LIF is a two-step process: absorption of a laser photon followed by emission of a fluorescence photon from the excited state. For absorption the laser wavelength λL must match an allowed energy transition of the LIF-active molecule (atom). Only a fraction of these excited molecules fluoresces, the rest relaxes without light emission. An optical filter selects the usually red-shifted fluorescence light at the emission wavelength λ. Only the fraction η of all emitted LIF-photons is detected and converted to the camera signal SF.

Imaging

A laser beam is formed to a light sheet (or volume) and intersects the fluid area of interest, e.g. in flames, sprays or thermal flows. The resulting fluorescence light from excited molecules in the light sheet is imaged through a selective filter onto a time-gated digital camera. For pulsed UV LIF applications usually an image intensifier amplifies the LIF signal. The conversion of LIF images into meaningful concentration or temperature fields is based on calibration measurements.

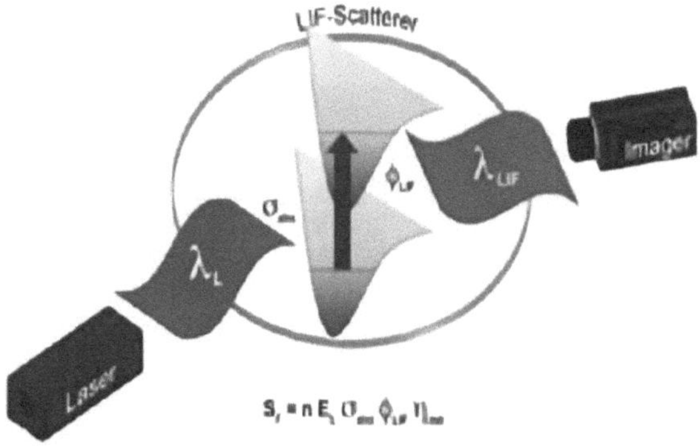

Figure 14.2: Set up.

Light Sources

Light sources of LIF are range from ultraviolet ray, visible ray, to infrared ray. Ultraviolet range is usually built up as the pulse laser, which cannot supply the stable output as the continuous-

wave (CW) exciting light source for LIF. The mostly utilized light sources for LIF are visible lasers from red ray to blue ray, even purple ray. Red diode laser, its main irradiation wavelength is 635 nm and was used for the detection of Cy-5-labeled anti-ovalbumin microfluidics capillary electrophoresis (CE). The gas laser, solid-state laser, dye laser, and diode laser have been utilized as exciting light sources for LIF integration with microfluidics/ Nano fluidics for the detection of molecules, particles, as well as cells

Types

It depends on the laser and detection system used.

(a)Excitation LIF spectroscopy

Lasers are employed to excite molecules from their ground state into an electronically excited state. As the molecules relax back into the ground state, fluorescence is detected by a photomultiplier tube (PMT).

The excitation wavelength is varied using a tunable laser which allows one to resolve the vibrational structure of the excited state. In a liquid sample, the molecules will fluoresce from the lowest vibrational level of their excited singlet state, decaying to a series of vibrational levels in the ground state, however the emission spectrum is not resolved by the detection system. A bandpass filter is placed between the sample and PMT to detect all the emissions from the sample whilst removing any scattered laser light.

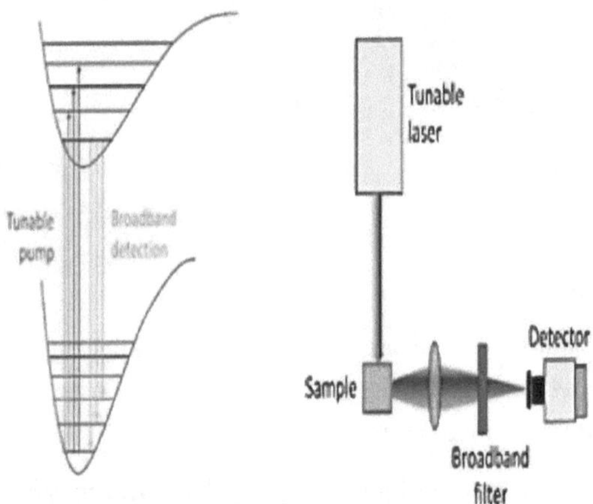

Figure 14.3: Excitation Spectroscopy bands and set up.

(b) Emission LIF - A fixed pump wavelength is used to excite the sample and the sample's emission spectrum is analysed utilising a monochromator to select the detection wavelength. Figure shows single-point detection with a PMT, but it is also possible to employ an array detector (CCD or CMOS) to capture the full spectrum in one shot.

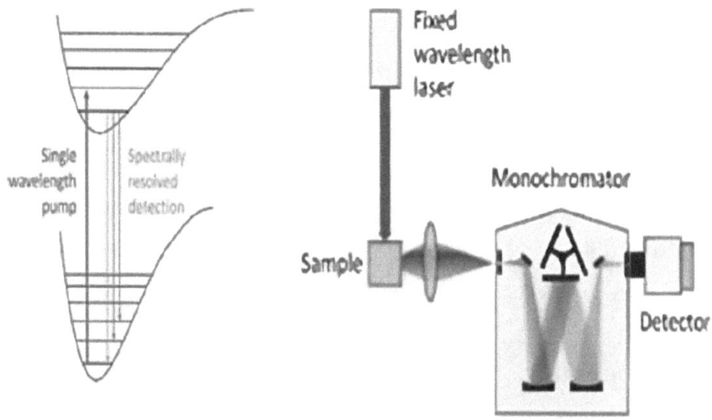

Figure 14.4: Emission Spectroscopy bands and set up.

(c) Continuous wave or time-resolved LIF – This utilizes a continuous laser for excitation and is employed when only spectral information is required.

(d) Time-resolved LIF- a pulsed laser is used to excite the sample and its emission (either a single wavelength or the full spectrum) is detected as a function of time. It provides valuable time- resolved information such as the lifetimes of chemical intermediates and their associated time- gated spectral evolution.

Applications

Detection of purity Optical tumor diagnosis

Imaging of paleontological specimens

Detection and quantification of biomolecules and biological processes (e.g DNA sequencing)

14.4 HOLOGRAPHY

Holography (whole+ write) is the science of producing holograms. It is an advanced form of photography that allows an image to be recorded in three dimensions. A method of producing a visual three-dimensional (3-D) image of an object by means of light wave patterns recorded on a photographic plate. The three measured dimensions are height, width, and depth. It is also known as Lensless Photography. It produces life like images.

Hologram is a photograph of interference patterns which, when suitably illuminated by laser light, produces a three-dimensional image. These images can be seen through naked eyes. The image floats in free space

Properties

Objects are visible from different perspectives

Divisible property i.e If you cut one in half, each half contains whole views of the entire holographic image.

Components

Laser light… usually helium-neon (HeNe) laser is used

Beam splitter…device that use mirrors and prisms to split laser beam into two beams - Object beam and Reference beam

Mirrors…Direct the beams of light to correct locations Holographic Film…to record image very high-resolution **Hologram Construction**

To create a hologram, a laser beam (coherent light) is split in two beams: Reference beam: that stays undisturbed

Object beam strikes the object and then bounces onto the plate Working of holography is divided into two phases:

Recording Reconstruction **Recording**

The first step is the recording of the interference pattern formed between the sample beam, which diffusely reflects from the object and the reference beam which is sent directly to the film. These two beams must be coherent and are normally obtained from a single laser by splitting its beam. The reflected, or scattered light, is directly mixed with the reference beam. When the film is developed (the developed film is called the hologram) and examined directly by eye, it does not look at all like a normal photograph but is simply a complex interference pattern of light and dark bands in complex shapes and bears no direct resemblance to the original objects.

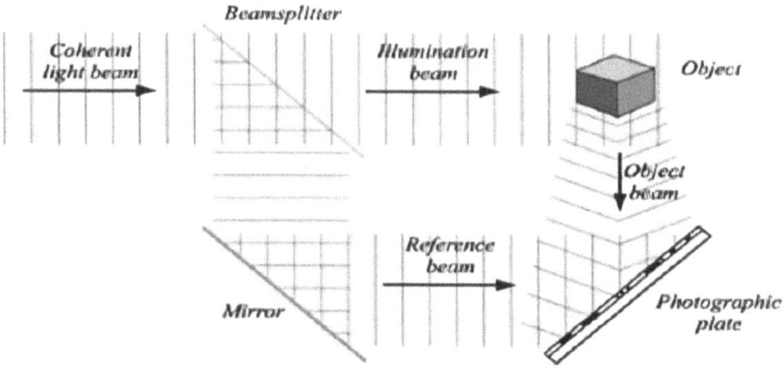

Optical arrangement of recording a hologram

Figure 14.5: Recording of Hologram.

Reconstruction

When a hologram is later illuminated with coherent light of the same frequency that created it, a three-dimensional image of the subject appears. Reconstruction is done by "playing back" the reference beam with the same orientation to the developed hologram was had when the hologram was made and viewing the image as shown below. The interference pattern on the film diffracts the reference beam - known as the reconstruction beam now - to produce a light wave that duplicates the original beam that was scattered from the real object, complete with all amplitude and phase information. Further, the developed hologram acts like a window glass so that if you move your eye around and examine different portions of the diffracted light you will see different views of the virtual image of the object, all in 3D.

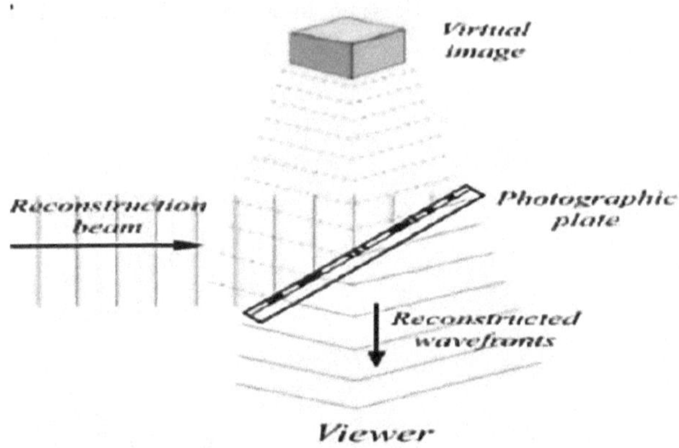

Figure 14.6: Reconstruction of Hologram.

Applications:

Endoscopy

X Ray Hologrpahy Cardiac

Dentistry Orthopedics Opthalomology

Advantages:

Cost effective

Higher storage capacity

Increased feasibility of objects(depth)

Enables the achievement of multiple images on a single plate and give 3-D images Ability to combine with other technologies.

14.5 SPECKLE APPLICATION OF LASER IN BIOLOGY AND MEDICINE

Speckle pattern is a pattern made up of irregularly spaced dots (specs). In optics, the speckle pattern is created by interference between a great number of wavelets with random phase values. These wavelets are formed when coherent light is reflected from a rough surface or transmitted through a diffusing media. Speckle is generally considered to be "optical noise". Speckle actually describes the microscopic details of the surface structure of the object. Optical interference can be observed when objects are illuminated with laser light. Effect is grainy in appearance, with light and dark "speckles" caused by constructive and destructive interference, respectively, of scattered laser light. Interference of elementary coherent beams of radiation from many secondary lights point sources is located on the rough surface of the object. Laser speckles offer the possibility of developing a full-field technique for velocity map imaging which produces an instantaneous map of velocities in real time: blood flow measurement in assessing condition such as inflammation, healing process, burn assessment, intra-operative measurement, dermatology (psoriasis, skin flap failure, skin irritation.

Imaging

Fast, full-field, cheap, and relatively simple imaging method that gives 2-D perfusion maps of large surfaces.

Principle is that the backscattered light from a tissue that is illuminated with coherent laser light forms a random interference pattern at the detector, the so-called speckle pattern. Movement of particles inside the tissue causes fluctuations in this speckle pattern resulting in blurring of speckle images when obtained with an exposure time equal to or longer than the speckle fluctuation time scale. This blurring can be related to blood flow if the fluctuations are caused by the movement of red blood cells.

Speckle image - static and dynamic speckles.

Static speckles are speckles that do not change over time, whereas dynamic speckles do change over time due to the optical Doppler effect.

Dynamic speckles contain information about movement of the object or motion of particles within the object.

Components

Low-powered laser diode Diffuser

Digital camera Processing software

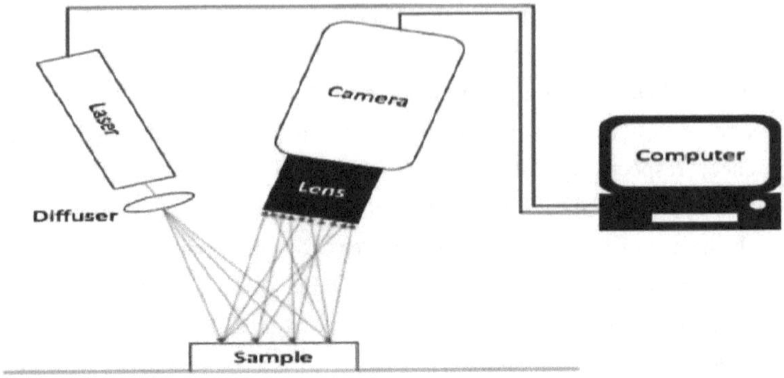

Figure 14.7: Speckle Imaging Model.

Speckle Size

To ensure proper sampling of the speckle pattern, the size of a single speckle should be approximately equal to the size of a single pixel in the image.

F-stop: the size of the aperture in a lens. Larger the F-stops give smaller lens openings. i.e. f2.8 gives a larger aperture (and more exposure) than f11.

$$\sigma \approx 1.2(1+M)\lambda F$$

Single speckle size — Magnification of lens — Wavelength of laser — Camera F-stop

Applications

Rheumatology Burns Dermatology Dentistry

Gastrointestinal Tract Surgery, Neurology and Opthalmology

Limitations

Bound to qualitative measurements Limited inter-patient comparability

Unwanted movement of tissues is the pitfall of the clinical application of laser speckles.

Needs Highly controlled environment.

14.6 RAMAN SPECTROSCOPY AND IMAGING

Raman spectroscopy was discovered by C. V. Raman in 1928

A spectroscopic technique used to observe vibration, rotational, and other low-frequency modes in a system. It is commonly used in chemistry to provide a fingerprint by which molecules can be identified.

When the radiation passes through the transparent medium the species present scatter a fraction of the beam in all directions. The difference in wavelength is between the incident and scattered visible radiation corresponds to wave length in mid IR region.

Principle

When monochromatic radiation is incident upon a sample then this light may get reflected, absorbed or scattered. Scattering gives information about molecular structure. When light is scattered from a molecule most photons are elastically scattered (Rayleigh). The scattered photons have the same energy (frequency/wavelength) as the incident photons. A small fraction of light (approximately 1 in 107photons) is scattered at optical frequencies usually lower than, the frequency of the incident photons. The process leading to this inelastic scattering is the termed Raman effect. Raman scattering can occur with a change in vibration, rotational or electronic energy of a molecule. The difference in energy between the incident photon and the Raman scattered photon is equal to the energy of a vibration of the scattering molecule. A plot of intensity of scattered light versus energy difference is a Raman spectrum. The spectrum is measured with the laser line as a reference. The peaks are measured as the shift from the laser line. Peak positions are determined by the vibrational energies associated with the bonds in the molecule(s) of which the sample is composed.

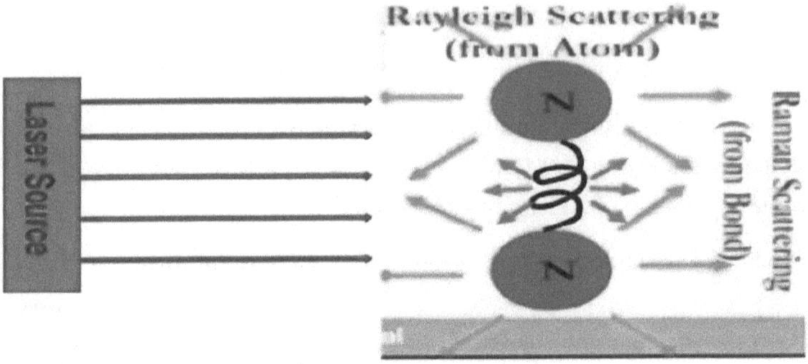

Figure 14.8: Scattering Mode.

Classification

Stokes- When the change in energy of the scattered photon is less than the incident photon, the scattering is called Stokes scatter.

Anti- Stokes- Some molecules may begin in a vibrationally excited state and when they are advanced to the higher energy virtual state, they may relax to a final energy state that is lower than that of the initial excited state. This scattering is called anti-Stokes.

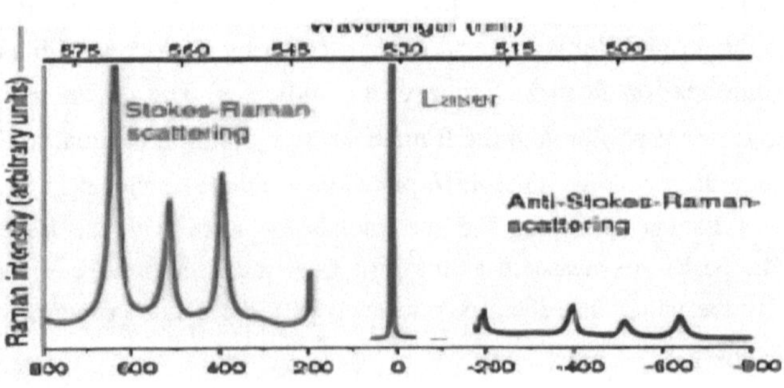

Figure 14.9: Types of Raman waveform.

Working Components

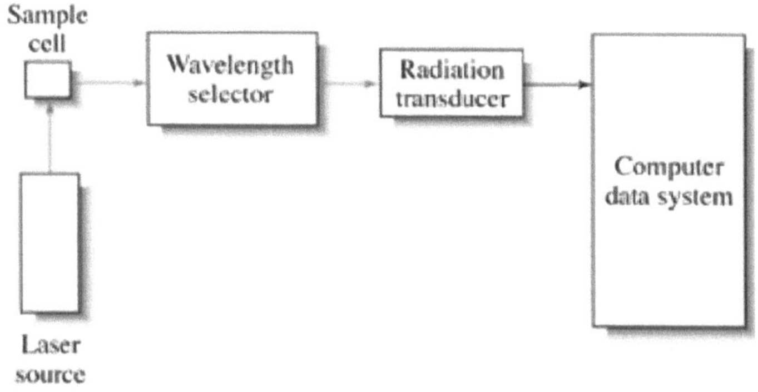

Figure 14.10: Spectrophotometer Block Diagram.

Instrumentation consists of three components:

Laser source

Sample illumination system Spectrometer.

Source:

Lasers are used because their high intensity is necessary to produce Raman

Because the intensity of Raman scattering varies as the fourth power of the frequency, argon and krypton ion sources that emit in the blue and green region of the spectrum have an advantage over the other sources. Nd-YAG, Argon ion, Krypton ion, Diode and He-Ne are used.

Sample Illumination System

Liquid Samples: Aqueous solutions can be studied by Raman spectroscopy but not by infrared. This advantage is particularly important for biological and inorganic systems and in studies dealing with water pollution problems.

Solid Samples: Raman spectra of solid samples are often acquired by filling a small cavity with the sample after it has been ground to a fine powder. Polymers can usually be examined directly with no sample pretreatment. Gas samples: Gas are normally contained in glass tubes, 1-2 cm in diameter and about 1mm thick. Gases can also be sealed in small capillary tubes. Raman spectrometers are either Fourier transform instruments equipped with cooled Germanium transducers or multichannel instruments based upon charge- coupled devices.

Raman Imaging

Raman imaging is a powerful technique for generating detailed chemical images based on a sample's Raman spectrum.

A complete spectrum is acquired at each pixel of the image and then interrogated to generate false color images based on material composition, phase, crystallinity and strain.

Standard point-by-point mapping affords the ultimate sensitivity for materials with extremely low Raman scattering properties, and additionally allows high resolution, large spectral range capability.

Typical acquisition times for such maps can be in the order of 1s-10s per point

Applications

Bio-compatibility DNA/RNA analysis Drug/cell interactions Photodynamic therapy (PDT) Disease diagnosis

Single cell analysis Characterisation of biomolecules

15 CHAPTER

THERAPEUTIC APPLICATIONS

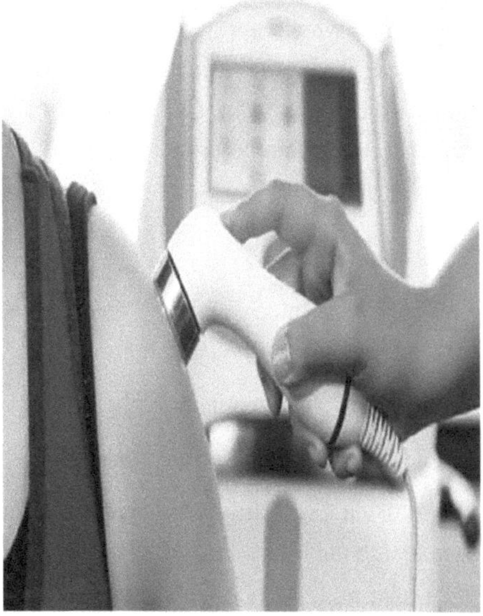

15.1 PHOTOTHERPAY

Phototherapy (light treatment) is the process of using light to eliminate bilirubin in the blood. Baby's skin and blood absorb these light waves. Light waves absorbed convert bilirubin into products, which can pass through their system. Lamps emitting light between the wavelengths of 400 - 500 nanometres (peak at 460nm) are specifically used for administering phototherapy as bilirubin absorbs this wavelength of light. Visible blue light is used.

Mechanism

Bilirubin are present in the interstitial spaces and superficial capillaries of the skin, subcutaneous tissues. During the phototherapy, these molecules are exposed to light. Photos of energy are absorbed by the pigment, bilirubin. This leads to a sequence of photochemical reactions; configurational isomerisation, structural isomerisation and photo-oxidation.

Energy converts bilirubin into its nontoxic isomers such as photobilirubin ,lumilirubin which are more polar and thus water soluble. Photo-isomers are eliminated from the body more easily without undergoing the process of conjugation in the liver. As formation of lumirubin is the rate limiting step, less amount of lumirubin is formed.

Lights

1. White Halogen lights -Positioned above the infant and can deliver 10 to 30 μ W/cm^2 /nm. Quartz halogen bulb

Tendency to become hot

It is positioned 52cm away from baby.

2. Blue and 2 White Fluorescent lights -blue light is the most effective light for reducing the bilirubin.

It delivers 12μW/cm^2 /nm.

Light should not be delivered from the side of the infant.

3. Biliblanket - Blue Halogen light -Uses a halogen bulb directed into a fiber optic mat. Filter removes the ultraviolet and infrared components, and the eventual light is a blue-green color.

Blanket to give double phototherapy and increases the surface area exposed.

4. Bilibed – Blue Fluorescent light -Blue fluorescent tube is fitted into a plastic crib with a stretched plastic cover over the top for the baby to lie on.

Baby is dressed in the Bilicombi baby suit and nursed on the soft plastic cover. Suit attaches to the crib by Velcro attachments.

Irradiance delivered is up to 40 μ W/cm^2 /nm.

Risks

Progressive and gradual damage to your skin on a molecular level Risk of developing skin cancer

Lead to immunosuppression.

Eyes become more sensitive to light

15.2 PHOTODYNAMIC THERAPY

A treatment that uses a drug, called a photosensitizer or photosensitizing agent, and a particular type of light. When photosensitizers are exposed to a specific wavelength of light, photoactivation causes the formation of singlet oxygen, which produces peroxidative reactions that can cause cell damage and death. Each photosensitizer is activated by light of a specific wavelength. This wavelength determines how far the light can travel into the body.

Steps

Three steps:

1. Application of photosensitizer drug
2. Incubation
3. Light activation

In the first step of PDT for cancer treatment, a photosensitizing agent is injected into the bloodstream. Agents are absorbed by cells all over the body but stay in cancer cells longer than they do in normal cells. Approximately 24 to 72 hours after injection, when most of the agent has left normal cells but remains in cancer cells, the tumor is exposed to light. Photosensitizers in the tumor absorb the light and produce an active form of oxygen that destroys nearby cancer cells

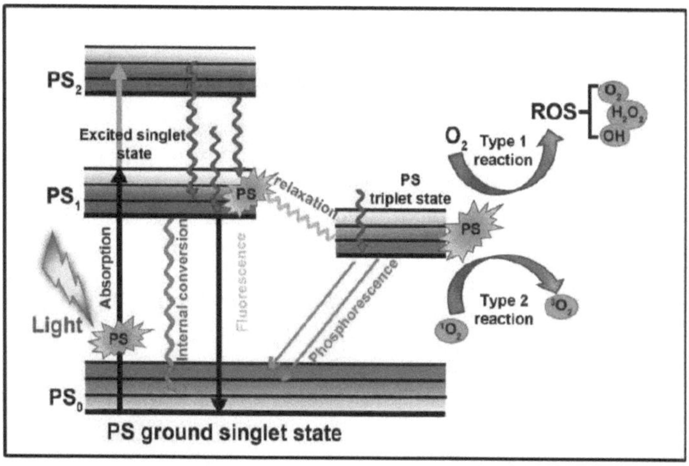

Figure 15.1: PDT Mechanism.

In addition to directly killing cancer cells, PDT appears to shrink or destroy tumors in two other ways. The photosensitizer can damage blood vessels in the tumor, thereby preventing the cancer from receiving necessary nutrients. PDT also may activate the immune system to attack the tumor cells. Light used for PDT include laser, intense pulsed light, light-emitting diodes (LEDs), blue light, red light, and many other visible lights (including natural sunlight). Laser light can be directed through fiber optic cables (thin fibers that transmit light) to deliver light to areas inside the body. A fiber optic cable can be inserted through an endoscope (a thin, lighted tube used to look at tissues inside the body) into the lungs or esophagus to treat cancer in these organs. Other light sources include light-emitting diodes (LEDs), which may be used for surface tumors, such as skin cancer.

Mechanism

Type I Reaction:

Direct reaction with substrate (cell membrane or molecule) Transfer of H atom to form radicals

Radicals react either O_2 to form oxygenated products Type II reaction:

Transfer of oxygen to form singlet oxygen

Drugs Used

Porfimer sodium

Benzoporphyrin derivative & Aminolevulinic acid Methyl ester of ALA-

Advantages

No long-term side effects when used properly. Less invasive than surgery. It takes only a short time and is most often done as an outpatient. Targeted very precisely.

PDT can be repeated many times at the same site if needed. Little or no scaring after the site heals.

Costs less than other cancer treatments.

Limitations

Light needed to activate most photosensitizers cannot pass through more than about one-third of an inch of tissue (1 centimeter).

PDT is usually used to treat tumors on or just under the skin or on the lining of internal organs or cavities.

PDT is also less effective in treating other tumors, because the light cannot pass far into these tumors.

PDT is a local treatment and generally cannot be used to treat cancer that has spread

Side Effects

Skin and eyes are sensitive to light for approximately 6 weeks after treatment

Photosensitizers tend to build up in tumors, and the activating light is focused on the tumor. As a result, damage to healthy tissue is minimal.

PDT can cause burns, swelling, pain, and scarring in nearby healthy tissue.

Other side effects include coughing, painful breathing, trouble swallowing, stomach pain, or shortness of breath; these side effects are usually temporary.

15.3 ONCOLOGICAL APPLICATIONS

1. Obstructive Esophageal Cancer-

Palliation of partially or totally obstructing tumors in the esophagus Photofrin powder, is dissolved in 5% dextrose for injection.

48 h post injection the photosensitizer localized to the tumor is activated by light at 630 nm (laser) that is directed via a single-quartz fiber optic and delivered to the tumor through the biopsy channel of an endoscope. Light is scattered laterally to the tumor on the wall of the esophagus, or the fiber may be inserted directly into the tumor. Experience mild to severe chest pain

2. Early-Stage Endobronchial Tumors –

Treatment of microinvasive, no small cell endobronchial tumors using Photofrin-PDT

Patients received 2 mg/kg Photofrin and 2 d later were treated endoscopically using a diffuser fiber (usually 1 to 2.5 cm) delivering 200 J/cm of diffuser length at 630 nm.

Because these lesions are very thin, the fiber was held in the lumen adjacent to the lesion. Patients were rescoped 2 days following treatment,and treated area was debrided.

3. Obstructing Endobronchial Tumors (Nonsmall Cell Lung Cancer)- Palliative treatment of obstructive endobronchial tumors.

Photofrin, 630 nm light treatment 48 h later

2 days following treatment, patients are re-endoscoped, and all necrotic tumor debris and exudate must be removed because they can further obstruct the airway.

Adverse reactions included photosensitivity reaction hemoptysis, cough, dyspnea, chest pain, and fever

4. Early-Stage Esophageal Cancer- Barrett's esophagus

Endoscopic PDT was applied using a specially designed balloon light applicator.

Balloon is inserted, deflated and then inflated in place to an appropriate pressure to allow "unfolding" of the esophageal wall without shutting down the blood flow.

5. Cholangiocarcinoma- Bile duct cancer

6. Head and Neck Cancer- adjuvant to surgery in an attempt to "clean up" the remaining cancer cells in the operative bed.

7. Brain Tumors- glioblastoma or astrocytoma.

8. Mesothelioma - asbestos-induced disease

15.4 BIOSTIMULATION EFFECTS

Biostimulation, also known as LILT or LLLT Low Intensity (Level) Laser Therapy, improves post-operative healing and yields excellent antalgic effects. It is also called photobiology. Biostimulation is obtained using a defocalised beam with low energy density. Light energy is absorbed by tissues and stimulates the metabolic processes inducing tissue regeneration. It emits no heat, sound, or vibration. Another name is cold laser therapy. Low levels of light do not heat the body tissue. Level of light is low when compared to other forms of laser therapy, such as those used to destroy tumors and coagulate tissue. Superficial tissue is commonly treated with wavelengths between 600 and 700 nanometers (nm). For deeper penetration, wavelengths between 780 and 950 nm are used. It generates light of a single wavelength. No temperature elevation within the tissue but rather produce their effects from photobiostimulation effect within the tissues. Low-level lasers do not cut or ablate the tissue.

LLLT devices include the gallium arsenide, gallium aluminum arsenide infrared semiconductor (gallium-aluminum-arsenide), and helium-neon lasers. Output powers range from 50 to 500 mW with wavelengths in the red and near infrared of the electromagnetic spectrum, from 630 to 980 nm with pulsed or continuous-wave emission.

Mechanism

Biostimulatory and inhibitory effects of LLLT are governed by the Arndt-Schulz law.

The law states that low dose will increase physiological processes, and strong stimulus will inhibit physiological activity. It represents a set of structural, biochemical and functional changes in living microorganisms. It acts directly on stimulating components of the so-called antenna pigments of the respiratory chain and manifest as an immediate effect cell vitalization by adenosine triphosphate (ATP) mitochondrial production increase. It Induces intracellular metabolic changes, resulting in faster cell division, proliferation rate, migration of fibroblasts and rapid matrix production.

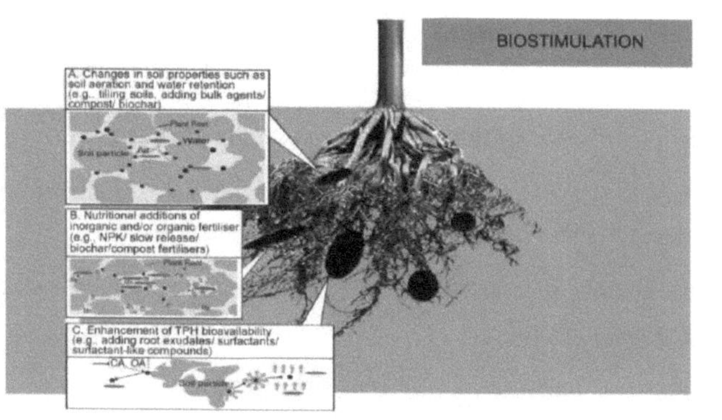

Figure 15.2: Mechanism of Biostimulation.

Benefits

Increases ATP synthesis Stimulates cell growth

Increases cell metabolism Improves cell regeneration

Invokes an anti-inflammatory response Promotes edema reduction

Reduces fibrous tissue formation Stimulates nerve function

Laser used

Previously helium-neon (HeNe) laser of <1 mW was used.

Limited by the need for an optic fiber, the size of the machine and the still rather low power option

Replaced by the indium-gallium-aluminum-phosphide laser, a diode producing red laser in the range 600-700 nm and able to deliver as much as 500 mW.

Frequently used in dentistry is the gallium-aluminum-arsenide laser.

Operates in the spectrum between 780 and 830 nm. The output is typically between 10 and 500 mW.

Advantage of the diode lasers is the small size and option for battery operation, making them rather handy and portable. Work in continuous mode, but can be mechanically or electronically pulsed.

Effects

Reduction of inflammation: It can occur within hours to days. Pain relief

Accelerated tissue regeneration: LLLT stimulates cell proliferation of fibroblasts, keratinocytes, endothelial cells and lymphocytes.

Wound healing in a range of sites, like surgical wounds, extraction sites, recurrent aphthous ulcerations – Dental

Applications

Minor injuries and sprains Inflammation

Aches and Pain Skin rejuvenation Wound healing

Acupuncture

15.5 LASER SAFETY PROCEDURES

Laser treatment increases the potential for laser accidents also increases.

Beam Hazards

Hazardous effects related to unintentional direct contact with the laser beam

- Eye related
- Interaction hazards (Plume and Fire)
- Skin related 1. Eye Related
- Corneal/Sclera Injury:caused by wavelengths that do not pass through fluid (roughly
- above 1400 nm and below 400 nm)
- Retinal Burns Injury: caused by wavelengths that do pass through fluid from (roughly 400-1400nm)

1. **Injury can result from exposure to:**
   - **a.** direct beam
   - **b.** mirror reflection (surgical instruments)
   - **c.** diffuse beam (tissue reflection)

- Damage dependent on:
- intensity - lens of eye can focus beam onto the retina
- wavelength - absorbed by different parts of the eye
- duration - fraction of second, before you can blink

2. **Interaction Hazards**

- Plume - Smoke from vaporization

Creates a visibility problem Can cause nausea

- Can be Carbon, Aerosolized blood, Gases – including benzene, toluene and formaldehyde with particle size - 0.1 microns. Smoking evacuators is the preferred control method

- Fire and explosion

- This can occur if the laser beam meets combustible or volatile materials, such as gauge pads, surgical drapes, gowns, alcohol, anesthetic gases

3. **Skin related**

- Thermal burn

- Laser effects on tissue are dependent on 4 factors: power density of laser beam, wavelength ,duration of exposure, effects of circulation and conduction

Non beam hazards

- Hazards associated with the generation of the laser beam

- Electrical - High voltage – many lasers require high voltage to generate the laser beam.

- Accidental exposure can result in electrical shock or death

- Chemical

- Dye lasers use hazardous dyes to generate the laser beam (hazardous waste)

Control Measure

- Engineering- control measures that are built into the laser system, such as: enclosing the electrical system, within a cabinet, enclosing the beam within fiber optics or mechanical arms

- Administrative Control

a. Controlled Entry- Closing doors and covering windows (when required), Posting of the PROPER "Laser in Use" signs outside all entries.

b. Education-All personnel that may be exposed to the laser shall be required to attend regular "in-services" on operating the laser and laser safety.

c. Standards- Each medical facility should develop their own set of operating standards

Personal Protection

- Eyewear - Each laser requires specific eyewear that can absorb laser light of that specific wavelength. Everyone in the laser OR must wear eye protection including the patient. Patient eyes can be protected by covering them with moist towels, goggles, and intra- ocular shields. The surgeon must have eye protection, even during microscopic and endoscopic procedures. Lens filters that fit over the eyepiece can be used.

- Skin Protection- Clothing, Gloves, Fire resistant gowns, Fire resistant surgical drapes, Moist gauze and drapes around surgical area. All gauze and drapes around the surgical area should be moistened with sterile saline. Smoke evacuators filter out the smallest particles (0.1 μ) found in the laser plume. Smoke evacuator suction tube must be placed as near to the site of laser ablation as possible

MEDICAL OPTICS

DHANALAKSHMI SRINIVASAN ENGINEERING PERAMBALUR
DEPARTMENT OF BIOMEDICAL ENGINEERING MEDICAL OPTICS

Part A

Unit-1

1. Define refractive index.
2. What are the properties involved in tissue?
3. Define optics.
4. Define absorption.
5. Define refraction.
6. Give two example of refraction.
7. Define fluorescence.
8. Define speckles
9. Explain light interaction with tissues.
10. Define optothermal interaction.
11. What is scattering.
12. Give the types of scattering.
13. Give the energy equation for luminescence.
14. Give the features of optothermal interaction.
15. How the optical properties of light is described.

Unit-2

1. Mention the instrumentation for absorption measurements.
2. Mention the instrumentation for scattering measurements.
3. Mention the instrumentation for emission measurements.
4. Give some examples of excitation light sources.
5. Write notes on high pressure arc lamp.
6. What are solid-state leds.
7. Define laser.
8. What are the principle of laser production.

9. Mention the properties of laser.

10. Name some optical filters.what do you mean by polarisers. Give example.

11. What are solid state detectors.

12. What are gratings.

13. What are monochromators.

14. Tabulate the various types of laser, wavelength and its application.

15. What are the time and phase resolved detectors.

16. Give the medical application of laser.

17. Define population inversion.

18. Define polarizer.

Unit-3

1. Draw the graph of wavelength Vs absorbance of hemoglobin, water, and melanin.

2. Give notes on skin optics.

3. Discuss laser skin interactions.

4. What are two factors that influence the laser resurfing.

5. What are three basic requirements of selective photothermolysis.

6. What do you mean by photomechanical interaction in laser.

7. Discuss the laser surgery of cornea.

8. What are the pathophysiologic considerations in laser surgery of posterior segment of the eye.

9. What are the five broad categories of short pulse tissue coagulation.

10. Name some optical filters

11. What are types of laser used in medical field?

12. Which laser is used for surgery of the cornea?

13. List any 2 treatment takes place in ophthalmology.

14. List any 2 treatment takes place in urology

15. List any 2 treatment takes place in laser tissue welding.

16. List the mechanism of laser tissue welding.

17. What are the chromophores present in skin.

18. What are the 3 basic effects takes place in laser skin interaction?

19. Why co2 laser is extensively used for surgical applications?

20. In the treatment of retinal detachment what type of laser is used and why?

21. What are the limitations of deuterium arc lamps?

22. What are the important properties of a solid state detector?

23. State the unique properties of laser?

24. State the technical specifications of laser used in medicine and in industry

25. What type of lasers are mainly used in ophthalmology?

26. Ruby and Co_2 lasers are mainly used in the clinical side for what applications respectively. Why?

Unit-4

1. Define optical hologram.
2. List the types of hologram.
3. What are the classifications of hologram?
4. Define interference.
5. Define wavefronts.
6. Define interference pattern.
7. List some medical application of hologram.
8. What are the components required to record hologram.
9. Give the difference between ordinary light and hologram.
10. List down the properties of hologram.
11. Write down the principle of an optical hologram.
12. Clinical laboratory instruments make use of holograms in what way?

Unit-5

1. What is near field imaging?
2. Give the features of near field imaging.
3. What is the principle involved in fluorescent spectroscopy?
4. Give the medical application of photo dynamic therapy.
5. What are the requirements of photodynamic therapy.
6. Define photosensitizer.
7. Define fluroscent spectroscopy.
8. Define vibrational relaxtion.
9. Give the medical application of fluroscent spectroscopy
10. Define in-vitro clinical diagnostic instrumentation.
11. Give the medical application of in-vitro clinical diagnostics.
12. What is near field imaging? State its features.
13. What is the principle of fluorescent spectroscopy?
14. List any 2 types of treatment carried out by otolaryngology?

Part B

Unit-1

1. i) with a experimental setup explain the measurement of scattering of tissues.

ii) what time resolved and phase resolved detectors.

2. How is light transported into the tissue?

i) What are the effects of light interaction with tissues? Discuss.

ii) Thermography is based on what properties of light? Explain.

3. i) outline the photon transport theory to explain the optical property of tissues.

ii) what are the optical properties of the tissues that can be measured.

4. with experimental setup explain the following measurement for the tissues:

a. absorption of light

b. scattering of light

c. emission of light

Unit-2

1) Explain the instrumentation for absorption measurements.

2) Discuss the Raman spectrophotometer in detail.

3) Explain the principle, theory & instrumentation of emission measurements.

4) Discuss various excitation light sources.

5) Write short notes on: high pressure arc lamp. Optical filters.

6) Explain the solid state LEDs

7) Write short notes on: Polarisers

Time and phase resolved detectors.

8) Give the characteristic features of absorption spectrophotometry

9) Compare the meaning of time resolved and phase resolved detectors

Unit-3

1. Explain in detail about the use of lasers in tissue welding.
2. Write about various applications of lasers in dermatology.
3. Discuss in detail about,

laser in ophthalmology laser in

otolaryngology laser in urology

4. List down the various types of laser used in the clinical side and their specific domain application.
5. explain in detail about application of laser in tissue welding
6. explain in detail about application of laser in urology.
7. explain in detail about application of laser in dermatology.
8. Give the clinical applications of lasers in urology and supplement why is it so successful in painless surgery?

Unit-4

1. i) explain the principle of operation of optical holographic interferometer.

ii) how hologram is classified. State the applications of hologram.

2. i) explain the operation of time average holographic interferometer.

ii) state the holographic optical components and their applications

3. i) compare the features of solid state LED and laser.

ii) explain the process of near field imaging in vitro clinical diagnostic.

4. i) what are the properties employed in hologram.

ii) explain in detail about precaution and requirements for recording a hologram.

Unit-5

1.i) what is the function of optical filter.

ii) explain the process of near field imaging of biological structure. 2.Enumerate the applications of optical holography in the medical side.

3 Explain the special technique used for near field imaging of biological structure.

4. Write brief notes on

i) Photodynamic therapy

ii) Fluorescent spectroscopy.

REFERENCES

1. Tuan Vo Dirh, Biomedical Photonics – Handbook, CRC Press, Bocaraton, 2003.
2. Paras.N. Prasad, Introduction to Biophotonics, Wiley Interscience, 2003
3. Tuan Vo Dirh, Biomedical Photonics – Handbook, CRC Press, Bocaraton, 2003.
4. Paras.N. Prasad, Introduction to Biophotonics, Wiley Interscience, 2003
5. Midgley HC III. Nd:YAG contact laser surgery. The scalpel of the future? Otolaryngol Clin North Am. 1990;23(1):99–105.
6. Li ZZ, Reinisch L, Van de Merwe WP. Bone abla- tion with Er:YAG and CO2 laser: study of ther- mal and acoustic effects. Lasers Surg Med. 1992;12(1):79–85.
7. Szyfter W, Mielcarek-Kuchta D, Miętkiewska- Leszniewska D, Młodkowska A, Łączkowska-Przybylska J. Comparison between 2 laser systems, Er-Yag and CO2, in stapes surgery. Otol Neurotol. 2013;34(1):29–35.
8. Philipp CM, Berlien HP. Basic principles of medical laser technology. In: Huttenbrink K, editor. Lasers in otorhinolaryngology. New York, NY: Thieme; 2005. p. 1–20.
9. Ossoff RH, Karlan MS. Safe instrumentation in laser surgery. Otolaryngol Head Neck Surg. 1984;92(6):644–8.
10. Ossoff R. Laser safety in otolaryngology – head and neck surgery: anesthetic and educational consider- ations for laryngeal surgery. Laryngoscope. 1989; 99(8):1–26.
11. Foth H-J. Endotracheal tubes for laser surgery: temperature rise and clinical experiences. SPIE Proc Med Appl Lasers III. 1996;2623:522–9.
12. Ungemach J. New laser tracheal tube. SPIE Proc Lasers Med Dent Diagn Treat. 1996;2887:129–32.
13. Foth HJ. Laser resistance of endotracheal tubes I: experimental results of a compound tube in comparison to a metallic tube. Lasers Med Sci. 1998;13(4):242–52.
14. Foth HJ. Laser resistance of endotracheal tubes II: observed temperature rise and theoretical explanation. Lasers Med Sci. 1999;14(1):24–31.
15. Coughlan CA, Verma SP. Evaluating the effects of a 532-nm fiber-based KTP laser on transoral laser surgery supplies. Otolaryngol Head Neck Surg. 2013;149(5):739–44.
16. Strong MS, Jako GJ. Laser surgery in the larynx. Early clinical experience with continuous CO2 laser. Ann Otol Rhinol Laryngol. 1972;81(6):791–8.
17. Strong MS, Jako GJ, Polanyi T, Wallace RA. Laser surgery in the aerodigestive tract. Am J Surg. 1973;126(4):529–33.
18. Steiner W, Ambrosch P. Endoscopic laser surgery of the upper aerodigestive tract. Stuttgart: Thieme; 2000.
19. Oswal VH. Laser surgery for benign laryngeal pathol- ogy. The Hague: Kugler Publications; 2002.
20. Steiner W. Experience in endoscopic laser surgery of malignant tumours of the upper aero-digestive tract. Adv Otorhinolaryngol. 1988;39:135–44.
21. BWS P Jr, Hinni ML. Transoral laser micro resection of advanced laryngeal tumors. In: Cummings CW, editor. Otolaryngology: head and neck surgery. 4th ed. St. Louis, MO: Mosby; 2005.
22. Rudert H. Larynx and hypopharynx cancers – endo- scopic surgery with laser: possibilities and limits. Arch Otorhinolaryngol Suppl. 1991;1:3–18.
23. Eckel HE, Thumfart WF. Laser surgery for the treat- ment of larynx carcinomas: indications, techniques, and preliminary results. Ann Otol Rhinol Laryngol. 1992;101(2 Pt 1):113–8.

24. Steiner W, Pfalz R. Laser surgery. HNO. 1993;41(8): A19–20.
25. Motta G, Esposito E, Cassiano B, Motta S. T1-T2-T3 glottic tumors: fifteen years experience with CO2 laser. Acta Otolaryngol Suppl. 1997;527:155–9.
26. Canis M, Martin A, Ihler F, Wolff HA, Kron M, Matthias C, Steiner W. Results of transoral laser microsurgery for supraglottic carcinoma in
27. 277 patients. Eur Arch Otorhinolaryngol. 2013; 270(8):2315–26.
28. Ansarin M, Zorzi S, Massaro MA, Tagliabue M, Proh M, Giugliano G, Calabrese L, Chiesa F. Transoral robotic surgery vs transoral laser microsurgery for resection of supraglottic cancer: a pilot surgery. Int J Med Robot. 2014;10(1):107–12.
29. Iro H, Waldfahrer F, Altendorf-Hofmann A, Weidenbecher M, Sauer R, Steiner W. Transoral laser surgery of supraglottic cancer: follow-up of
30. 141 patients. Arch Otolaryngol Head Neck Surg. 1998;124(11):1245–50.
31. Rudert HH, Werner JA, Hoft S. Transoral carbon dioxide laser resection of supraglottic carcinoma. Ann Otol Rhinol Laryngol. 1999;108(9):819–27.
32. Vaughan CW. Transoral laryngeal surgery using the CO2 laser: laboratory experiments and clini- cal experience. Laryngoscope. 1978;88(9 Pt 1): 1399–420.
33. Vaughan CW, Strong MS, Jako GJ. Laryngeal carcinoma: transoral treatment utilizing the CO2 laser. Am J Surg. 1978;136(4):490–3.
34. Laccourreye O, Lawson G, Muscatello L, Biacabe B, Laccourreye L, Brasnu D. Carbon dioxide laser debulking for obstructing endolaryngeal carcinoma: a 10-year experience. Ann Otol Rhinol Laryngol. 1999;108(5):490–4.
35. Eckel HE. Lasers for benign diseases of the larynx, hypopharynx and trachea. In: Huttenbrink K, edi- tor. Lasers in otorhinolaryngology. New York, NY: Thieme; 2005. p. 96–105.
36. Mahnke CG, Fröhlich O, Lippert BM, Werner JA. Recurrent laryngeal papillomatosis. Retrospective analysis of 95 patients and review of the literature. Otolaryngol Pol. 1996;50(6):567–78.
37. Koufman JA, Rees CJ, Frazier WD, et al. Office- based laryngeal laser surgery: a review of 443 cases using three wavelengths. Otolaryngol Head Neck Surg. 2007;137(1):146–51.
38. Pransky SM, Canto C. Management of subglottic hemangioma. Curr Opin Otolaryngol Head Neck Surg. 2004;12(6):509–12.
39. Waner M, Suen JY. Hemangiomas and vascular mal- formations of the head and neck. New York, NY: Wiley; 1999.
40. Zeitels SM, Akst LM, Bums JA, Hillman RE, Broadhurst MS, Anderson RR. Pulsed angiolytic laser treatment of ectasias and varices in singers. Ann Otol Rhinol Laryngol. 2006;115(8):571–80.
41. Sternberg, P. Subfoveal neovascular lesions in age-related macular degeneration. Guidelines for evaluation and treatment in the macular photocoagulation study. Arch. Ophthalmol. 109, 1242–1257 (1991).
42. Tanzi, E. L., Lupton, J. R. & Alster, T. S. Lasers in dermatology: four decades of progress. J. Am. Acad. Dermatol. 49, 1–34 (2003).
43. Anderson, R. R. & Parrish, J. A. Selective photothermolysis: precise microsurgery by selective absorption of pulsed radiation. Science 220, 524–527 (1983).
44. Anderson, R. R. & Parrish, J. A. Microvasculature can be selectively damaged using dye lasers: a basic theory and experimental evidence in human skin. Lasers Surg. Med. 1, 263–276 (1981).
45. Nelson, J. S. et al. Dynamic epidermal cooling during pulsed laser treatment of port-wine stain. A new methodology with preliminary clinical evaluation. Arch. Dermatol. 131, 695–700 (1995).
46. Fitzpatrick, R. E., Goldman, M. P., Satur, N. M. & Tope, W. D. Pulsed carbon dioxide laser

resurfacing of photo-aged facial skin. Arch. Dermatol. 132, 395–402 (1996).
47. Manstein, D., Herron, G. S., Sink, R. K., Tanner, H. & Anderson, R. R. Fractional photothermolysis: a new concept for cutaneous remodeling using microscopic patterns of thermal injury. Lasers Surg. Med. 34, 426–438 (2004).
48. Sherling, M. et al. Consensus recommendations on the use of an erbium- doped 1,550-nm fractionated laser and its applications in dermatologic laser surgery. Dermatologic Surg. 36, 461–469 (2010).
49. Kositratna, G., Evers, M., Sajjadi, A. & Manstein, D. Rapid fibrin plug formation within cutaneous ablative fractional CO2 laser lesions. Lasers Surg. Med. 48, 125–132 (2016).
50. Kilmer, S. L. & Anderson, R. R. Clinical use of the Q-switched ruby and the Q-switched Nd:YAG (1064 nm and 532 nm) lasers for treatment of tattoos. J. Dermatol. Surg. Oncol. 19, 330–338 (1993).
51. Brauer, J. A. et al. Successful and rapid treatment of blue and green tattoo pigment with a novel picosecond laser. Arch. Dermatol. 148, 820–823 (2012).
52. Grossman, M. C., Dierickx, C., Farinelli, W., Flotte, T. & Anderson, R. R. Damage to hair follicles by normal-mode ruby laser pulses. J. Am. Acad. Dermatol. 35, 889–894 (1996).
53. Metelitsa, A. I. & Green, J. B. Home-use laser and light devices for the skin: an update. Semin. Cutan. Med. Surg. 30, 144–147 (2011).
54. Jackson, S. D. Towards high-power mid-infrared emission from a fibre laser.
55. Nat. Photon. 6, 423–431 (2012).
56. Gilling, P., Cass, C., Cresswell, M. & Fraundorfer, M. Holmium laser resection of the prostate: preliminary results of a new method for the treatment of benign prostatic hyperplasia. Urology 47, 48–51 (1996).
57. Malek, R. S., Kuntzman, R. S. & Barrett, D. M. High-power
58. potassium-titanyl-phosphate (KTP/532) laser vaporization prostatectomy: 24 hours later. Urology 51, 254–256 (1998).
59. Sofer, M. et al. Holmium:YAG laser lithotripsy for upper urinary tract calculi in 598 patients. J. Urol. 167, 31–34 (2002).
60. Ell, C., Lux, G., Hochberger, J., Müller, D. & Demling, L. Laser lithotripsy of common bile duct stones. Gut 29, 746–751 (1988).
61. Wazni, O. et al. Lead extraction in the contemporary setting: the LExICon study: an observational retrospective study of consecutive laser lead extractions. J. Am. Coll. Cardiol. 55, 579–586 (2010).
62. Wilkoff, B. L. et al. Pacemaker lead extraction with the laser sheath: results of the pacing lead extraction with the excimer sheath (PLEXES) trial. J. Am. Coll. Cardiol. 33, 1671–1676 (1999).
63. Grundfest, W. S. et al. Laser ablation of human atherosclerotic plaque without adjacent tissue injury. J. Am. Coll. Cardiol. 5, 929–933 (1985).
64. Min, R. J., Khilnani, N. & Zimmet, S. E. Endovenous laser treatment of saphenous vein reflux: long-term results. J. Vasc. Interv. Radiol. 14, 991–996 (2003).
65. Proebstle, T. M., Moehler, T. & Herdemann, S. Reduced recanalization rates of the great saphenous vein after endovenous laser treatment with increased
66. energy dosing: definition of a threshold for the endovenous fluence equivalent.
67. J. Vasc. Surg. 44, 834–839 (2006).
68. Mccoppin, H. H., Hovenic, W. W. & Wheeland, R. G. Laser treatment of superficial leg veins. Dermatologic Surg. 37, 729–741 (2011).
69. Hibst, R. & Keller, U. Experimental studies of the application of the Er:YAG laser on dental hard substances: I. Measurement of the ablation rate. Lasers Surg. Med. 9, 338–344 (1989).

70. Wigdor, H. A. et al. Lasers in dentistry. Lasers Surg. Med. 16, 103–133 (1995).
71. Strong, M. S. & Jako, G. J. Laser surgery in the larynx. Early clinical experience with continuous CO_2 laser. Ann. Otol. Rhinol. Laryngol. 81, 792–798 (1972).
72. Amin, Z. et al. Hepatic metastases: interstitial laser photocoagulation with
73. real-time US monitoring and dynamic CT evaluation of treatment. Radiology
74. 187, 339–347 (1993).
75. Mellow, M. H. & Pinkas, H. Endoscopic laser therapy for malignancies affecting the esophagus and gastroesophageal junction: analysis of technical and functional efficacy. Arch. Intern. Med. 145, 1443–1446 (1985).
76. Wahidi, M. M., Herth, F. J. F. & Ernst, A. State of the art: interventional pulmonology. Chest 131, 261–274 (2007).
77. Maisels, M. J. & McDonagh, A. F. Phototherapy for neonatal jaundice.
78. N. Engl. J. Med. 358, 920–928 (2008).
79. Schwarz, T. & Beissert, S. Milestones in photoimmunology. J. Invest. Dermatol.
80. 133, E7–E10 (2013).
81. Gläser, R. et al. UV-B radiation induces the expression of antimicrobial peptides in human keratinocytes in vitro and in vivo. J. Allergy Clin. Immunol. 123, 1117–1123 (2009).
82. Liu, P. T. et al. Toll-like receptor triggering of a vitamin D-mediated human antimicrobial response. Science 311, 1770–1773 (2006).
83. Kripke, M. L. Antigenicity of murine skin tumors induced by ultraviolet light.
84. J. Natl Cancer Inst. 53, 1333–1336 (1974).
85. Stapelberg, M. P. F., Williams, R. B. H., Byrne, S. N. & Halliday, G. M. The alternative complement pathway seems to be a UVA sensor that leads to systemic immunosuppression. J. Invest. Dermatol. 129, 2694–2701 (2009).
86. Lim, H. W. et al. Phototherapy in dermatology: a call for action. J. Am. Acad. Dermatol. 72, 1078–1080 (2015).
87. Johnson-Huang, L. M. et al. Effective narrow-band UVB radiation therapy suppresses the IL-23/IL-17 axis in normalized psoriasis plaques. J. Invest. Dermatol. 130, 2654–2663 (2010).
88. Stern, R. S. Psoralen and ultraviolet A light therapy for psoriasis.
89. N. Engl. J. Med. 357, 682–690 (2007).
90. Norval, M. & Halliday, G. M. The consequences of UV-induced immunosuppression for human health. Photochem. Photobiol. 87, 965–977 (2011).
91. Becklund, B. R., Severson, K. S., Vang, S. V & DeLuca, H. F. UV radiation suppresses experimental autoimmune encephalomyelitis independent of vitamin D production. Proc. Natl Acad. Sci. USA 107, 6418–6423 (2010).
92. Geldenhuys, S. et al. Ultraviolet radiation suppresses obesity and symptoms of metabolic syndrome independently of vitamin D in mice fed a high-fat diet. Diabetes 63, 3759–3769 (2014).
93. Slusher, T. M. et al. A randomized trial of phototherapy with filtered sunlight in African neonates. N. Engl. J. Med. 373, 1115–1124 (2015).
94. Anderson, J. L., Glod, C. A., Dai, J., Cao, Y. & Lockley, S. W. Lux vs. wavelength in light treatment of seasonal affective disorder. Acta Psychiatr. Scand. 120, 203–212 (2009).
95. LeGates, T. A., Fernandez, D. C. & Hattar, S. Light as a central modulator of circadian rhythms, sleep and affect. Nat. Rev. Neurosci. 15, 443–454 (2014).
96. Golden, R. N. et al. The efficacy of light therapy in the treatment of mood disorders: a review and meta-analysis of the evidence. Am. J. Psychiatry 162, 656–662 (2005).
97. Lockley, S. W., Brainard, G. C. & Czeisler, C. A. High sensitivity of the human circadian

melatonin rhythm to resetting by short wavelength light. J. Clin. Endocrinol. Metab. 88, 4502–4505 (2003).
98. Lam, R. W. et al. Efficacy of bright light treatment, fluoxetine, and the combination in patients with nonseasonal major depressive disorder. JAMA Psychiatry 73, 56–63 (2015).
99. Dai, T. et al. Blue light rescues mice from potentially fatal Pseudomonas aeruginosa burn infection: efficacy, safety, and mechanism of action. Antimicrob. Agents Chemother. 57, 1238–1245 (2013).
100. Dai, T. et al. Blue light for infectious diseases: Propionibacterium acnes, Helicobacter pylori, and beyond? Drug Resist. Updates 15, 233–236 (2012).
101. Wu, P. C., Tsai, C. L., Wu, H. L., Yang, Y. H. & Kuo, H. K. Outdoor activity during class recess reduces myopia onset and progression in school children. Ophthalmology 120, 1080–1085 (2013).
102. Smith, E. L., Hung, L. F. & Huang, J. Protective effects of high ambient lighting on the development of form-deprivation myopia in rhesus monkeys. Investig. Ophthalmol. Vis. Sci. 53, 421–428 (2012).
103. Wang, J., Li, B. & Wu, M. X. Effective and lesion-free cutaneous influenza vaccination. Proc. Natl Acad. Sci. USA 112, 5005–5010 (2015).
104. Avci, P., Gupta, G. K., Clark, J., Wikonkal, N. & Hamblin, M. R. Low-level laser (light) therapy (LLLT) for treatment of hair loss. Lasers Surg. Med. Surg. Med. 46, 144–151 (2014).
105. Chung, H. et al. The nuts and bolts of low-level laser (light) therapy.
106. Ann. Biomed. Eng. 40, 516–533 (2012).
107. Chow, R. T., Johnson, M. I., Lopes-Martins, R. A. & Bjordal, J. M. Efficacy of low-level laser therapy in the management of neck pain: a systematic review and meta-analysis of randomised placebo or active-treatment controlled trials. Lancet 374, 1897–1908 (2009).
108. Naeser, M. A. et al. Significant improvements in cognitive performance post-transcranial, red/near-infrared light-emitting diode treatments in chronic, mild traumatic brain injury: open-protocol study. J. Neurotrauma 31, 1008–1017 (2014).
109. Arany, P. R. et al. Photoactivation of endogenous latent transforming growth factor-β1 directs dental stem cell differentiation for regeneration. Sci. Transl. Med. 6, 238ra69 (2014).
110. Shapiro, M. G., Homma, K., Villarreal, S., Richter, C.-P. & Bezanilla, F. Infrared light excites cells by changing their electrical capacitance. Nat. Commun.
111. 3, 736 (2012).
112. Jenkins, M. W. et al. Optical pacing of the embryonic heart. Nat. Photon.
113. 4, 623–626 (2010).
114. Teudt, I. U., Nevel, A. E., Izzo, A. D., Walsh, J. T. & Richter, C.-P. Optical stimulation of the facial nerve: a new monitoring technique? Laryngoscope 117, 1641–1647 (2007).
115. Wollensak, G., Spoerl, E. & Seiler, T. Stress-strain measurements of human and porcine corneas after riboflavin-ultraviolet-A-induced cross-linking.
116. J. Cataract Refract. Surg. 29, 1780–1785 (2003).
117. Lang, N. et al. A blood-resistant surgical glue for minimally invasive repair of vessels and heart defects. Sci. Transl. Med. 6, 218ra6 (2014).
118. Roche, E. T. et al. A light-reflecting balloon catheter for atraumatic tissue defect repair. Sci. Transl. Med. 7, 306ra149 (2015).
119. Du, Y., Lo, E., Ali, S. & Khademhosseini, A. Directed assembly of cell-laden microgels for fabrication of 3D tissue constructs. Proc. Natl Acad. Sci. USA 105, 9522–9527 (2008).
120. Hillel, A. T. et al. Photoactivated composite biomaterial for soft tissue restoration in rodents and in humans. Sci. Transl. Med. 3, 93ra67 (2011).

121. Castano, A. P., Mroz, P. & Hamblin, M. R. Photodynamic therapy and anti- tumour immunity. Nat. Rev. Cancer 6, 535–545 (2006).
122. Agostinis, P. et al. Photodynamic therapy of cancer: an update. CA Cancer J. Clin. 61, 250–281 (2011).
123. Spring, B. Q., Rizvi, I., Xu, N. & Hasan, T. The role of photodynamic therapy in overcoming cancer drug resistance. Photochem. Photobiol. Sci. 14, 1476–1491 (2015).
124. Wan, M. T. & Lin, J. Y. Current evidence and applications of photodynamic therapy in dermatology. Clin. Cosmet. Investig. Dermatol. 7, 145–163 (2014).
125. Lozano, M., Cid, J. & Müller, T. H. Plasma treated with methylene blue and light: clinical efficacy and safety profile. Transfus. Med. Rev. 27, 235–240 (2013).
126. Yang, Y. et al. Thienopyrrole-expanded BODIPY as a potential NIR photosensitizer for photodynamic therapy. Chem. Commun. 49, 3940–3942 (2013).
127. Idris, N. M. et al. In vivo photodynamic therapy using upconversion nanoparticles as remote-controlled nanotransducers. Nat. Med.
128. 18, 1580–1585 (2012).
129. Kim, Y. R. et al. Bioluminescence-activated deep-tissue photodynamic therapy of cancer. Theranostics 5, 805–817 (2015).
130. Hildebrandt, B. The cellular and molecular basis of hyperthermia. Crit. Rev. Oncol. Hematol. 43, 33–56 (2002).
131. Jin, C. S., Lovell, J. F., Chen, J. & Zheng, G. Ablation of hypoxic tumors with dose-equivalent photothermal, but not photodynamic, therapy using a nanostructured porphyrin assembly. ACS Nano 7, 2541–2550 (2013).
132. Huang, X., El-Sayed, I. H., Qian, W. & El-Sayed, M. A. Cancer cell imaging and photothermal therapy in the near-infrared region by using gold nanorods. J. Am. Chem. Soc. 128, 2115–2120 (2006).
133. Cheng, L., Yang, K., Chen, Q. & Liu, Z. Organic stealth nanoparticles for highly effective in vivo near-infrared photothermal therapy of cancer. ACS Nano 6, 5605–5613 (2012).
134. Lovell, J. F. et al. Porphysome nanovesicles generated by porphyrin bilayers for use as multimodal biophotonic contrast agents. Nat. Mater. 10, 324–332 (2011).
135. Shaikh, N., Hoberman, A., Kaleida, P. H., Ploof, D. L. & Paradise, J. L. Diagnosing otitis media — otoscopy and cerumen removal. N. Engl. J. Med. 362, e62 (2010).
136. Thangaratinam, S., Brown, K., Zamora, J., Khan, K. S. & Ewer, A. K. Pulse oximetry screening for critical congenital heart defects in asymptomatic newborn babies: a systematic review and meta-analysis. Lancet
137. 379, 2459–2464 (2012).
138. Boas, D. A., Elwell, C. E., Ferrari, M. & Taga, G. Twenty years of functional near-infrared spectroscopy: introduction for the special issue. Neuroimage 85, 1–5 (2014).
139. Schwarz, R. A. et al. Noninvasive evaluation of oral lesions using depth- sensitive optical spectroscopy. Cancer 115, 1669–1679 (2009).
140. Humeau-Heurtier, A., Guerreschi, E., Abraham, P. & Mahé, G. Relevance of laser doppler and laser speckle techniques for assessing vascular function: state of the art and future trends. IEEE Trans. Biomed. Eng. 60, 659–666 (2013).
141. Bolay, H. et al. Intrinsic brain activity triggers trigeminal meningeal afferents in a migraine model. Nat. Med. 8, 136–142 (2002).
142. Boppart, S. A. & Richards-Kortum, R. Point-of-care and point-of-procedure optical imaging technologies for primary care and global health. Sci. Transl. Med. 6, 253rv2 (2014).

143. Greenbaum, A. et al. Wide-field computational imaging of pathology slides using lens-free on-chip microscopy. Sci. Transl. Med. 6, 267ra175 (2014).
144. Shen, L., Hagen, J. A. & Papautsky, I. Point-of-care colorimetric detection with a smartphone. Lab Chip 12, 4240–4243 (2012).
145. R. Haglund, The properties of light, ed. by F. Träger, in Springer Handbook of Lasers and Optics (Springer, New York, 2007), pp. 3–32
146. O. Svelto, S. Longhi, G. Valle, S. Kück, G. Huber, M. Pollnau, H. Hillmer, S. Hansmann, R. Engelbrecht, H. Brand, J. Kaiser, A. Peterson, R. Malz, S. Steinberg, G. Marowsky, U. Brinkmann, D. Lo, A. Borsutzky, H. Wähter, M. Sigrist, E.
147. Saldin, E. Schneidmiller, M. Yurkov, K. Midorikawa, J. Hein, R. Sauerbrey, and J. Helmcke, Lasers and coherent light sources, ed. by F. Träger, in Springer Handbook of Lasers and Optics (Springer, New York, 2007), pp. 583–936
148. N. Lindlein, G. Leuchs, Wave optics, ed. by F. Trägerin, in Springer Handbook of Lasers and Optics (Springer, New York, 2007), pp. 87–156
149. W. Koechner, Optical resonator, in Solid-State Laser Engineering. Springer Series in Optical Sciences, vol. 1 (Springer New York, 2006), pp. 210–299
150. M. Niemz, Laser-tissue Interactions (Springer, Berlin, 2004)
151. M. Allmen, Laser-Beam Interactions with Materials: Physical Principles and Applications, Springer Series in Materials Science (Springer, Berlin, 2012)
152. D. Bäuerle, Laser Processing and Chemistry (Springer, Berlin, 2011)
153. M. Brinkmann, J. Hayden, M. Letz, S. Reichel, C. Click, W. Mannstadt, B. Schreder, S. Wolff, S. Ritter, M. Davis, T. Bauer, H. Ren, Y.-H. Fan, S.-T. Wu, K. Bonrad, E. Krätzig, K. Buse, R. Paquin, Optical materials and their properties, ed. by F. Träger, in Springer Handbook of Lasers and Optics (Springer, New York, 2007), pp. 249–372
154. A. Vogel, V. Venugopalan, Mechanisms of pulsed laser ablation of biological tissues. Chem. Rev. 103(2), 577–644 (2003)
155. S.L. Jacques, Optical properties of biological tissues: a review. Phys. Med. Biol. 58(11), R37 (2013)
156. L. Fichera, D. Pardo, L. Mattos, Modeling tissue temperature dynamics during laser exposure, ed. by I. Rojas, G. Joya, J. Cabestany, in Advances in Computational Intelligence. Lecture Notes in Computer Science, vol. 7903 (Springer, Berlin, 2013), pp. 96–106. http://dx.doi.org/10.1007/978-3-642-38682-4_12 (Online)
157. R. Steiner, Laser-tissue interactions, in Laser and IPL Technology in Dermatology and Aesthetic Medicine, ed. by C. Raulin, S. Karsai (Springer, Berlin, 2011), pp. 23–36
158. M. Rubinstein, W. Armstrong, Transoral laser microsurgery for laryngeal cancer: a primer and review of laser dosimetry. Lasers Med. Sci. 26(1), 113–124 (2011)
159. W. Steiner, P. Ambrosch, Endoscopic laser surgery of the upper aerodigestive tract: with special emphasis on cancer surgery. Thieme (2000)
160. V. Oswal, M. Remacle, Transoral laser laryngeal surgery, in Principles and Practice of Lasers in Otorhinolaryngology and Head and Neck, 2nd edn., ed. by O. Vasant, R. Marc (Kugler Publications, Amsterdam, The Netherlands, 2014), pp. 99–116
161. C. Apel, R. Franzen, J. Meister, H. Sarrafzadegan, S. Thelen, N. Gutknecht, Influence of the pulse duration of an er: yag laser system on the ablation threshold of dental enamel. Lasers Med. Sci. 17(4), 253–257 (2002)
162. Gai, X., Choi, D.-Y., Madden, S., and Luther-Davis, B., Materials and Structures for Nonlinear Photonics, Chapter 1 in All-Optical Signal Processing—DataCommunication and Storage

Applications. Springer Se-ries in Optical Sciences, Editors: Wabnitz, Stefan, Eggleton, Benjamin J. (Springer, New York, USA 2015)
163. Armstrong, S., All-Optical Storage. Nature Photonics 6, 636–637 (2012)
164. Sugioka, K. and Cheng, Y., Ultrafast lasers—reliable tools for advanced materials processing. Light: Science & Applications 3, e149, doi:10.1038 (2014)
165. Diddams, S.A., Jones, D.J., Ye, J., Cundiff, S.T., Hall, J.L., Ranka, J.K., Windeler, R.S., Holzwarth, R., Udem, Th., and Hänsch, T.W.,Direct Link between Microwave and Optical Frequencies with a 300 THz Femtose-cond Laser Comb. Phys. Rev. Lett. 84, 5102 (2000)
166. Hell, S.W., Nanoscopy with focused Light (Nobel Lecture). Angew. Chem. Int. Ed. 54,
167. 8054-8066 (2015)
168. Betzig, E., Patterson, G.H., Sougrat, R., Lindwasser, O.W., Olenych, S., Bonifacino, J.S., Davidson, M.W., Schwartz, J.L., and Hess, H.F., Im-aging Intracellular Fluorescent Proteins at Nanometer Resolution. Science 313, 1642 (2006)
169. Goldsmith, R.H., Moerner, W.E., Watching conformational- and photo-dynamics of single fluorescent proteins in solution. Nature Chemistry 2, 179–186 (2010)
170. Bloembergen, N., Nonlinear Optics and Spectroscopy. Nobel Lectures, Physics 1981-1990, Editor-in-Charge Tore Frängsmyr, Editor Gösta Eks-pong(World Scientific Publishing Co., Singapore, 1993)
171. Zewail, A. H., Femtochemistry: Ultrafast Dynamics of the Chemical Bond, Vols. 1 and 2 (World Scientific, Singapore 1994)
172. Goswami, D., Optical pulse shaping approaches to coherent control. Phys. Rep. 374(6), 385-481 (2003)
173. Katzir A (1990) Selected papers on optical fibers in medicine, SPIE milestone
174. United Nations DESA (2015) World population prospects: the 2015 revision. United Nations, New York
175. Bradbury S (1967) The evolution of the microscope. Pergamon Press, Oxford
176. Bozzini P (1806) Lichtleiter, eine Erfindung zur Anschauung innerer Teile und Krankheiten. J Prakt Heilkunde 24:107–124
177. Von Helmholtz HLF (1856) Handbuch der physiologischen Optik. L. Voss, Leipzig
178. History of ASLMS. American Society for Laser Medicine and Surgery. http://www.aslms.org/aslms/history.shtml
179. Choy DS (1988) History of lasers in medicine. Thorac Cardiovasc Surg 36(Suppl 2):114–117
180. Mignani AG, Baldini F (1979) Fibre-optic sensors in health care. Phys Med Biol 42(5):967–979
181. Fujimoto JG et al (2002) Optical coherence tomography: an emerging technology for biomedical imaging and optical biopsy. Neoplasia 2(1–2):9–25
182. Cusano A, Consales M, Crescitelli A, Ricciardi A (eds) (2015) Lab-on-fiber technology. Springer, Berlin
183. Lakshminarayanan V et al (2015) Smartphone science in eye care and medicine. Opt Photonics News 26:45–51, Optical Society of America
184. Maamari RN et al (2014) Novel telemedicine device for diagnosis of corneal abrasions and ulcers in resource-poor settings. JAMA Ophthalmol 132:894–895
185. Breslauer DN et al (2009) Mobile phone based clinical microscopy for global health applications. PLoS One 4, e6320
186. Hett JH (1969) Medical optical instruments. In: Kingslake R (ed) Applied optics and optical engineering, Vol. 5, optical instrument. Academic, New York
187. Devroey D et al (2000) Do general practitioners use what's in their doctor's bag? Scand J Prim

Health Care 20:242–243
188. Kravetz RE (2002) The otoscope. Am J Gastroenterol 97:470
189. Feldmann H (1996) History of the ear speculum. Images from the history of otorhinolaryngology, highlighted by instruments from the collection of the German Medical History Museum in Ingolstadt. Laryngorhinootologie 75:311–318
190. Millodot M (2009) Dictionary of optometry and visual science, 7th edn. Butterworth-Heinemann, Edinburgh
191. Millodot M (1973) A centenary of retinoscopy. J Am Optom Assoc 44:1057–1059
192. Koltai PJ, Nixon RE (1989) The story of the laryngoscope. Ear Nose Throat J 68(7):494–502
193. García M (1855) Observations on the Human Voice. Proc R Soc Lond 7:399–410
194. Hirsch NP, Smith GB, Hirsch PO (1986) Alfred Kirstein Pioneer of direct laryngoscopy. Anaesthesia 41(1):42–45
195. Kawahara I, Ichikawa H (1987) Fiberoptic Instrument technology. In: Sivak MV (ed) Gastrointestinal endoscopy. W. B. Saunders, Philadelphia, pp 201–241
196. Hirschowitz B (1979) A personal history of the fiberscope. Gastroenterol 76;(4):864–869
197. Sulewski JG. Historical survey of laser dentistry. Dent Clin North Am. 2000;44(4):717–52. [PubMed] [Google Scholar]
198. Asnaashari M, Mohebi S, Paymanpour P. Pain reduction using low level laser irradiation in single-visit endodontic treatment. J Lasers Med Sci. 2011;2(4):139–43. [Google Scholar]
199. Asnaashari M, Moeini M. Effectiveness of Lasers in the Treatment of Dentin Hypersensitivity. J Lasers Med Sci. 2013;4(1):1–7. [PMC free article] [PubMed] [Google Scholar]
200. Convissar RA. Principles and practice of laser dentistry. Mosby. 2010 [Google Scholar]
201. Paghdiwala AF. Application of the erbium: YAG laser on hard dental tissues; Measurement of the temperature changes and depth of cut. Lasers Med Surg Dent. 1988;64:192–201. [Google Scholar]
202. Kawczyk-Krupka A, Waskowska J, Raczkowska-Siostrzonek A, Kosciarz-Grzesiok A, Kwiatek S, Straszak D. et al. Comparison of cryotherapy and photodynamic therapy in treatment of oral leukoplakia. Photodiagnosis Photodyn Ther. 2012;9(2):148–55. [PubMed] [Google Scholar]
203. Shafirstein G, Friedman A, Siegel E, Moreno M, Baumler W, Fan CY. et al. Using 5-aminolevulinic acid and pulsed dye laser for photodynamic treatment of oral leukoplakia. Arch Otolaryngol Head Neck Surg. 2011;137(11):1117–23. [PubMed] [Google Scholar]
204. Montebugnoli L, Frini F, Gissi DB, Gabusi A, Cervellati F, Foschini MP. et al. Histological and immunohistochemical evaluation of new epithelium after removal of oral leukoplakia with Nd:YAG laser treatment. Lasers Med Sci. 2012;27(1):205–10. [PubMed] [Google Scholar]
205. Yang SW, Tsai CN, Lee YS, Chen TA. Treatment outcome of dysplastic oral leukoplakia with carbon dioxide laser--emphasis on the factors affecting recurrence. J Oral Maxillofac Surg. 2011;69(6):12. [PubMed] [Google Scholar]
206. Misra N, Chittoria N, Umapathy D, Misra P. Efficacy of diode laser in the management of oral lichen planus. BMJ Case Rep. 2013;15(10):2012–007609. [PMC free article] [PubMed] [Google Scholar]
207. Agha-Hosseini F, Moslemi E, Mirzaii-Dizgah I. Comparative evaluation of low-level laser and CO(2) laser in treatment of patients with oral lichen planus. Int J Oral Maxillofac Surg. 2012;41(10):1265–9. [PubMed] [Google Scholar]
208. Fornaini C, Raybaud H, Augros C, Rocca JP. New clinical approach for use of Er:YAG laser in the surgical treatment of oral lichen planus: a report of two cases. Photomed Laser Surg. 2012;30(4):234–8. [PubMed] [Google Scholar]
209. de Magalhaes-Junior EB, Aciole GT, Santos NR, dos Santos JN, Pinheiro AL. Removal of oral

lichen planus by CO2 laser . Braz Dent J. 2011;22(6):522–6. [PubMed] [Google Scholar]
210. Hegde R, Padhye A, Sumanth S, Jain AS, Thukral N. Comparison of surgical stripping; erbium-doped:yttrium, aluminum, and garnet laser; and carbon dioxide laser techniques for gingival depigmentation: a clinical and histologic study. J Periodontol. 2013;84(6):738–48. [PubMed] [Google Scholar]
211. Simsek Kaya G, Yapici Yavuz G, Sumbullu MA, Dayi E. A comparison of diode laser and Er:YAG lasers in the treatment of gingival melanin pigmentation. Oral Surg Oral Med Oral Pathol Oral Radiol. 2012;113(3):293–9. [PubMed] [Google Scholar]
212. Baeder FM, Pelino JE, de Almeida ER, Duarte DA, Santos MT. High-power diode laser use on Fordyce granule excision: a case report. J Cosmet Dermatol . 2010 Dec;9(4):321–4. [PubMed] [Google Scholar]
213. Jerjes W, Upile T, Hamdoon Z, Al-Khawalde M, Morcos M, Mosse CA. et al. CO2 laser of oral dysplasia: clinicopathological features of recurrence and malignant transformation . Lasers Med Sci. 2012;27(1):169–79. [PubMed] [Google Scholar]
214. Deppe H, Mucke T, Hohlweg-Majert B, Hauck W, Wagenpfeil S, Holzle F. Different CO2 laser vaporization protocols for the therapy of oral precancerous lesions and precancerous conditions: a 10-year follow-up . Lasers Med Sci. 2012;27(1):59–63. [PubMed] [Google Scholar]
215. Luna-Ortiz K, Campos-Ramos E, Pasche P, Mosqueda-Taylor A. Oral mucosal melanoma: conservative treatment including laser surgery. Med Oral Patol Oral Cir Bucal. 2011;16(3):e381–5. [PubMed] [Google Scholar]
216. Lopez-Jornet P, Camacho-Alonso F. Comparison of pain and swelling after removal of oral leukoplakia with CO(2) laser and cold knife: a randomized clinical trial. Med Oral Patol Oral Cir Bucal. 2013;18(1):e38–44. [PMC free article] [PubMed] [Google Scholar]
217. Fornaini C, Rocca JP, Merigo E, Meleti M, Manfredi M, Nammour S. et al. Low energy KTP laser in oral soft tissue surgery: A 52 patients clinical study. Med Oral Patol Oral Cir Bucal. 2012;17(2):e287–91. [PMC free article] [PubMed] [Google Scholar]
218. Boj JR, Poirier C, Espasa E, Hernandez M, Espanya A. Lower lip mucocele treated with an erbium laser. Pediatr Dent. 2009;31(3):249–52. [PubMed] [Google Scholar]
219. Yague-Garcia J, Espana-Tost AJ, Berini-Aytes L, Gay-Escoda C. Treatment of oral mucocele-scalpel versus CO2 laser . Med Oral Patol Oral Cir Bucal. 2009;14(9):e469–74. [PubMed] [Google Scholar]
220. Lai JB, Poon CY. Treatment of ranula using carbon dioxide laser--case series report. Int J Oral Maxillofac Surg. 2009;38(10):1107–11. [PubMed] [Google Scholar]
221. Lindenmuller IH, Noll P, Mameghani T, Walter C. CO2 laser-assisted treatment of a giant pyogenic granuloma of the gingiva . Int J Dent Hyg. 2010;8(3):249–52. [PubMed] [Google Scholar]
222. Asnaashari M, Azari-Marhabi S, Alirezaei S, Asnaashari N. Clinical Application of 810nm Diode Laser to Remove Gingival Hyperplasic Lesion. J Lasers Med Sci. 2013;4(2):96–8. [PMC free article] [PubMed] [Google Scholar]
223. Monteiro LS, Mouzinho J, Azevedo A, Camara MI, Martins MA, La Fuente JM. Treatment of epulis fissuratum with carbon dioxide laser in a patient with antithrombotic medication. Braz Dent J. 2012;23(1):77–81. [PubMed] [Google Scholar]
224. 28. Iseri U, Ozcakir-Tomruk C, Gursoy-Mert H. Treatment of epulis fissuratum with CO2 laser and prosthetic rehabilitation in patients with vesiculobullous disease . Photomed Laser Surg. 2009;27(4):675–81. [PubMed] [Google Scholar]
225. Arslan A, Gursoy H, Cologlu S. Treatment of lymphangioma with CO2 laser in the mandibular

alveolar mucosa . J Contemp Dent Pract. 2011;12(6):493–6. [PubMed] [Google Scholar]
226. Genovese WJ, dos Santos MT, Faloppa F, de Souza Merli LA. The use of surgical diode laser in oral hemangioma: a case report. Photomed Laser Surg. 2010;28(1):147–51. [PubMed] [Google Scholar]
227. Singh GB, Tiwari M, Shukla HS, Pandey M. Nd:YAG laser therapy of carcinoma lip (stage I squamous cell carcinoma): a retrospective evaluation. Indian J Otolaryngol Head Neck Surg. 2009;61(3):179–84. [PMC free article] [PubMed] [Google Scholar]
228. Canis M, Ihler F, Martin A, Wolff HA, Matthias C, Steiner W. Enoral laser microsurgery for squamous cell carcinoma of the oral cavity. Head Neck. 2013;25(10):23365. [PubMed] [Google Scholar]
229. Hakeem AH, Tubachi J, Pradhan SA. Significance of anterior commissure involvement in early glottic squamous cell carcinoma treated with trans-oral CO2 laser microsurgery . Laryngoscope. 2013;123(8):1912–7. [PubMed] [Google Scholar]
230. De Santis D, Gerosa R, Zanotti G, Cigikov N, Cenzi A, Chiarini L. et al. Experimental analysis about the evaluation of tungsten carbide-bur, piezoelectric and laser osteotomies. Minerva Stomatol. 2013;1:1. [PubMed] [Google Scholar]
231. Gabric Panduric D, Bago I, Katanec D, Zabkar J, Miletic I, Anic I. Comparison of Er:YAG laser and surgical drill for osteotomy in oral surgery: an experimental study. J Oral Maxillofac Surg 2012;70(11):2515–21. [PubMed] [Google Scholar]
232. Luna-Ortiz K, Gomez-Pedraza A, Mosqueda-Taylor A. Soft palate preservation after tumor resection with transoral laser microsurgery. Med Oral Patol Oral Cir Bucal. 2013;18(3):e445–8. [PMC free article] [PubMed] [Google Scholar]
233. Jerjes W, Upile T, Hamdoon Z, Alexander Mosse C, Morcos M, Hopper C. Photodynamic therapy outcome for T1/T2 N0 oral squamous cell carcinoma. Lasers Surg Med. 2011;43(6):463–9. [PubMed] [Google Scholar]
234. Gargari M, Autili N, Petrone A, Ceruso FM. Using laser diodes for the removal of a lesion of the oral mucosaCase report. Oral Implantol. 2011;4(1-2):10–3. [PMC free article] [PubMed] [Google Scholar]
235. Suter VG, Altermatt HJ, Dietrich T, Reichart PA, Bornstein MM. Does a pulsed mode offer advantages over a continuous wave mode for excisional biopsies performed using a carbon dioxide laser? J Oral Maxillofac Surg 2012; 70(8):1781-8. Does a pulsed mode offer advantages over a continuous wave mode for excisional biopsies performed using a carbon dioxide laser? J Oral Maxillofac Surg. 2012;70(8):1781–8. [PubMed] [Google Scholar]
236. Shires CB, Saputra JM, King L, Thompson JW, Heck DH, Sebelik ME. et al. Histopathological and postoperative behavioral comparison of rodent oral tongue resection: fiber-enabled CO2 laser versus electrocautery . Otolaryngol Head Neck Surg. 2012;147(4):716–21. [PMC free article] [PubMed] [Google Scholar]
237. Tuncer I, Ozcakir-Tomruk C, Sencift K, Cologlu S. Comparison of conventional surgery and CO_2 laser on intraoral soft tissue pathologies and evaluation of the collateral thermal damage . Photomed Laser Surg. 2010;28(1):75–9. [PubMed] [Google Scholar]
238. Crockett DJ, Meier JD, Wilson KF, Grimmer JF. Treatment of Oral Cavity Venous Malformations with the Nd:YAG Laser Using the Underwater Technique. Otolaryngol Head Neck Surg. 2013;19:19. [PubMed] [Google Scholar]
239. Miyazaki H, Romeo U, Ohshiro T, Kudo T, Makiguchi T, Kawachi N. et al. Treatment strategies for large oral venous malformations using intralesional laser photocoagulation. Lasers Med Sci. 2013;28:28. [PubMed] [Google Scholar]

240. Miyazaki H, Ohshiro T, Watanabe H, Kakizaki H, Makiguchi T, Kim M. et al. Ultrasound-guided intralesional laser treatment of venous malformation in the oral cavity. Int J Oral Maxillofac Surg. 2013;42(2):281–7. [PubMed] [Google Scholar]
241. Alvarez-Camino JC, Espana-Tost AJ, Gay-Escoda C. Endoluminal sclerosis with diode laser in the treatment of orofacial venous malformations. Med Oral Patol Oral Cir Bucal. 2013;18(3):e486–90. [PMC free article] [PubMed] [Google Scholar]
242. Glade RS, Buckmiller LM. CO2 laser resurfacing of intraoral lymphatic malformations: a 10-year experience . Int J Pediatr Otorhinolaryngol. 2009;73(10):1358–61. [PubMed] [Google Scholar]
243. Atalay B, Yalcin S, Emes Y, Aktas I, Aybar B, Issever H. et al. Bisphosphonate-related osteonecrosis: laser-assisted surgical treatment or conventional surgery? Lasers Med Sci 2011; 26(6):815-23. laser-assisted surgical treatment or conventional surgery? Lasers Med Sci. 2011;26(6):laser–assisted surgical treatment or conventional surgery? Lasers Med Sci 2011; 26(6). [PubMed] [Google Scholar]
244. Vescovi P, Meleti M, Merigo E, Manfredi M, Fornaini C, Guidotti R. et al. Case series of 589 tooth extractions in patients under bisphosphonates therapyProposal of a clinical protocol supported by Nd:YAG low-level laser therapy. Med Oral Patol Oral Cir Bucal. 2013;18(4):e680–5. [PMC free article] [PubMed] [Google Scholar]
245. Rugani P, Acham S, Truschnegg A, Obermayer-Pietsch B, Jakse N. Bisphosphonate-associated osteonecrosis of the jaws: surgical treatment with ErCrYSGG-laserCase report. Oral Surg Oral Med Oral Pathol Oral Radiol Endod. 2010;110(6):013. [PubMed] [Google Scholar]
246. Kan B, Altay MA, Tasar F, Akova M. Low-level laser therapy supported teeth extractions of two patients receiving IV zolendronate. Lasers Med Sci. 2011;26(5):569–75. [PubMed] [Google Scholar]
247. Scoletta M, Arduino PG, Reggio L, Dalmasso P, Mozzati M. Effect of low-level laser irradiation on bisphosphonate-induced osteonecrosis of the jaws: preliminary results of a prospective study. Photomed Laser Surg. 2010;28(2):179–84. [PubMed] [Google Scholar]
248. Vescovi P, Manfredi M, Merigo E, Meleti M, Fornaini C, Rocca JP. et al. Surgical approach with Er:YAG laser on osteonecrosis of the jaws (ONJ) in patients under bisphosphonate therapy (BPT) Lasers Med Sci. 2010;25(1):101–13. [PubMed] [Google Scholar]
249. Lopez-Ramirez M, Vilchez-Perez MA, Gargallo-Albiol J, Arnabat-Dominguez J, Gay-Escoda C. Efficacy of low-level laser therapy in the management of pain, facial swelling, and postoperative trismus after a lower third molar extractionA preliminary study. Lasers Med Sci. 2012;27(3):559–66. [PubMed] [Google Scholar]
250. Paschoal MA, Santos-Pinto L. Therapeutic effects of low-level laser therapy after premolar extraction in adolescents: a randomized double-blind clinical trial. Photomed Laser Surg. 2012;30(9):559–64. [PubMed] [Google Scholar]
251. Aras MH, Gungormus M. Placebo-controlled randomized clinical trial of the effect two different low-level laser therapies (LLLT)--intraoral and extraoral--on trismus and facial swelling following surgical extraction of the lower third molar. Lasers Med Sci. 2010;25(5):641–5. [PubMed] [Google Scholar]
252. Bodrumlu E, Keskiner I, Sumer M, Sumer AP, Telcioglu NT. Temperature variation during apicectomy with Er:YAG laser. Photomed Laser Surg. 2012;30(8):425–8. [PubMed] [Google Scholar]
253. Angiero F, Benedicenti S, Signore A, Parker S, Crippa R. Apicoectomies with the erbium laser: a complementary technique for retrograde endodontic treatment. Photomed Laser Surg. 2011;29(12):845–9. [PubMed] [Google Scholar]

254. Junior RM, Gueiros LA, Silva IH, de Albuquerque Carvalho A, Leao JC. Labial frenectomy with Nd:YAG laser and conventional surgery: a comparative study. Lasers Med Sci. 2013;22:22. [PubMed] [Google Scholar]
255. De Santis D, Bertossi D, Zanotti G, Rossetto A, Farronato G, Gelpi F. et al. Nd-YAP laser assisted frenulectomy: a case series on 23 patients. Minerva Stomatol. 2013;1:1. [PubMed] [Google Scholar]
256. Pie-Sanchez J, Espana-Tost AJ, Arnabat-Dominguez J, Gay-Escoda C. Comparative study of upper lip frenectomy with the CO2 laser versus the Er, Cr:YSGG laser . Med Oral Patol Oral Cir Bucal. 2012;17(2):e228–32. [PMC free article] [PubMed] [Google Scholar]
257. Lee JW, Park KH, Chung JH, Kim SJ. Effects of laser-aided circumferential supracrestal fiberotomy on root surfaces. Angle Orthod. 2011;81(6):1021–7. [PMC free article] [PubMed] [Google Scholar]
258. Kim SJ, Paek JH, Park KH, Kang SG, Park YG. Laser-aided circumferential supracrestal fiberotomy and low-level laser therapy effects on relapse of rotated teeth in beagles. Angle Orthod. 2010;80(2):385–90. [PMC free article] [PubMed] [Google Scholar]
259. Aras MH, Goregen M, Gungormus M, Akgul HM. Comparison of diode laser and Er:YAG lasers in the treatment of ankyloglossia. Photomed Laser Surg. 2010;28(2):173–7. [PubMed] [Google Scholar]

FSC
www.fsc.org
MIX
Papier | Fördert
gute Waldnutzung
FSC® C083411

Kolibri 360 GmbH
Ferdinand-Jühlke-Straße 7
99095 Erfurt, Deutschland
produktsicherheit@kolibri360.de

Druck:
CPI Druckdienstleistungen GmbH
im Auftrag der
Kolibri 360 GmbH
Ferdinand-Jühlke-Str. 7
99095 Erfurt